Talking Cures and Placebo Effects

International Perspectives in Philosophy and Psychiatry

Series editors: Bill (K.W.M.) Fulford, Katherine Morris, John Z Sadler, and Giovanni Stanghellini

Volumes in the series:

Mind, Meaning, and Mental Disorder
Bolton and Hill

What is Mental Disorder?
Bolton

Postpsychiatry
Bracken and Thomas

The Philosophical Understanding of Schizophrenia
Chung, Fulford, and Graham (ed.)

Nature and Narrative: An Introduction to the New Philosophy of Psychiatry
Fulford, Morris, Sadler, and Stanghellini

The Oxford Textbook of Philosophy and Psychiatry
Fulford, Thornton, and Graham

Dementia: Mind, Meaning, and the Person
Hughes, Louw, and Sabat

Body-Subjects and Disordered Minds
Matthews

Talking Cures and Placebo Effects
Jopling

Schizophrenia and the Fate of the Self
Lysaker and Lysaker

Rationality and Compulsion: Applying action theory to psychiatry
Nordenfelt

The Metaphor of Mental Illness
Pickering

Trauma, Truth, and Reconciliation: Healing Damaged Relationships
Potter (ed)

The Philosophy of Psychiatry: A Companion
Radden

Feelings of Being
Ratcliffe

Values and Psychiatric Diagnosis
Sadler

Disembodied Spirits and Deanimated Bodies: The Psychopathology of Common Sense
Stanghellini

Essential Philosophy of Psychiatry
Thornton

Empirical Ethics in Psychiatry
Widdershoven, McMillan, Hope and Van der Scheer (eds)

Forthcoming volumes in the series:

Philosophical Perspectives on Psychiatry and Technology
Phillips (ed)

Talking Cures and Placebo Effects

David A. Jopling

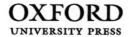

OXFORD
UNIVERSITY PRESS

OXFORD

UNIVERSITY PRESS

Great Clarendon Street, Oxford OX2 6DP

Oxford University Press is a department of the University of Oxford.
It furthers the University's objective of excellence in research, scholarship,
and education by publishing worldwide in

Oxford New York

Auckland Cape Town Dar es Salaam Hong Kong Karachi
Kuala Lumpur Madrid Melbourne Mexico City Nairobi
New Delhi Shanghai Taipei Toronto

With offices in

Argentina Austria Brazil Chile Czech Republic France Greece
Guatemala Hungary Italy Japan Poland Portugal Singapore
South Korea Switzerland Thailand Turkey Ukraine Vietnam

Oxford is a registered trade mark of Oxford University Press
in the UK and in certain other countries

Published in the United States
by Oxford University Press Inc., New York

A catalogue record for this title is available from the British Library

Data available

Library of Congress Cataloging in Publication Data

Data available

Typeset by Cepha Imaging Private Ltd., Bangalore, India
Printed in Great Britain
on acid-free paper by
Biddles Ltd., King's Lynn.

ISBN 978–0–19–923950–4

10 9 8 7 6 5 4 3 2 1

Whilst every effort has been made to ensure that the contents of this book are as
complete, accurate and up-to-date as possible at the date of writing, Oxford
University Press is not able to give any guarantee or assurance that such is the case.
Readers are urged to take appropriately qualified medical advice in all cases. The
information in this book is intended to be useful to the general reader, but should
not be used as a means of self-diagnosis or for the prescription of medication.

For Jeremy and Julia

Contents

Acknowledgments

Above all I would like to thank my parents, Alan and Rhoda Jopling. I would like to thank Paul Antze, Greg Dubord, Les Greenberg, Barbara Held, Edwin Hersch, Jon Mills, Ulric Neisser, Henry Pietersma, John Sadler, and Duff Waring for their encouragement and philosophical input during the writing of this book. For their inspiration and philosophical guidance in the years leading up to the start of this research, I would like to thank Christina Howells and Mary Warnock. The late John Macquarrie and the late Stuart Hampshire were also inspirational. I would also like to acknowledge my gratitude to Nadia Halim, Slava Sadovnikov, Burcu Gurkan, Paula Popovici, Serife Tekin, Hakam al Shawi, Sara Applebaum, and Pearl Jacobson for their assistance with research. The late Greg Jacobs, of the Office of Research Administration at York University, kindly assisted with research funding opportunities. Thanks are especially owing to the Canadian Institutes of Health Research, which provided me with a three-year operating grant to carry out research. Finally, my sincerest thanks go to my wife Rebecca Wells Jopling.

Preface

Memorials of Credulity

What pledge can be afforded that the boasted remedies of the present day will not, like their predecessors, fall into disrepute, and in their turn serve only as a humiliating memorial of the credulity and infatuation of the physicians who recommended and prescribed them?

John Ayrton Paris, *Pharmacologia*, 9th ed, 1843: 4–5

Crocodile Dung

For centuries, the history of medicine was witness to a succession of remedies whose only lasting impact was to supply later generations of physicians and medical researchers with what John Ayrton Paris politely called 'humiliating memorials of the credulity and infatuation of physicians'. It was a history of medical explanations that were celebrated as genuine advances in medical knowledge, but were in fact little more than explanatory fictions; of diagnostic strategies that revealed more about the fertile imaginations, superstitions, and reasoning biases of the physicians who invented them, than about the actual nature of symptoms; of theories of etiology that were enthusiastically endorsed by the leading physicians of the day, but were in fact based upon entirely fictitious causal pathways and causal forces; of theories of pathology that were arrived at more by a prioristic speculation than careful observation or experimentation; of medical reasoning strategies that were rife with obscurities, inconsistencies, and logical fallacies; of *materia medica* and pharmacological agents that were in many cases nothing short of bizarre; and of treatment methods that were irrelevant, ineffective, or just plain toxic. Behind this history of humiliating memorials of credulity was another history, much less visible to physicians and medical researchers of the day, and much more difficult to decode: a history of placebo effects, self-limiting diseases, autonomous responses, as well as nocebo effects, dangerous side effects, and iatrogenic diseases.

Consider, for example, the many pharmacological agents regarded by physicians of different eras and medical cultures as possessing curative powers, but now known to be inert or dangerous. Almost every available substance has been prescribed at one time or another to unsuspecting patients: crocodile dung, teeth of swine, hooves of asses, spermatic fluid of frogs, eunuch fat, fox lung, lozenges of dried vipers, powder of precious stones, bricks, Gascoyne's powder (a mix of bezoar, amber, pearls, crabs' eyes, coral, and black tops of crabs' claws), fur, feathers, hair, human perspiration, oil of ants, earthworms, spiders, animal blood, excreta of all forms, moss scraped from the skulls of victims of violent death, and so on (Garrison 1921). Supported by medical reasoning strategies that relied upon analogy, speculation, intuition, or unquestioned authority, these substances were justified as curative by background therapeutic theories that hooked up the putatively unique causal powers of the relevant substances with the hypothesized etiology of the relevant ailment. Most of the etiologies were wildly off track, and most of the substances simply did not work. Some proved to be fatal.

But this is not the end of the story. While many of these substances were pharmacologically inert, they sometimes played an important role as therapeutically beneficial explanatory fictions. Some patients experienced therapeutic improvement, not because of the substances themselves, but because the physicians who dispensed the substances supplied patients with a rationale, conceptual scheme, or myth that offered an explanation for otherwise puzzling and frightening symptoms, and because they prescribed to patients manageable but progressively more difficult procedures for treating symptoms (Frank and Frank 1991). Moreover, the physicians who treated patients displayed high levels of confidence in their explanations and treatments, and they appeared to be authorities in the treatment of diseases. Bear fat, for example, was thought to cure baldness, since the bear is a hirsute animal; and oak leaves were thought to cure dizziness, since the oak tree never falls. (Neither of these treatments worked.) What appeared to physician and patient to be an effective treatment was really a treatment consisting of explanatory fictions that served as vehicles for the delivery of a variety of unacknowledged therapeutic processes: namely, placebo effects, self-limiting disorders, autonomous responses, suggestion, and expectancy effects. Much of the history of pharmacology is a history of pharmacologically inert substances being endowed with what are really non-existent causal powers, and being hooked up by means of non-existent causal pathways with other non-existent entities or forces—the putative pathogens.

Consider, again, the long history of ineffective clinical interventions that were once thought to have been capable of exerting unique therapeutic benefits for a variety of ailments. A bewildering variety of invasive treatment procedures have been performed on patients' bodies, justified by some empirically impoverished therapeutic theory as curative, and endorsed by physicians who were overly confident in their medical abilities. Patients have been subjected to purging, poisoning, puncturing, cutting, cupping, blistering, bleeding, leeching, heating, freezing, sweating, and shock, among other invasive treatments (Shapiro 1971). Most of these treatment procedures were later proven to be medically ineffective. In some cases they proved fatal. Nevertheless, some of them have played an important role as therapeutically beneficial—but fictional—clinical interventions, because they triggered the placebo effect. They count as fictional, because non-existent entities or forces constituting the perceived target disorders are subjected to real interventions (e.g. cutting, purging, or bleeding) to produce real but misunderstood effects (e.g. blood loss, surgical incisions, or cauterized tissue), which are then explained by means of fictional causal pathways. The explanatory entities and clinical procedures that were regarded by patients and physicians as fitting the target disorder like a key fitting a lock were, respectively, theoretical and performative fictions that supported—and at the same time masked—the rallying of the body's natural self-healing powers.

Finally, consider the long history of explanatory theories and medical research paradigms that across history have represented the cutting edge of medical knowledge: theories, for example, of the humors, animal magnetism, demon possession, tutelary spirits, astrology, alchemy, and occult forces (Radden 2000). Explanatory theories integrating what was taken to be the most advanced nosological, etiological, and symptomatological understanding of the day, and the most advanced methods of medical reasoning (e.g. explanation by analogy and similarity), came imbedded within more general models of the functioning of the human body, that were themselves imbedded within still more general models of normalcy and pathology. But what was taken as indisputable medical knowledge in one era was regarded in subsequent—and ostensibly more enlightened—eras as incomplete or unfounded.

What is striking about the history of explanatory theories and medical research paradigms is its sheer variety; a lasting testament to the unbounded creativity of healers and medical researchers. But there is something even more striking: its astonishing transience. Almost nothing from this rich past has lasted, other than humiliating memorials of credulity.[1]

*

---

[1] The passage from Paris' *Pharmacologia* from which this is excerpted is as follows:
'To the medical philosopher there exist but few objects of deeper interest than an extensive and well-arranged cabinet of Materia Medica. What lessons of practical wisdom lie stored within its narrow recesses! How many reminiscences may the contemplation of it call forth, and how many beacons for future guidance may it not afford! Its records are the symbols of medical history—the accredited registers of departed systems, founded on ideal assumptions, and of superstitions engendered by fear and nurtured by ignorance. In its earlier specimens, as from a collection of antique medals, we read the revolutions of the past, and in the space of a few minutes recall the exploded theories of as many centuries, for to these archives have the various sects, which from time to time have held dominion, bequeathed some striking memorial, or left some characteristic trace of their vain and transient existence. With no less interest than instruction will the young practitioner,

Is the situation any better in the history of psychological treatments? Have psychological remedies somehow been spared the fate of ending up as little more than the humiliating memorials of the credulity and infatuation of the psychologists who recommended them? Have they, unlike their medical cousins, somehow escaped the confounding interference of placebo effects, self-limiting diseases, autonomous responses, nocebo effects, dangerous side effects, and iatrogenic diseases? It seems not.

First, consider the colorful history of psychological treatments, with its roots in ancient soul doctoring, mesmerism, shamanism, religio–magical practices, hypnotism, quackery, and suggestion therapy (Torrey 1986; Frank and Frank 1991; Radden 2000). Like the history of medical remedies, the history of psychological therapies has been witness to a succession of spurious treatment methods, etiologies based on causal pathways and causal forces that turn out to be non-existent, empirically impoverished theories of pathology and nosology, and dubious reasoning strategies. Successive therapeutic systems have risen up to occupy centre stage briefly, greeted by the fanfare of so-called experts in human psychology, attracting clients who are eager to attest to a treatment's efficacy, and boasting of unparalleled treatment successes, only to have fallen on hard times, and to have been replaced by yet other treatment methods that have met the same fate a short time later. If the dominant psychological remedies of yesterday are now relics in the museum of quaint ideas, then it seems likely that the same fate lies in store for many of the dominant psychological remedies of today. Certainly this fate is all but inevitable for the fringe psychotherapies: for instance, neuro-linguistic programming, thought field therapy, emotional freedom technique, rage reduction therapy, primal scream therapy, Sedona method, entity depossession therapy, eye movement desensitization, body-centered psychotherapy, rebirthing therapy,

---

entering upon his professional career, regard such a collection. In casting his eyes over so extensive and motley an assemblage of substances, he will be forcibly impressed with the palpable absurdity of some—the disgusting and loathsome nature of others—the total inactivity of many—and the uncertain and precarious reputation of all; and he will be naturally impelled by an eager and laudable curiosity to inquire, how it can have happened that substances, at one period in the highest esteem, and of generally acknowledged utility, should have ever fallen into total neglect or disrepute?—why others, of humble pretensions and little significance, should have maintained their ground for so many centuries; and by what caprice or accident, materials of no energy whatever should have continued to receive the indisputable sanction and unqualified support of the best and wisest practitioners of the age; and, above all, he will inquire, by what necromantic spell certain medicinal substances, after having run their appointed course of trial, and been fairly denounced as inert or useless, could ever again have been raised into especial favour, as if but to sink once more into deeper and more lasting discredit?' (Paris 1843: 3–4)

and past lives therapy (Beyerstein 2001; Lilienfeld *et al.* 2003a, 2003b; Singer and Nievod 2003). But over the course of time, even the more scientifically credentialled psychotherapies—those that disavow the obscurantism, high-sounding technical jargon, and 'strategies of dissimulation' (van Rillaer 1991) of their fringe cousins—may end up as relics in the museum of quaint ideas.

Second, consider the vigorous history of attempts to assess the efficacy of psychological treatments. Fifty years ago, for instance, shortly after the time when placebo controls were first called for in the study of psychotherapy out-comes (Meehl 1955; Rosenthal and Frank 1956), Eysenck (1960, 1965, 1969, 1985, 1994) raised radical doubts about the field of psychotherapy as a whole: there is, he argued, no clear scientific evidence that *any* particular form of psy-chotherapy is effective. This challenge generated a wealth of rebuttals and con-trolled studies that continue to this day. Only a few years after this challenge, more confusion about the field as a whole was raised by what appears to be the very opposite finding to Eysenck's: namely, that *all* forms of psychotherapy *are* effective, and moreover, *equally* effective (Luborsky *et al.* 1975; Smith, Glass, and Miller 1980; Hunsley and Di Guilio 2002). The confusion was further compounded by the subsequent finding, based on a re-analysis of the results of Smith, Glass, and Miller's meta-analysis (1980), that psychotherapy in general is no more effective than a credible placebo (Prioleau *et al.* 1983). The state of confusion and uncertainty afflicting the field of psychotherapy as a whole was not helped by the further claim that psychotherapy *is* none other than a placebo (Frank 1983; Frank and Frank 1993).

And yet, despite what is indisputably a state of deep uncertainty surround-ing therapeutic effectiveness, the nature of clinical evidence, and the scientific status of psychotherapy, many schools of psychotherapy have continued to make bold and unsubstantiated claims about therapeutic effectiveness and explanatory power. So grandiose are these 'claims of unbounded dominion over all disorders and the miseries of the human condition... that the psycho-logical therapies continue to have difficulty defining not what they are but, more importantly, what they are not. The very fact that unchallenged claims to profound and undifferentiated therapeutic benefit are regularly made by an ever-proliferating, theoretically and procedurally inconsistent set of schools (and by their divergently trained practitioners) raises serious doubts about the scientific status of the flourishing enterprises of psychotherapeutic practice and education' (Parloff 1986a: 521).

Coming from psychologists and psychotherapy researchers, these are just a small subset of the internal criticisms of the field of psychotherapy (see also Torrey 1986; Dawes, Faust and Meehl 1989; Albee 1990; Crews 1990; Dawes 1994; Watters and Ofshe 1999). To add to the general state of confusion and uncertainty surrounding psychotherapy, there is also a robust history of external criticisms of psychology, coming from sociology, anthropology, philosophy, and literary criticism, among other quarters. The primary target of most of these criticisms has been the talking cures. Of the philosophers weighing in on the debate, for instance, Popper's criticism is one of the most damning (although it is restricted mainly to psychoanalysis, rather than to the field of psychotherapy as a whole). Psychoanalysis, Popper argued (1963: 37–38), is a pseudo-science rather than a genuine science (but see Grünbaum 1984, 1993; Crews 1990; Cioffi 1998). Its central theoretical claims are as unfalsifiable as the theoretical claims of astrology. 'Psychoanalytic theories... are simply nontestable, irrefutable. There was no conceivable human behavior which could contradict them. [T]hose 'clinical observations' which analysts naively believe confirm their theory cannot do this any more than the daily confirmations which astrologers find in their practice'. Popper (1963: 38 footnote 3) also advanced a tentative and mostly undeveloped version of the suggestion theory that was first raised by Freud's critic and friend Fleiss, and later developed by Farrell (1981) and Grünbaum (1984, 1993): 'How much headway has been made in investigating the question of the extent to which the (conscious or unconscious) expectations and theories held by the analyst influence the 'clinical responses' of the patient? (To say nothing about the conscious attempts to influence the patient by proposing interpretations to him, etc.) Years ago I introduced the term Oedipus effect to describe the influence of a theory or expectation or prediction *upon the event which it predicts* or describes: it will be remembered that the causal chain leading to Oedipus' parricide was started by the oracle's prediction of this event. This is a characteristic and recurrent theme of such myths, but one which seems to have failed to attract the interest of the analysts, perhaps not accidentally'.

If any tentative observations can be made about the *whole* of the history of psychological treatments, with its transient successes and lasting failures, they are the following: There have been few—if any—durable and powerful psychological explanations about why people succumb to psychological troubles (such as depression, anxiety, fear, sadness, phobias, interpersonal troubles, obsessions, mood swings, general unhappiness, as well as to more serious difficulties such as psychoses and personality disorders). Concomitantly, there have been few—if any—durable and powerful psychological treatments for psychological troubles. Nothing, in other words, lasts long. And yet, despite this, there have been many more people who *claim* expertise in understanding human psychology and behavior, and in treating psychological disorders, than there are genuine experts.

From these tentative observations about the past, it is not a far step to make some tentative observations about the present. Erwin (1997; see also

Erwin 1994) takes this step. He argues that there is little to differentiate the pervasive explanatory and treatment failures of physical medicine in the nineteenth century from the explanatory and treatment failures of contemporary psychotherapy.

> First, how effective were most medical treatments at that time [in nineteenth century medicine]? According to some commentators, most, if not all, were no more effective than a credible placebo.... Second, what did medical expertise consist of? It did not consist of the ability to use medical treatments more effectively than credible placebos; for there were generally no such treatments.... How analogous is the current state of psychotherapeutic knowledge to the medical knowledge of 100 years ago? On both of the criteria that I have mentioned, the analogy is almost exact. Most of the various forms of psychotherapy, as far as anyone knows, are not more effective than credible placebos; psychotherapeutic expertise, as far as anyone knows, does not generally consist of knowledge about how to wield techniques that can routinely outperform a credible placebo (Erwin 1997: 144–5).

Erwin concludes from this that psychotherapy is currently in a state of theoretical crisis, just as physical medicine was a hundred years ago. However profound the crisis may be, few people are aware of it. Psychotherapy is flourishing: it has never been more popular, more available, and more in demand, than it is today.

Erwin's analogy is plausible. First, some of the basic principles of psychotherapeutic theories of personality, development, behavior, and psychopathology have only limited empirical, clinical, and experimental support. In this respect, they bear more than superficial similarities to theories of human physiology and pathology that persisted throughout ancient, medieval, and early modern medicine. Theories, that is, where the relation between explanatory theory and empirical evidence resembled an inverted pyramid, with empirical evidence located at a narrow base, and a theoretical superstructure extended far above it and sharply away from it. Second, just as physicians of the past continued to exert a hold over the popular imagination as expert healers, and as sole guardians of esoteric knowledge about physical maladies, despite a long history of explanatory and treatment failures, so psychotherapists of today have continued to exert a hold over the popular imagination as expert healers of minds, and as sole guardians of esoteric knowledge about psychological maladies—despite a long history of explanatory and treatment failures. Moreover, as in physical medicine, clients have continued to invest their hopes in the latest psychotherapeutic treatments, overlooking the procession of short-lived treatment methods that make up the history of psychotherapy, and unaware of the fact that the treatments to which they are submitting themselves are likely bound to become museum relics. Ignorant of this history, and ignorant of treatment success rates, comparative outcome studies, and baseline rates for the natural history of psychological disorders, clients have had few opportunities to be skeptical in the face of extravagant claims about the beneficial therapeutic effects of what may in actuality be weak, worthless, or dangerous treatment methods.

Suppose that Paris' and Erwin's diagnoses of the efficacy of psychological explanations and treatments are more or less correct. Suppose, following Paris, that the history of psychological treatments is a history of treatments that were so clinically ineffective and explanatorily impoverished that they stand now as little more than humiliating memorials of the credulity of the psychologists who recommended them. Suppose further, with Erwin, that even most contemporary psychological treatments are roughly about as effective as the treatments of nineteenth century physical medicine. *Does this really matter?* That is, does it matter whether or not psychological treatments are effective, or whether or not they are successful in explaining the nature and causes of psychological disorders, or whether or not they outperform placebos? Common sense, after all, would suggest that the clinical, predictive, and explanatory failures of psychological treatments do not have consequences that are nearly as serious as the failures of physical medicine; and that the psychological disorders treated by the passing show of psychological remedies are not nearly as serious, costly, or debilitating as physical diseases. The situation may be embarrassing, particularly given the often extravagant claims of the psychotherapies, but it is hardly a serious crisis.

There are a number of reasons why these issues do matter. Erwin, for example, cites three important ones: cost effectiveness, psychotherapist training, and public policy. And there are others.

First, if a psychological treatment is therapeutically effective not because of its presumed characteristic or active ingredients, but because of other nonspecific factors such as expectancy, suggestion, placebo responsiveness, and so forth, then it is likely that there are cheaper, easier, and briefer ways to ensure the delivery of these treatment factors than through expensive psychotherapeutic or psychopharmacological means. A pill placebo plus minimal therapist contact, for example, is one cost effective and more or less successful way that some of these nonspecific factors can be delivered, and it has the advantage of avoiding many of the potentially harmful side effects of drug or psychological treatments. 'If for a certain problem, such as non-psychotic depression, the pill placebo procedure is just as effective, what are the grounds for not using it? ... It might be preferable to drugs and standard psychotherapies for certain depressed clinical populations, such as the spinal cord injured, who must take a variety of other medications that sometimes interact with drugs for depression' (Erwin 1997: 158). Brown (1994) has also argued for the use of placebos for the treatment of psychological disorders such as depression.

Second, if psychological treatments do not outperform inexpensive and easy to deliver placebos, then there is little justification for having expensive and time-consuming psychotherapy training programs, and for placing such great emphasis on therapist expertise (Erwin 1997: 158).

Third, the public and private costs of providing psychotherapeutic (or psychopharmacological) services to the population are huge, while the public and private funding for treatment of mental health problems is limited. There is, Erwin suggests, no good reason why states or third party insurers should pay for expensive treatments such as psychotherapy, the clinical and explanatory successes of which are at best questionable, if there are alternative ways of treating psychological disorders that are less costly, easier to dispense, more widely available, and less prone to side effects. Erwin (1997: 158) suggests that pill placebos and minimal therapist contact would qualify as one of these alternative treatments.

Fourth, if Paris and Erwin's doubts about the clinical, predictive, and explanatory failures of psychological treatments are correct, then it is unethical for psychotherapists to deceive the public with false, exaggerated, or unsupported claims about therapeutic effectiveness and explanatory success. If, for example, clients are told that the psychological theories used by their psychotherapists successfully explain the nature and causes of their psychological disorders, and yet there are insufficient grounds for these explanatory claims—indeed, if many psychological theories are likely to end up as museum relics just as their forebears have—then clients are the victims of deception and false advertising. Clients have the right to be fully informed about the validity of the psychological explanations they are given, just as much as they have the right to be fully informed about the actual effectiveness of the treatments they are receiving. In the psychodynamic psychotherapies, for example, clients who are led to believe that the insights acquired during treatment and the psychodynamic interpretations given by therapists, are true, are deceived if the logical and epistemic grounds for psychodynamic insights and interpretations are questionable. It is unethical to deceive clients in this way.

Finally, consider the common sense claim that the clinical, predictive, and explanatory failures of psychological treatments have not had social, economic, and political consequences that are nearly as devastating as the clinical, predictive, and explanatory failures of physical medicine. This is a gross distortion of the facts, and it borders on mythmaking. Disorders such as depressions, anxieties, phobias, substance abuse, bipolar disorders, and mood disorders create a huge burden upon any society; and by implication, a huge burden upon global resources. The less successful the treatment or prevention of these disorders, the heavier the social burden; and the heavier the social burden, the more the overall state of a society's health and well-being is diminished. If Paris' and Erwin's (and Eysenck's and Albee's) criticisms are valid, then the persistent failures of psychological treatments over the course of history have not helped to significantly reduce the global and social burdens of psychological disorders.

This may appear to be overstated. Psychological disorders do not seem to be nearly as deleterious to a society's health and well-being as afflictions such as cancers, heart and lung diseases, transmissible diseases, famines, epidemics, wars, and accidents. Certainly the more traditional approaches to measuring global health and well-being do not rank psychological disorders as among the leading impediments of a society's overall health and well-being. Typically, these measures rely on metrics that identify the number of *deaths* in a population, and the leading causes of death. And the leading causes of death are rarely of a psychological or psychiatric nature.

In a radical departure from these traditional approaches—one that casts an entirely new light on the social costs of psychological and psychiatric disorders, and the urgent need to find effective treatments and credible explanations for them—Murray and Lopez (1996) have argued that death rates alone could not adequately define the quality of a society's overall health and well-being. Their claim is that it is really *disability* that is the leading burden on any given society's overall health status. And yet disability goes largely unrecognized and unmeasured; and the leading *causes* of disability, which are also overlooked, diverge widely from the leading causes of death. What Murray and Lopez mean is that any one disease, injury, or disorder has multiple disabling effects. When the amount of time that people must live with each of the various disabling sequelae of diseases and injuries is quantified, and when the disabling effects are weighted for severity, an entirely different picture of a society's overall health and well-being emerges. This approach, known as 'burden of disability analysis', allows researchers to measure the gap between current health status and an ideal situation where everyone lives into old age, free of disease and disability (Murray 1996).

Burden of disability analysis diverges from traditional approaches by using a single measure of health status that combines three factors: the number of deaths, the impact of premature death, and disability. The new metric for measuring health status through the impact of the burden of disease is what Murray and Lopez call the Disability Adjusted Life Year (DALY). The DALY combines in one indicator an estimate of the years of life that are *lost* from premature death and the years of life that are lived *with* disabilities. Clearly, then, the concept of *potential* health plays a central role in this measure: that is, potential years of life that are lost due to premature death, as well as potential years of healthy life that are lost by virtue of being in states of poor health and disability. One DALY can be thought of as one lost year of healthy life.

When the burden of disability approach is adopted, it becomes clear that the impact of psychological and psychiatric disorders on the overall quality of a population's health has been severely underestimated. While these disorders are responsible for a mere one percent of deaths globally, they are (in Murray and Lopez's estimate) responsible for almost 11% of the global burden of disease. Half of the top ten leading causes of disability worldwide are psychological or psychiatric conditions: namely, depression, alcohol abuse, bipolar affective disorder, schizophrenia, and obsessive compulsive disorder. Depression ranks fourth in terms of the global burden of disease, and for women in developing and first world countries it ranks as the leading cause of disease burden. When projected to the year 2020, psychological and psychiatric disorders are expected to contribute even more significantly to the global burden of disease, increasing in proportion from 10.5% in 1990 to 15% by 2020 (see also Andrews *et al.* 2000).

Burden of disability analysis demonstrates what some have known all along: that psychological disorders are both more pervasive and more taxing to social resources than is commonly acknowledged. It also demonstrates the pressing need for durable, tested, and effective psychological treatments, and the need for public health policies that take seriously the importance of public funding of research into the prevention and treatment of psychological and psychiatric disorders.

To conclude, it does matter whether or not psychological treatments are effective, or whether or not they are successful in explaining the nature and causes of psychological disorders, or whether or not they outperform placebos, or whether or not they are little more than placebos. The stakes are high.

Range of Inquiry

Two preliminary points about the range of inquiry of the work that follows are in order. First, for reasons of economy and conceptual precision, the focus of this work will not be psychotherapy in all its manifold guises, but only the so-called talking cures. More specifically from this large group, it will only be the psychodynamic psychotherapies: that is, the psychotherapies that place a premium on psychological exploration, and the importance of insight to psychological well-being. These are the quintessential talking cures, and they include psychoanalysis in its many incarnations, Jungian analysis, short-term psychodynamic psychotherapy, and the newer psychodynamic theories of ego psychology, object relations theory, self psychology, and interpersonal psychology. Not only do these psychotherapies make strong claims about therapeutic effectiveness, often coupled with robust theoretical claims about human nature, the nature of the mind, and the causation of psychopathology; they also make strong *epistemic* claims about the nature of psychotherapists' and clients' knowledge, belief, and insight. In particular, they make strong epistemic claims about helping clients to make important *discoveries* about themselves—that is, claims about achieving self-growth, or actualization, or psychological maturity through the acquisition of *insight* or *self-understanding*. The psychodynamic psychotherapies promote themselves as being in the exploration business—the business of helping clients find out who they are, why they are as they are, and why they are experiencing psychological problems.

The main focus of the work that follows can be summed up in the following questions. Is there any credible evidence that psychological exploration is in fact what the talking cures, and especially the psychodynamic psychotherapies, are up to? Is there any credible evidence that psychological discovery is what they are in fact achieving? Are the *epistemic* claims warranted? To paraphrase John Ayrton Paris, is there any guarantee that the boasted remedies of present day psychodynamic psychotherapies will not, like their predecessors, fall into disrepute, and in their turn serve only as a humiliating memorial of the credulity and infatuation of the psychologists who recommended them?

There are a number of other psychotherapeutic systems that also accord an important role to insight and depth-psychological exploration, even though they are not strictly psychodynamic in theoretical orientation or clinical practice: person-centered psychotherapy, process-experiential psychotherapy, emotionally focused psychotherapy, gestalt psychotherapy, feminist psychotherapy, and narrative psychotherapy. For reasons of economy and conceptual precision, however, these psychotherapies will not be the focus of discussion here. This does not mean that the guiding questions and conclusions of this work cannot be extrapolated to these other psychotherapeutic systems; there may indeed be very good grounds for extrapolation, since they are all, in some form or other 'cures' involving talking, but they will not be explored here. There is little doubt that there are some psychodynamic psychotherapies that do not adhere strictly in practice to psychodynamic principles; there is also little doubt that some non-psychodynamic psychotherapies import psychodynamic methods, claims, and goals into their clinical practice. While it is beyond the scope of this work, it is likely that a detailed survey of the vast number of psychotherapies that fall under the broad and diffuse category of talking cures would reveal a significant number that in practice encourage self-exploration and insight, even though in principle they are not centrally committed to these goals. Psychotherapeutic systems, in other words, do not occupy discrete, theoretically well-bounded domains. Their day to day application in the clinic strays easily across theoretical borders, and what clients take away from them is not always what the outcome measures and effectiveness studies track. Thus the analyses and arguments about insight that follow in this work may apply to many types of insight-oriented psychotherapy.

Finally, for reasons of economy, there will be no discussion of the diluted versions of the psychodynamic psychotherapies that are found in what is commonly known as 'pop psychology;' nor will there be any discussion of the fringe psychotherapies that happen to emphasize the importance of insight to psychological healing.

What distinguishes the psychodynamic psychotherapies from the other psychotherapies? There is no easy answer here. Along with the massive proliferation of psychotherapeutic systems—over 400 by one standard of counting—there are also multiple ways to distinguish psychotherapies one from another: for instance, in terms of their theories, goals, or clinical practices. No single way is definitive and final. However, one of the distinguishing features of the psychodynamic psychotherapies that shows up both in theory and clinical practice concerns the etiology of psychological disorders. The psychodynamic psychotherapies are distinguished from many other psychotherapies in holding the view that the causes of many psychological disorders are to be found in the rapid and often turbulent psychological developments occurring in infancy and early childhood. It is thought that the emotionally charged conflicts and interpersonal relations of infancy and early childhood exert powerful influences over adult thoughts, feelings, and behaviors, mainly in the form of defense mechanisms and neurotic complexes. Childhood wishes and fears do not weaken with age, but tend to go underground, persisting 'despite later experiences that might be expected to alter them. Repression ... does not merely prevent the individual from being aware of what is being repressed; it also prevents the repressed desire from 'growing up', from changing in the course of development as do unrepressed desires or fantasies' (Wachtel 1977: 27). These powerful influences go unrecognized and unnamed: they are outside the range of conscious awareness. They are also dynamic and stealthy, and flourish only to the extent that they remain unrecognized. So pervasive are these unconscious influences that there are many instances of interpersonal and intrapersonal behaviors in which people are ignorant of what they are really doing, despite their claims to authoritative self-knowledge, and despite the fact that their behaviors display a robust (and often self-destructive) sense of purpose and direction. If the psychodynamic model of mind is correct, then there is a valid sense in which people can be described as strangers to themselves. One of the primary goals of psychodynamic psychotherapy is thus to help clients recognize and understand the forces that shape their behavior. Whatever freedom they enjoy in changing their behaviors through an enlarged self-understanding is based on identifying motives that have not been recognized before, and tracing their causal histories back into childhood and infancy.

Another of the many important distinguishing features of the psychodynamic psychotherapies is the use made of deep theoretical explanations of psychological phenomena. These explanations diverge, often sharply, from common sense or folk psychological explanations, as well as from first-person explanations. Psychodynamic explanations are typically framed in terms of what Geertz (1983) calls experience-distant concepts, which stand in sharp opposition to experience-near concepts.

> An experience-near concept is, roughly, one that someone—a patient, a subject— might himself naturally and effortlessly use to define what he or his fellows see, feel, think, imagine, and so on, and which he would readily understand when similarly applied by others. An experience-distant concept is one that specialists of one sort or another—an analyst, an experimenter, an ethnographer, even a priest or an ideologist—employ to forward their scientific, philosophical, or practical aims. 'Love' is an experience-near concept, 'object cathexis' is an experience-distant one. 'Social stratification' and for most peoples in the world even 'religion' (and certainly 'religious system') are experience-distant; 'caste' and 'nirvana' are experience-near, at least for Hindus and Buddhists... Confinement to experience-near concepts leaves an ethnographer awash in immediacies, as well as entangled in vernacular. Confinement to experience-distant ones leaves him stranded in abstractions and smothered in jargon (Geertz 1983: 57).

Geertz notes that the distinction between the two types of concepts is fluid and evolving. What is regarded as an experience-distant concept at one time is experience-near at another; and what is considered to be an experience-distant explanatory concept at one time in the history of the social sciences is at another considered to be an antiquated piece of speculative metaphysics. Some psychoanalytic concepts that were experience-distant in the early 1900s, for example, have become incorporated into late twentieth century common sense psychology.

Experience-distant concepts in psychodynamic psychotherapy include concepts such as unconscious forces, resistance, repression, denial, regression, transference, reaction formation, displacement, reversal, sublimation, and splitting. These concepts come to play a central role in interpretations and insights. Clients learn to think of themselves in terms of these new concepts, so much so that what they first encounter as an experience-distant concept upon first entering treatment may evolve into an experience-near concept.

The second point about the range of inquiry of the work that follows concerns the relation between the placebo effect and the mind–body problem. The placebo effect, which will serve as one of the main points of discussion here, might seem to offer a unique window onto the mind–body problem. When freed of the many myths and misconceptions that surround it, it seems to provide 'real world' illustrations and suggestive analogies that are more compelling than the many arguments and thought experiments used by philosophers, neuroscientists, and cognitive scientists to defend theoretical positions about the mind–body problem. It is also a definitional litmus test. The placebo effect is typically defined in ways that already, and sometimes illicitly, embody substantive theoretical positions—or, worse, substantive myths and misconceptions. It is defined, for instance, as a purely 'subjective' or psychological phenomenon that has no 'real' influence on the so-called non-negotiable 'objective' properties of the body; as a psychological cause of objective physical effects; as a physical (neurophysiological) event with psychological effects; as a subjective epiphenomenon, like 'oil on water;' as a 'meaning response' that somehow translates into physical effects; and so on. Each of these definitions is freighted with assumptions about the relation between mind and body, about psychosomatic causal pathways and interactions, and about multidisciplinary research agendas linking up the behavioral and social scientific approach to placebos with the neurobiological approach.

But scientific advances in the understanding of the placebo effect will not, of themselves, solve the mind–body problem; that is, they will not supply compelling evidence for the truth (or evidence for the falsity) of any philosophical position about the nature of the mind–body relation (e.g. substance dualism, property dualism, reductive materialism, non-reductive materialism, eliminativist materialism, functionalism, substance monism, anomalous monism, and so on). Placebo phenomena may help to *illustrate* philosophical positions about the nature of the mind–body relation, and may help to nudge intuitions in one theoretical direction or another, but those positions are defended on grounds that are largely independent of the phenomena. What they provide is color, not argumentative substance. The following work is therefore not about the mind–body problem, with its ongoing history of valiant theoretical struggles and repeated failures; nor does not it take any principled stand on what the mind is, or what it is ultimately made of, or what it can and cannot do.

Chapter 1

Placebos and Psychotherapy

Placebo Effects

The following examples illustrate the placebo effect.

- '...A tale [was] told me by one of my late father's servants who was an apothecary. He was a simple man—a Swiss (a people little given to vanity and lying). He had had a long acquaintance with a sickly merchant in Toulouse who suffered from the stone; he had frequent need of enemas and made his doctors prescribe him various kinds, depending on the symptoms of his illness. When the enemas were brought in, none of the usual formalities were omitted: he often used to finger them to see if they were hot. There he was, lying down and turned on his side; all the usual preliminaries were gone through... except that no clyster was injected! After this ceremony the apothecary withdrew; the patient was treated as though he had taken the clyster and the result was the same as for those who had. If the doctor found that the treatment did not prove effective he gave him two or three other enemas—all of the same kind! Now my informant swears that the sick man's wife (in order to cut down expenses, since he paid for these clysters as though he had really had them) assayed simply injecting warm water; that proved to have no effect: the trickery was therefore discovered but he was obliged to return to the first kind. There was a woman who believed she had swallowed a pin in her bread; she yelled and screamed as though she felt an insufferable pain in her throat where she thought she could feel it stuck; but since there was no swelling nor external symptoms, one clever fellow concluded that it was all imagination and opinion occasioned by a crust that had jabbed her on the way down; he made her vomit and secretly tossed a bent pin into what she had brought up. That woman believed she had vomited it out and immediately felt relieved of the pain'. (Montaigne 2003: 117)

- B, a 46-year-old interior designer who had suffered from 30 years of depression, volunteered at UCLA's Neuropsychiatric Institute for a large randomized controlled trial of one of the new generation of antidepressant drug, venlafaxine (Effexor®) (Greenberg 2003; see also Kirsch *et al.* 1998; Kirsch *et al.* 2002; Greenberg 2007). B received a neuropsychiatric assessment to establish her baseline brain activity, signed a consent form acknowledging her participation in the study, and then was given a bottle of pills, not knowing whether they contained the drug or placebo. Within two weeks she reported that she was feeling significantly improved, and her scores on a battery of weekly measures (e.g. interviews, tests, EEGs) indicated this improvement. During the study, she experienced some of the side effects that are associated with the new generation of SSRI antidepressants (nausea), and she guessed (along with a nurse conducting some of the weekly interviews and tests) that she must have been assigned to the group receiving the drug. By the end of the study, B was dramatically improved, and credited her improvement to the drug. She was astonished to learn that she was given the placebo and not the drug. B's improvement could not possibly be attributed to the pharmacological effects of the pills she was assigned in the study.

- In an experiment on placebos and pain reduction (Montgomery and Kirsch 1996), experimental participants were told that they would be given a new local anesthetic called Trivaricane, which in previous clinical testing had proven to be effective in reducing pain. While it looked and smelled like a real medication, Trivaricane was in fact a placebo, consisting only of iodine, oil of thyme, and water. In the experiment, Trivaricane was applied to participants' index fingers by an experimenter who wore a physician-like lab coat and surgical gloves. A minute later, after the 'anesthetic' had 'taken effect', a sharp painful force was applied to the treated index finger, and then to other nontreated fingers. Participants were then asked to rate the pain on a scale of 0 ('no pain') to 10 ('pain as intense as one can imagine'). Several variations in experimental design were used. Participants consistently reported that the intensity and unpleasantness of the pain were less on the finger treated with Trivaricane than on fingers without it.

- One hundred children diagnosed with upper respiratory tract infections, and who had been coughing for an average of more than three days, took part in a double-blind randomized controlled study of pediatric cough medication (Paul *et al.* 2004). The children were randomly assigned to one of three groups: a group treated with a well-known over-the-counter brand name cough syrup (containing dextromethorphan), a group treated with another well-known over-the-counter cough syrup (containing diphenhydramine), and a group treated with a placebo cough syrup (flavored water). Children in all three groups improved in terms of cough frequency, but those assigned to the placebo condition showed the best results. The authors concluded that time and proper hydration are the best treatment for most respiratory infections, and that the benefits that come from medicated cough syrups are likely psychological.

- In one study of placebo pacemakers (Linde *et al.* 1999, cited in Moerman 2002a), 81 people who had received surgery for hypertrophic cardiomyopathy (abnormal thickening of the heart muscle) had pacemakers implanted. Half of the pacemakers were turned on, and half were turned off, without the recipients knowing this fact. Those with working pacemakers had better overall results than those with the nonworking pacemakers, but the patients in the latter group were still significantly better than when they began the study, reporting fewer symptoms than before (e.g. less chest pain, less shortness of breath, less dizziness, and fewer heart palpitations).

- In a large double-blind randomized controlled study of the treatment of headaches, 835 British women who regularly used aspirin to treat their headaches were given packets of headache tablets, with instructions to take two tablets at the onset of their headaches (Braithwaite and Cooper 1981). They were told that the study was conducted on behalf of a well known manufacturer of pharmaceutical products, and that the goal of the study was to compare the effectiveness of two kinds of headache tablet already on the market. The participants were asked to complete a questionnaire one hour after the onset of their headaches, answering questions about how much the pain had changed on a six-point scale. The women were divided into four groups, and none knew who got which tablets. Group A received placebo pills that were identified with the simple generic label 'Analgesic tablets'. Group B received placebo pills that were labeled with the brand name of a popular aspirin that is widely available in Great Britain. Group C received aspirin tablets that were identified with the simple generic label 'Analgesic tablets' (of the same appearance as the tablets in Group A). Group D received aspirin tablets that were labeled with the brand name of the same popular and widely available aspirin (the same appearance as the tablets in Group B). The results showed that placebo tablets were effective in reducing headache pain for most women in Groups A and B. Since these were the placebo groups, it appears that the very fact of taking a pill brought about significant pain relief. Curiously, participants who took branded placebos reported more pain relief in one hour than those who took placebos with the generic label. In general, however, placebos did not work as well at relieving pain as *bona fide* aspirin tablets. But branded aspirin tablets worked better at relieving pain than generically labeled aspirin tablets (cited in Moerman 2002a).

- In one highly publicized and commonly misunderstood randomized placebo-controlled study of the effectiveness of arthroscopic surgery for osteoarthritis of the knee (Moseley *et al.* 2002), it was found that sham surgery performed just as well as actual surgery. At a VA hospital in

Houston, Texas, 180 patients were randomly assigned to groups receiving either arthroscopic débridement, arthroscopic lavage (a knee wash-out), or placebo surgery (in which patients received skin incisions and underwent a simulated débridement without insertion of the arthroscope). Neither patients nor assessors of outcome knew who had been assigned to which group. The outcomes of the study were assessed at several points over a two-year period using five self-reported scores (three scores using scales for pain and two using scales for function), and one objective test of walking and stair climbing. The authors of the study concluded that at no point did either of the intervention groups report less pain or better function than the placebo group: 'the outcomes after arthroscopic lavage or arthroscopic débridement were no better than those after a placebo procedure'. The authors of the study did not conclude that arthroscopic surgery does not work; nor did they conclude that arthroscopic surgery does not work for such problems as cartilage tears and other specific conditions. The study lends support to the view that arthritis is not a good reason to perform arthroscopic surgery.

♦ In a well-known study conducted by the psychotherapy researcher Hans Strupp (1979), male college students with similar psychological problems (depression, anxiety, social introversion) were assigned to one of two treatment groups: highly experienced professional psychotherapists, or college professors with no psychological training, but skilled at forming understanding relationships. No specific psychological treatment method was used in the latter group. Therapy sessions were twice weekly for three to four months, for a total of 25 hours. Multiple measures of assessment were used to detect therapeutic improvement: client and psychotherapist ratings of fundamental change, psychological test scores, and self-reported changes in specific target complaints. Strupp also conducted a follow-up of the clients one year later. The results of the study were surprising. Clients who were 'treated' by the college professors on average showed as much improvement on most measures as clients treated by professional psychotherapists. The most significant therapeutic changes happened during the treatment period, but therapeutic benefits were still evident at the one-year follow-up. Strupp concluded that beneficial therapeutic change is attributable more to the healing effects of a benign human relationship (trust, warmth, understanding), than to the specific characteristics of any one treatment method, or to the level of training and expertise of the psychotherapist. Strupp's view is that almost all psychotherapeutic approaches are more or less equally effective, with no single approach generally outperforming all others.

♦ People diagnosed with mild to moderate depression were enrolled in a 16-week clinical study designed to compare the effectiveness of a relatively new short-term psychodynamic psychotherapy (Psychotherapy A) against what they were told was an older short-term psychodynamic psychotherapy (Psychotherapy B). A total of 60 participants were randomly assigned to one of the two groups. They received full psychological assessments to establish their baseline psychological states, signed consent forms acknowledging participation in the study, and were assigned to psychotherapists for weekly psychotherapy sessions of one hour each. Neither participants nor experiment coders knew who had been assigned to which group. By the end of the study, 80% of all participants reported feeling significantly improved: that is, their scores in interviews, self-report scales, and standard depression inventories indicated clinically significant improvement. Participants assigned to Psychotherapy A showed slightly greater overall therapeutic improvement over those assigned to B. Participants assigned to B were surprised to learn that they were assigned not to a "real" psychodynamic psychotherapy, but to a sham psychotherapy. Their "psychotherapists" were actors with no psychological training or experience; and the interventions consisted of sham empathy, play-acted professional behaviors, and nearly vacuous one-size-fits-all therapeutic comments based on rehearsed scripts. The 'psychotherapists' posed one-size-fits-all questions ('Tell me about your childhood,' 'What are your feelings about x?' 'Why do you have these feelings?' 'Tell me about your dreams,' 'What do you think your dreams mean?'), with scripted follow-up questions requesting clarification ('what do you mean?'); and they supplied clients with one-size-fits-all interpretations, consisting of trivial claims such as 'you have had trouble being intimate with people,' 'you have certain complex issues from your childhood that have not been worked out,' and 'you have sometimes felt that you were misunderstood.'

The first eight cases illustrate the placebo effect. The first one dates from around 1575; the rest are contemporary. Each case is real—except for the last one, which is entirely fictional. Ethics regulations in most countries would prevent such an overtly deceptive clinical trial from taking place. But the comparison this case invites is obvious. If there is a placebo effect in the first eight cases, then would there not also be a placebo effect in the last case? If placebo pills and placebo surgeries can somehow rally the body's native self-healing powers, then might a placebo psychotherapy somehow rally the mind's native self-healing powers? Are the same kinds of mechanisms at work in the latter case as in the former cases? Moreover, would the statistical trends that document the incidence and frequency of placebo responses in the various branches of physical medicine be expected to hold for placebo responses in the various branches of psychotherapy?

In 1955, in one of the groundbreaking scientific papers on the placebo effect, the Harvard-based physician Henry Beecher (1955) estimated that 30–40% of *any* treatment group responded to placebo, and that 55% of any treatment group responded to placebo pain relief. These were extraordinary claims, supported by what appeared to be the first solid clinical and experimental evidence in the history of placebo research. Beecher's paper served to synthesize an emerging but until then disparate research trend that began with the 1946 and 1954 Cornell-based Conferences on Therapy (1946, 1954), which focused on placebos and double-blind clinical trial design (Kiene 1993a, 1993b; Kaptchuk 1998a, 1998b). Not surprisingly, his one-size-fits-all estimates have been subjected to increasingly precise refinements from one medical subdiscipline to another, and from one medical condition to another: the 30–40% estimate is now considered to be a 'vintage number', at least in the words of one medical historian (Kaptchuk 1998a, 1998b). Moreover, Beecher's claims about the 'powerful placebo' were not helped by the fact that his own meta-analysis of the original data was flawed in a number of significant respects (Kienle and Kiene 1997). There is considerably wider variation in the placebo response in individuals from one time to another, and from one condition to another, than Beecher's estimates suggest. There is also wider variation within groups of individuals diagnosed with the same disease or disorder; across clinical trials; within any one disease condition; and with any one drug or medical procedure. There is even some evidence to suggest that the rate of placebo responsivity in clinical trials of antidepressant drugs is not fixed, but is slowly increasing over time (Walsh *et al.* 2002).

Despite these problems, however, the general intuition behind Beecher's estimates is not off the mark: when confounding factors are eliminated or controlled for, and unsupported inferences are corrected, there is good reason to believe that there is *some* determinate and measurable statistical average for placebo response for a significant number of medical conditions, patient populations, and medical procedures. The placebo is not, as some have proclaimed, *merely* a medical myth (Kienle and Kiene 1997; Hróbjartsson and Gøtzsche 2001).

If Beecher's general intuition is correct, then it would also seem reasonable to expect that just as there is *some* determinate and measurable statistical average for placebo response for specific physical conditions in response to specific medical treatments, so there is *some* determinate and measurable statistical average for placebo response for specific psychological conditions in response to specific psychological treatments. The placebo response, in other words, is not restricted to physical medicine alone.

Consider now the following twist to the imaginary case.

♦ A 50-year-old technical writer suffering from depression and anxiety volunteers at a university-based psychotherapy clinic for a 24-week controlled clinical trial designed to compare the effectiveness of a new short-term psychodynamic psychotherapy against that of an older short-term psychodynamic psychotherapy. A placebo control consisting of a dummy pill, wait list, and minimal psychotherapist contact is also included in the study. A total of 75 participants with similar psychological problems are randomly assigned to one of the three groups. After signing a consent form acknowledging participation in the study, the writer receives a psychological assessment to establish his baseline psychological state and several neuro-psychiatric tests to establish his baseline neurological state. He is assigned to a psychotherapist for weekly psychotherapy sessions of one hour each. Immediately after the baseline testing, he has reservations and decides to back out of the trial. He seeks no professional help for his problems. Twenty-four weeks later he is contacted by the director of the study and is asked to volunteer three hours of his time, for a follow-up session. He agrees, and at the clinic receives a full psychological assessment to establish his psychological state, as well as a battery of neuro-psychiatric tests to establish his neurological state. In the interview he reports feeling significantly improved over his last visit to the clinic weeks ago. Many of his presenting symptoms have remitted. His scores on standard depression inventories and standard neuropsychiatric tests indicate clinically significant improvement, although it is not as marked as in those who received either form of psychotherapy, nor as in those who received the placebo.

This last case, also fictional, illustrates what in physical medicine is known as the autonomous response. This is distinct from the placebo response, although it is quite often conflated with it. Untreated physical diseases and disorders that evoke the body's autonomous immunological responses often tend to display a natural history: that is, depending on the pre-existing physiopathological conditions of the host, and pre-existing environmental conditions, they tend to follow regular patterns of onset, course, duration, and symptom remission. It can be expected, for example, that the symptoms of an untreated common cold in an otherwise healthy host in an otherwise normal environment will follow a predictable course, remitting within (say) six to seven days. Hence the saying 'if you treat a cold it will last a week, and if you don't treat it, it will last seven days'. The symptoms of colds, and many other diseases and disorders, are self-limiting. (The autonomous response has sometimes been called spontaneous remission, but this term, deployed by Eysenck (1960, 1965; see also Strupp and Luborsky 1962; Strupp 1973) in his critique of the effectiveness of psychotherapy, is fuzzy, and liable to give the mistaken impression that no causal agent is involved.)

In addition to the conventional two-arm clinical trials that include the experimental group and the placebo control group, a relatively small number of clinical trials have included no-treatment control groups. Participants assigned to these groups receive no treatment at all: after baseline measures are taken, they are (for example) placed on wait lists, and contacted for follow-up measures weeks or months later. The crucial assumption behind this controversial methodological strategy (see Chapter 5) is that in the no-treatment condition, the natural patterns of onset, course, duration, and symptom remission of the untreated disease or disorder would be clearly observable, and would yield to objective measurement: no-treatment groups, in other words, would reveal the *actual* natural history of the disease or disorder (rather than, for instance, experimental or measurement artifacts). With this information in hand, experimenters would have an objective baseline against which the performance of the experimental drug *and* placebo could be measured. This information would also serve the goals of medical statistics and biostatistics, which aim to determine baseline averages for the success rates of treatment interventions for specific diseases and disorders in specific patient populations. If no-treatment controls provide viable measures of the natural history of diseases and disorders, then medical statistics and biostatistics could also develop statistically reliable baseline averages for them. Once both sets of baseline averages are known, clinicians would have at their disposal powerful actuarial methods of diagnosis and prediction that would not be vulnerable to the pervasive biases in reasoning that afflict clinical methods of diagnosis and prediction (Meehl 1953; Arkes 1981; Faust 1986; Dawes 1988; Dawes *et al.* 1989; Garb 1989, 1996; Grove and Meehl 1996; Koehler 1996).

Do psychological and psychiatric disorders also follow a natural history like many of their physical cousins? Will they remit if left untreated? Could there be a psychological analog of medical statistics and biostatistics, the goal of which would be to establish statistically reliable baseline averages of the natural history of (untreated) psychological disorders for well-defined patient populations? While there is relatively scant information on these topics, there is emerging evidence to suggest that some psychological and psychiatric disorders follow a natural history (see Kleinman, in Harrington 1997: 217-219; Barsky, in Harrington 1997: 217; Kleinman *et al.* 2002: 15; Moerman 2002a: 26). Beneath its manifold sociocultural and individual variations, for instance, depression appears to display the broad outlines of a natural history. Two recent studies show that episodes of major depressive disorder with specific patient populations tend to remit within six to ten weeks. McLeod *et al.* (1992), for example, studied a sample of married persons with untreated depression, and observed that the median duration of depressive episodes (according to *DSM-III-R* criteria) was ten weeks, with 75% of the sample having episodes of under 22 weeks. Kendler *et al.* (1997) studied a sample of women and observed that the median time to recovery was six weeks, with 75% recovering within twelve weeks.[1]

The last imaginary case discussed illustrates a crucial distinction: namely, the distinction between placebo interventions, medically active (nonplacebo) interventions, and no-treatment conditions (where the disease or disorder follows its natural history). Diseases or disorders that are treated with active interventions tend to follow a different history (in terms of onset, course, duration, and symptom remission) from those that are treated with placebos, which in turn tend to follow a different history from those that are left untreated. It is a common mistake, however, to confound the effects of a medical or psychological intervention with the natural history of a disease, or with random fluctuations in the course of symptoms, or with other factors: that is, to give credit to a treatment intervention for changes that would have occurred anyways, or that are caused by other factors that have been over-looked or not controlled for. Similarly, it is a common mistake—one that even Beecher fell prey to—to give credit to a placebo intervention for changes that would have occurred anyways, or changes that have been caused by other disguised or uncontrolled-for factors, and then to make unsupported conclusions about the so-called powerful placebo. The response that is seen in the placebo arm of a clinical trial, for instance, is often taken to be the true placebo effect: but without controlling for the effects of a number of disguised or neglected therapeutic agents, this is a mistaken inference (Kiene 1993a, 1993b; Ernst and Resch 1995; Kienle and Kiene 1997; Kaptchuk 1998a, 1998b; Bootzin and Caspi 2003). The comparisons this last imaginary case invites should be obvious.

First, if autonomous responses and self-limiting diseases play an important role in physical medicine, then it seems reasonable to suppose that they also play a role in psychological medicine. Psychological disorders such as depression, anxiety, and phobia may follow a natural history, and display regular patterns of onset, course, duration, and symptom remission. The idea that self-limiting diseases and disorders belong exclusively to the province of bodily phenomena presumes a sharp and problematic dichotomy between mind and body.

Second, if autonomous responses and self-limiting diseases need to be factored in as a third control arm when designing randomized controlled studies of medical interventions or pharmaceutical drugs, then it is reasonable to suppose that they also need to be factored in when designing controlled studies of the effectiveness of psychotherapies. One of the first calls for controls in psychotherapy outcome studies was from Meehl in 1955 (Meehl 1955), followed shortly by Rosenthal and Frank (1956). Since then, placebo-controlled studies have come to occupy a respected if methodologically controversial place in clinical psychology, psychotherapy and psychopharmacology. The rise to prominence of placebo-controlled studies, however, has been matched by an equally noticeable absence of studies and trials using no-treatment controls, coupled with a noticeable absence of conceptual, methodological, and ethical reflection on no-treatment controls.

Finally, it seems reasonable to suppose that just as there are statistically determinate trends for the incidence, onset, course, duration, and symptom remission of self-limiting diseases in physical medicine, so there may be statistically determinate trends for the incidence, onset, course, duration, and symptom remission for self-limiting disorders of a psychological nature. And just as physical medicine has benefited from actuarial methods that complement or overrule clinical methods in the diagnosis and prognosis of disease (Dawes *et al.* 1989), and that help physicians to decide whether treatment is required at all, so psychology may benefit from actuarial methods that complement or overrule clinical methods in the diagnosis and prognosis of psychological disorders.

Self-Exploration, Insight, and Healing

The more obvious an idea seems, the more difficult it is to see around it, test it, and call it into question. Consider what seems obvious about the talking cures, and in particular about the psychodynamic psychotherapies. First, it seems obvious that the psychodynamic psychotherapies help clients by encouraging them to explore themselves and acquire a deeper understanding of their feelings, memories, desires, interpersonal relationships, personality, and childhood. The goal of treatment is not primarily behavioral modification, crisis intervention, emotional support, or short-term symptom relief: it is, among other things, the exploration of the psyche and its depths, with a view to helping clients acquire insight or self-knowledge. It seems obvious that insight matters to psychological well-being, and to what is variously called self-growth, self-actualization, or psychological maturity. Without insight, psychological problems tend to recur, and psychological well-being remains a distant goal. Second, it seems obvious that clients who are engaged in such difficult exploratory work should, and in fact do, emerge from treatment improved—assuming that the treatment has been carried out properly. Among other achievements, they have made valid discoveries about themselves. They enjoy a greater clarity about their psychological make-up, personality, past, and behaviors than they had at the outset of the treatment. Third, it seems obvious that the newly-won insights claimed by clients in the psychodynamic psychotherapies somehow constitute an improvement to their lives, and serve the ends of psychological healing.

These appear to be good assumptions, not only because the clinical evidence and outcome studies supplied by the psychodynamic psychotherapies *seems* to bear them out, but because it is hard for us to imagine what else clients and psychotherapists engaged in these treatments could possibly be doing if they were *not* engaged in psychological exploration. The link between self-exploration, insight, and healing seems natural and obvious to us. It is reinforced by the persuasive and confident claims used by many psychodynamic psychotherapists to characterize their practice: for example, the psychodynamic psychotherapies are claimed to help clients acquire self-knowledge; they are claimed (by some psychoanalysts at least) to proceed by a kind of archaeological excavation of hidden layers of psychological sediment; or they are claimed to help clients 'get in touch' with an 'inner' or 'core' or 'authentic' self (see Chapter 2, section 2, for a survey of relevant positions). The link between self-exploration, insight, and healing is further reinforced by the testimonials of satisfied and purportedly insightful clients (despite the fact that every psychological therapy that has ever been devised has found supporters willing to provide sincere testimony).

A number of substantive assumptions about the etiology of psychological disorders also come into play to help reinforce the obviousness of the link between self-exploration, insight, and healing. It seems obvious, for example, that childhood traumas and conflicts are among the leading causes of psychological disorders. Many people, it seems, never fully escape their childhood, but are destined to repeat their childlike responses to ancient conflicts over and over again. It also seems obvious that emotions such as anger, hostility, and hatred, if unexpressed, will build up like steam in a kettle until they explode. This is the hydraulic model of mind. Robust causal assumptions such as these tend to be accompanied by a number of assumptions about the nature of memory. It seems obvious—at least to many—that most traumatic memories from childhood are repressed; that hypnosis is a reliable means of recovering repressed memories; and that memory is like a video recorder that starts at birth. Yapko (1994) for instance surveyed nearly 1000 psychotherapists and found that more than half believed that 'hypnosis can be used to recover memories from as far back as birth'; that one-third agreed that 'the mind is like a computer, accurately recording events that actually occurred'; and that one-third agreed that 'someone's feeling certain about a memory means the memory is likely to be correct'. Highlighting the scientist–practitioner gap that afflicts a great deal of psychotherapy (Lilienfeld *et al.* 2003b), Yapko notes that none of these statements is supported by sound scientific evidence. In fact, the scientific research on memory confabulation, distortion, and error tends to undermine each of these beliefs.

Is the link between self-exploration, insight, and healing epistemically and logically cogent? Why assume in the first place that what occurs in the exploratory psychotherapies is *bona fide* exploration that leads to *veridical* insight, rather than something that *looks* like *bona fide* exploration but is in fact something else? Why assume that the exploration of the psyche—rather than (for example) the exploration of one's society, or the exploration of one's brain and central nervous system, or the exploration of one's values, or the exploration of the logic of one's concepts—is essential to psychological healing and well-being? Why assume that therapeutic improvement is caused (among other things) by the acquisition of insight, and not by other causal factors that are masked by and yet coincident with the acquisition of insight? Why assume that the kind of psychological exploration that occurs in the psychodynamic psychotherapies is truth-tracking, rather than something that merely gives the *appearance* of being truth-tracking? Is it possible that the activity of therapeutic exploration might *appear* to uncover the deep layers of the psyche, while it is in fact doing something else altogether? And finally, why assume that clients' insights refer to anything—or if they do refer at all, why assume that what they *appear* to refer to, or what they are claimed to refer to, is what they *really* refer to? Is it possible that the long-standing philosophical distinction between appearance and reality applies in some form to psychodynamic insights?

These are philosophical—and specifically *epistemological*—questions. They are informed by a moderately skeptical and nominalist approach that refuses to take allegedly obvious ideas at face value. They are to be distinguished from the kinds of questions that might be answered satisfactorily by appeal to empirical data: that is, by the accumulation of clinical case studies, by client self-reports, by the pursuit of greater methodological fine-tuning in insight measures and tests, or by the development of more accurate measures for outcome studies. It is a fallacy to assume that once all the relevant empirical data are in, the epistemological questions will simply take care of themselves.

To cast light on these questions about the logical and epistemological foundations of the psychodynamic psychotherapies, and to coax the questions into more manageable format, the focus here will be trained on one primary question: does truth matter in the psychodynamic psychotherapies—and if so, how? This question will be rephrased and reiterated from a number of different perspectives throughout the work that follows: is it the case in the psychodynamic psychotherapies that clients' putative discoveries and insights, as well as the interpretations offered by psychotherapists to clients during the course of the therapy, must be true in order to be therapeutically effective? Are they in fact true? To what degree are deliberate or inadvertent explanatory fictions therapeutically beneficial? Do insights and interpretations matter to psychological well-being—and if so, do they have to be true?

Despite quite wide-ranging disagreements about the *nature* of truth and the *nature* of clinical evidence, most of the psychodynamic psychotherapies defend some form of commitment to the *ideal* of truth as it pertains to psychodynamic explanations, interpretations, and insights. First, most are committed to the idea that truth (whatever it is) matters; that is, the psychodynamic psychotherapies do not trade in mere fictions, artifacts, or useful tools. And most are committed to the idea that it is possible—somehow—to validate, prove, test, or find objective support for psychodynamic explanations, interpretations, and insights. Few psychodynamic psychotherapies are committed to the epistemic position that anything goes in matters pertaining to explanations, interpretations, and insights. Second, and more basically, most of the psychodynamic psychotherapies defend some type of *distinction* between truth and falsity. Something makes one psychodynamic interpretation true and another one false, or one insight closer to the truth and another more distant. Whatever it is that fulfills this role, it is not arbitrary, or a matter of mere convention, or a matter of how a client simply feels about it, or a matter of political power or persuasion. With these two basic epistemic commitments, then, most psychodynamic psychotherapies are opposed to poststructuralist attempts to deconstruct the very distinction between truth and falsity, or to show that the distinction is illusory (Held 1995; Held 2007). Moreover, it is these two basic epistemic commitments that serve to distinguish the psychodynamic psychotherapies from therapeutic charlatanism and pseudo-science. If these commitments were abandoned, and if it were granted that false interpretations and insights are just as effective as (or no more than) true ones, or that all interpretations and insights are on equal footing with regards to their truth value, then there would be no reliable way of telling the psychodynamic psychotherapies apart from bogus treatment methods. Commitment to the ideal of truth is one of the crucial planks in the psychodynamic psychotherapies' project to be scientific (see also Lilienfeld *et al.* 2003a; Held 1995; Held 2007).

But these two commitments are on shaky epistemic and logical ground. They are jeopardized by a number of unwarranted inferential leaps, inconsistencies, and logical gaps in the theories of the psychodynamic psychotherapies, as well as in the broad principles supporting these theories. Iterations of these problems are found in psychoanalysis, Jungian analysis, and short-term psychodynamic psychotherapy, as well as in the newer psychodynamic theories. For reasons of economy and precision, however, there is no need to analyze each and every logical and epistemic problem in each and every psychodynamic theory: some other strategy is called for. In what follows, a robust *generic* model of the relevant *epistemic* portions of the theory and principles of psychodynamic psychotherapy will be developed. This will of necessity overlook the theoretical and methodological idiosyncrasies that differentiate one school from another. Such a strategy may seem to be unwarrantedly reductionist: it may seem to leave out too much in the way of important theoretical differentiae. This generic model, however, is simple enough to be compatible with most forms of psychodynamic psychotherapy. It is a skeleton that can be fitted with different layerings of flesh and muscle, without the skeleton itself becoming unduly distorted. In order to show how this fitting is possible—how to move from abstract model to instantiation and back again—a number of examples from specific psychodynamic psychotherapies will be called upon at each major move in the analysis of the logical and epistemic problems.

It might be argued that the question 'does truth matter in the psychodynamic psychotherapies?' can be answered quite simply: truth (in psychodynamic insight, interpretation, and explanation) matters sometimes, and sometimes it does not. True insights sometimes matter to a client's psychological well-being, and sometimes they do not. Similarly, true interpretations sometimes matter for therapeutic progress, and sometimes they do not. Any demand for a more principled answer is a demand that ought to be jettisoned, because the assumption on which it rests—that there *is* a determinate answer—is incoherent. This is what might be called (for lack of a better term) the deflationary approach to the epistemology and logic of psychodynamic psychotherapy. If this approach is valid and cogent, then the epistemological questions raised above lose their force: they are not solved, but dissolved. According to the deflationary approach, the explorations and insights of clients, and the interpretations of psychotherapists, are sometimes therapeutically effective *because* they are true. And sometimes their truth-value has nothing to do with their therapeutic effectiveness. Conversely, the explorations and insights of clients, and the interpretations of psychotherapists, are sometimes therapeutically effective *because* they are false or incomplete; and sometimes their falsity or incompleteness have nothing to do with their therapeutic effectiveness. Nothing beyond particularist description of the facts—that is, nothing 'philosophical'—can be said.

The deflationary approach is unconvincing. First, it is philosophically uninteresting because it is compatible with any state of affairs that might occur in psychodynamic psychotherapy; and it is compatible with any therapeutic outcome. Second, it is uninformative, because it merely pushes the central question ('does truth matter?') back one step: if it is true that therapeutic improvement can be attributed *either* to veridical interpretations and insights *or* to false ones, then there must be something else that explains why this epistemic bivalency—or the conditions of possibility of bivalency—is therapeutically effective. Third, the deflationary approach fails to set out normative epistemic guidelines about what the psychodynamic psychotherapies *should* aim at, and what epistemic norms are worth preserving, especially in those difficult cases where decisions about truth and falsity, and evidentiary validity, actually do matter because of their weighty legal and moral consequences: for instances, in cases of false versus repressed memory. Fourth, if the deflationary account is true, then it is unclear why psychotherapists invest so much time in training in a specific therapeutic orientation, why they appeal to effectiveness studies as supportive evidence for their theoretical claims, and why they so often try to differentiate their own therapeutic modalities from those of competitors.

Finally, the deflationary approach leaves clients in the dark about what to count as the goal of treatment. Suppose they approach psychodynamic psychotherapy with the expectation of learning something important about who they are, and connecting this new self-understanding with an adequate explanation of why they are experiencing psychological or behavioral difficulties. The deflationary answer would be as unsatisfactory as a car mechanic explaining to a car owner that the repairs just completed are guided by mechanical principles that may or may not be valid. It is doubtful if there is any point in pursuing something as difficult and time-consuming as psychodynamic psychotherapy if the outcome (in terms of truth-value) is so indeterminate, particularly if such ambivalent outcomes could equally well be achieved through alternative means, including not seeking therapeutic help at all.

Truth, in other words, matters. To clients, it matters that what they learn about themselves in exploratory psychotherapy is what is *really* the case, rather than what a psychological theory or psychological expert *says* is the case; and it matters that their therapeutic explorations aim at the psychological and historical facts of the matter, rather than at theoretical fictions, artifacts, subjectively satisfying stories, or useful cognitive tools. If the treatment is to help them deal successfully with their problems, and to help them reach a point where they can formulate viable plans for the future without the interference of the problems that first drove them to seek help, then they need a genuine truth-tracking explanation of their behaviors, psychological makeup, and the causes of their problems. Even if a robustly validated psychological explanation is not actually available, they must still believe that such an explanation could, with further investigation, be achieved. That is, they must believe that their personalities, behaviors, and psychological make-up consist of some definite set of facts that have specific consequences for their future, and that knowledge of these facts has specific consequences for their future-directed intentions and actions. Without this, they would have no reason to think that who they currently are, and what they currently do, has consequences for who they will be and what they will do.

There is also an ethical dimension to the idea that truth matters. False, bogus, or fictional psychodynamic interpretations and insights can be as psychologically harmful as false memories. Like false memories, they can lead to the break-up of families, the dissolution of marriages or partnerships, the radical alteration of life plans, the erosion of religious faith, or the morally self-serving rewriting of the past. What looks like *bona fide* insight, or self-knowledge, or a genuine realization, or a new and more empowering way of looking at oneself, may in fact be ethically calamitous. This theme will be picked up in the last chapter.

An Alternative Hypothesis

There is no doubt that a certain subset of clients in the psychodynamic psychotherapies improves during the course of treatment: their symptoms disappear, their behaviors improve, or their personalities are changed in positive directions. But therapeutic effectiveness is not what is at issue here. What is, is the question of what could possibly explain these changes. Is it because of the agency of a unique set of characteristic ingredients (such as insights, interpretations, and transference) that are found only in the treatment methods of the psychodynamic psychotherapies? Is it because of the unique expertise of psychotherapists? Is it because some psychological problems simply go away on their own after a certain amount of time, with or without treatment? Is it a function of the placebo effect? Or could there be other, perhaps less obvious, factors at play?

Three broad models of explanation of therapeutic change have emerged across 2500 years of medical history:

Model 1: Therapeutic improvement occurs because of the agency of some specific or characteristic set of features of the treatments given to patients. These features can be examined, isolated, and predicted within the context of contemporary medical theory (Brody 1985: 42; Brody 1986). In contemporary medicine, patients' responses to these features are sometimes called specific responses: for example, the responses of the human body to the antibiotic properties of penicillin.

Model 2: Therapeutic improvement occurs because diseases or disorders have run their natural course, at least in patients whose native healing or recuperative powers are not impaired. In ancient times these powers were attributed to a special force, the *vis medicatrix naturae* (the tendency of nature to heal) (Neuberger 1932), which itself was a function of a more comprehensive natural force, *conatus*, or the drive to self-preservation that is inherent in each living creature. (Versions of the concept of conatus have been defended by the Stoics, Cicero, St. Augustine, Duns Scotus, Dante, Hobbes, and Spinoza; and more recently by Damasio (2003)). Contemporary scientific medicine has dropped the concept of the *vis medicatrix naturae*, and replaced it with the concept of autonomous responses, which include the panoply of immunological processes and other biological systems used by organisms to restore and maintain health.

Model 3: Therapeutic improvement occurs because the treatments patients receive have powerful symbolic effects on their imagination, beliefs, emotions, and feelings of hope and expectation. This has been interpreted variously as the placebo response, the meaning response, the expectancy effect, and the suggestion hypothesis. It is constituted by patients' total interaction with their healing context, which is rich in shared symbols and metaphors (Hahn and Kleinman 1983; Moerman 1983; Moerman 2002a).

The precise relation between these models is open to dispute (Brody 1985). In some cases all three may work together to enhance a patient's return to health; in some cases they may be mutually exclusive. The fact that there are these three categories and not others illustrates an important tension in the way disease has been conceptualized across history. According to the ancient Hippocratic and Galenic model of disease, the body (under normal conditions) was considered capable of ridding itself of most noxious elements naturally, an elimination process that occurred through symptoms such as fevers, vomiting, and diarrhea. Symptoms, in other words, were the natural response of the body to toxic stimuli, and this made the task of physicians quite simple: namely, to respect and stimulate the body's natural recuperative mechanism (the *vis medicatrix naturae*) (Neuberger 1932). In the early nineteenth century, however, with the emergence of scientific approaches to medicine, the concept of disease went through an unusually rapid transformation. Symptoms were reconceptualized as manifestations of disease itself, rather than as natural responses of the body fighting off noxious threats. The task of physicians was thus to suppress symptoms, since the body's own responses were insufficient, and in need of active intervention to fight the pathological effects of the disease.

Contemporary psychotherapy has inherited a version of model 1. Psychotherapists intervene with special treatment methods in order to combat symptoms and to aid a psyche that is considered incapable of healing itself. Positive therapeutic change, it is typically claimed, is not merely a function of the native healing powers of clients, or the self-limiting nature of psychological disorders (model 2); nor is it merely a function of the symbolic effects of the treatment (model 3): it is a function of the characteristic ingredients of the treatment methods (model 1). This interventionist model is found in many of the 400 forms of psychotherapy available today, including psychodynamic psychotherapy. There is (so the claim goes) something about the unique interpersonal dynamics (one of the characteristic ingredients) and the unique exploratory processes (another of the characteristic ingredients) of dynamic psychotherapy that works to bring about therapeutic changes that would not otherwise have occurred. Clients improve because the psychodynamic treatment methods allow them to make important affect-discharging or personality-restructuring discoveries about their psychology, behavior, emotions, development, and personality. In addition to taking credit for cases of successful therapeutic change, most psychodynamic psychotherapies offer explanations of why such changes occur. These explanations are framed in terms of the relevant theory of the psychotherapy which, as theories go, is robust and freighted with complex explanatory entities. Clinical evidence is adduced to support these explanations and to validate the theories.

There are a number of unquestioned epistemic and logical assumptions at work here. Perhaps the most basic assumption here is that *talking* about psychological problems, and developing some form of *insight* into their causes, is necessary to overcoming them. Talking is therapeutic, and insight is liberating. This assumption is so pervasive that it is rarely called into question: it is as close to an axiom in psychology as one can get (Borch-Jacobsen 1996).

Accompanying this is another basic assumption: there is a crucial difference between the psychologically manifest and the psychologically latent. The latter is considered to be written in mysterious code, and inaccessible to all but a few experts. Powerful techniques of exploration—the psychological equivalent of exploratory surgery—are called for to gain access to this dimension of the psyche, to decipher its code, and to help to weave it together with the psychologically manifest for the sake of the client's well-being. This assumption too is hardly ever questioned.

Accompanying this is yet another basic assumption: the methods of the exploratory psychotherapies somehow put clients in touch with an 'inner' or 'true' or 'core' or 'authentic' self (or, as some of the popular dynamically-inclined psychotherapies might phrase it, one's 'inner child', 'inner free spirit', and so on). This discovery, it is assumed, is profound and transformative. It is not merely a matter of clients learning mildly interesting facts about themselves. It is a kind of deep self-knowledge, enabling clients to *be* themselves more fully.

Taken together, these assumptions are so pervasive and so obvious that they form a rigid template, beyond which we cannot think.

In the work that follows each of these assumptions will be analyzed and evaluated. It will be argued that neither the psychodynamic explanations of therapeutic change, nor the clinical evidence that putatively validates such explanations, should be taken at face value. Psychodynamic explanations, it will be argued, are in some cases empirically impoverished and speculative—perhaps hopelessly so. The clinical evidence that putatively supports them is, at least in some cases, suspect and contaminated—again, perhaps hopelessly so. An alternative explanation of therapeutic change will be presented as an hypothesis to be tested. It is an explanation that has remained largely unexplored in the psychodynamic psychotherapy literature (Jopling 2001):

Hypothesis: *Some therapeutic changes in psychodynamic psychotherapy are not attributable to the specific active ingredients that are hypothesized to be unique to the treatment methods of the psychodynamic psychotherapies, but are instead functions of powerful placebos that rally the mind's native healing powers in much the same way that sugar pills and placebo surgeries rally the body's native healing powers. One of these placebos—and there may be many others at work in the psychodynamic psychotherapies—is the explanatory fiction: that is, explanations of clients' psychology, emotions, behavior, and personality that are false or fictitious, but when offered as interpretations or acquired as insights are powerful enough to rally the mind's native healing powers. In other words, certain interpretations and insights that appeal to dynamic unconscious forces (including such forces as resistance, repression, denial, regression, transference, reaction formation, displacement, reversal, sublimation, and splitting), inferred childhood events, the field of infantile and childhood sexual experience, and the unity or disunity of the self, may trigger the placebo response, and may help to treat psychological disorders, even though they are false or fictitious.*

To avoid the risk of overstatement and misinterpretation, four important qualifications need to be added to this hypothesis.

First, this hypothesis is not committed to the grandiose universal claim that *all* psychodynamic psychotherapies trade in placebos; nor to the narrower universal claim that some psychodynamic psychotherapies *always* trade in placebos; nor to the grandiose reductionist claim that *all* psychodynamic insights and interpretations are placebos. These are empirical claims, and unlikely ones at that. The hypothesis presented here is primarily a *conceptual hypothesis*: that is, an hypothesis about the cogency of the *concept* of placebo effects in psychodynamic psychotherapy, with a special focus on the concept of insight placebos and interpretation placebos. If psychodynamic placebos are a *conceptual* possibility—that is, if the *very idea* of psychodynamic placebos makes sense—then empirical studies would need to be designed to determine precisely how and when these placebos arise, and how they function.

Second, even if psychodynamic interpretations and insights may on occasion be placebos, it does not follow that *all* claims to insight or self-understanding are similarly compromised: that is, claims to moral, psychological, or existential insight made by persons in contexts other than exploratory psychotherapy (Jopling 2000). Psychodynamic insight is a species of the broader phenomenon of self-knowledge. But the methods by which it is attained, the functions it serves, and the epistemic liabilities from which it suffers due to its highly specific context, do not always carry across to non-psychotherapeutic forms of self-knowledge. It may be that the exploratory techniques of psychodynamic psychotherapy have the potential to interfere with the kinds of reflective self-inquiry and reflective self-evaluation that would otherwise lead to veridical self-knowledge.

Third, even if the psychodynamic psychotherapies sometimes trade in insight and interpretation placebos, it does not follow that they are, *qua* treatment methods, illusory, sham, or bogus—the psychological equivalent of snake oil; nor does it follow that psychodynamic psychotherapists who elicit the placebo response are charlatans or unethical con artists. Such views are based upon an outdated and pejorative model of the placebo response, the myths and misconceptions of which are slowly being replaced by new scientific understandings of how the brain, central nervous system, cognition, language, emotions, and social interactions interact to create the placebo response.

Fourth, explanatory fictions are not arbitrary and fanciful fictions on a par with some of the more questionable theoretical entities postulated by the fringe psychotherapies. They are pseudo-explanations that give the appearance of explanation (Skinner 1971). That is, they pick out just the right set of powers, forces, or entities to explain the phenomena in question, but these powers, forces, or entities are not themselves explained; the explanation, in other words, terminates prematurely and arbitrarily. Explanatory fictions are typically taken as valid, but they reflect our ignorance of the actual causal machinery underlying the phenomena in question. Free will, for example, is a pre-scientific explanatory fiction that is called upon to explain action and behavior; but, as Spinoza, Nietzsche, and others have argued, it is a cover for our ignorance of the actual causes underlying human behavior. 'Men believe that they are free, precisely because they are conscious of their volitions and desires; yet concerning the causes that have determined them to desire and

will, they have not the faintest idea, because they are ignorant of them'
(Spinoza 1677/1992: 57).

With these four qualifications in mind, it should be obvious that this
alternative explanation of therapeutic change is sharply at odds both with
common sense assumptions about the talking cures, and with conventional
psychodynamic explanations of therapeutic change. It is usually assumed that
the interpretations and explanations offered by psychotherapists to clients are
psychologically accurate (if the treatment method has been adhered to
properly). And it is usually assumed that clients' explorations during
psychotherapy are authentic, and their insights are truth-tracking and transformative. The hypothesis that is explored here turns these claims upside
down. It may be that the psychodynamic psychotherapies sometimes trade in
precisely the *opposite* of authentic and truth-tracking insights and interpretations: that is, they trade in elaborate explanatory fictions. As potent placebos,
however, these fictions may serve to rally the mind's native self-healing powers.

Underlying this alternative explanation of therapeutic change are three
broad guiding assumptions. The first assumption, supported by emerging
research in the medical, behavioral, and neurosciences on placebo effects, is
that the placebo response is a function of the human organism's powerful
innate capacity to heal itself, to restore itself to equilibrium, and to repair
damage (Harrington 1997; Guess *et al.* 2002; Humphrey 2002). This response
calls for complex cells, organs, nerve pathways, and immune systems to work
together synergistically to repair damage to the organism and to protect
against external threats (Wilentz and Engel 2002: 284). What is striking about
this capacity for self-repair is the sheer variety of endogenous and exogenous
triggers that stimulate it to action: not only the pharmaceutical and surgical
interventions that engage the biological processes of patients, but widely
divergent symbolic, cultural, and interpersonal interventions that engage their
hopes, expectations, and beliefs. The capacity for self-repair is not limited to
biological processes alone. Just as human beings are endowed with complex
multi-level biological systems to protect against and repair damage, so they are
endowed with complex psychological, cognitive, and emotional systems to
protect against and repair psychological damage. These too are activated by
symbolic and interpersonal interventions, as well as by more specific treatment interventions, such as those supplied by psychological treatments.

The placebo response that is a function of this innate capacity for self-
repair does not suddenly make its appearance in the life of a patient fully
formed and fully operational. Developmentally, the first placebo response
occurs at some point in early childhood at the caregiver's knee, with the band-
aid or spoonful of sugar presented as a treatment for some minor ailment.

This is an enculturated event, requiring the multidimensional interactive scaffolding of cognition, language, symbolism, interpersonal understanding, and social learning. Following this first event is a series of graduated developmental markers for placebo responsivity, corresponding to organism-wide changes in neuroimmunological, behavioral, linguistic, social, and cognitive capacity. (It is an open question whether other species, particularly the non-human primates, can respond to placebos.)

If the alternative hypothesis that is defended here is correct, then the psychodynamic psychotherapies may be effective, at least sometimes, not because of the agency of the presumed specific active ingredients of their treatment methods, but because they tap this innate capacity for self-healing. Other treatment methods may be just as effective in unleashing the potential of self-healing.

The second guiding assumption is that genuine insight—the sort of deep psychological insight clients in psychodynamic psychotherapy often *claim* to achieve, and that psychodynamic psychotherapists often cite as evidence for the success of their treatment methods—is much more difficult to achieve than is commonly assumed. This derives from the broader view that reality is always much richer and much more complex than our knowledge of it. From the first person point of view, there are countless ways to be wrong, confused, ignorant—or even deceived—about things as complexly configured as one's behavior, personality, motivational structure, psychological make-up, developmental history, emotions, and psychological pathology. Indeed, there are many *more* ways to be wrong, confused, ignorant, or deceived about these things than there are ways to be knowledgeable. As a general rule, self-ignorance, self-misunderstanding, and self-opacity, rather than truth-tracking self-awareness and self-understanding, constitute a broad cognitive baseline condition. If this general rule is valid, then the burden of proof is on the psychodynamic psychotherapies to show that they have the resources to overcome this condition, rather than to simply generate yet one more instantiation of it.

The former half of this assumption is relatively uncontroversial. Across human history, false, trivial, or pseudo-explanations of psychology, behavior, and personality have been the norm rather than the exception: explanations, for instance, that appeal to entities such as humors, demons, astrological forces, or magnetic fields. The poverty of these explanations is even more pronounced in the case of the abnormal behaviors and psychological states that constitute the target disorders identified by the various schools of psychotherapy. Why has there been such explanatory poverty? One reason is that the causes of behaviors, personality structures, and psychological states are not given *in* those behaviors, personality structures, and psychological states. The causation of behavior is not something obvious: it is not easily read off the phenomena. Mere observation of the phenomena, for example, says nothing about how environmental and social factors causally influence psychological well-being; how personality causally influences behavior, and vice versa; and how the relative mismatch or coherence of the different aspects of an individual's psychological make-up causally influences psychological disorders. Psychological reality is always richer and more complex than our knowledge of it.

The latter half of the guiding assumption—that the psychodynamic psychotherapies may be instances of the general rule about the broad cognitive baseline rather than exceptions to it—remains to be determined. This is especially important given the strong epistemic claims made in the psychodynamic psychotherapies about the attainability and validity of insight.

The third guiding assumption, supported by emerging research in social psychology on positive illusions and creative self-deception, and research in cognitive psychology on the constitutional limits of cognition and memory, is that in some cases it is more *psychologically adaptive* to be deceived, misinformed, or ignorant about oneself than it is to be knowledgeable; that is, to live with an understanding of one's psychology, behavior, and personality that is shaped by 'user-friendly' explanatory fictions. If this assumption is valid, then it may be that therapeutic improvement sometimes amounts to acquiring workable explanatory fictions rather than deep truth-tracking insights. Truth-tracking insight may not be as essential to psychological well-being as pseudo-insight, or an insight placebo.

The idea that human beings are vulnerable to illusions and deceptions because they are subject to a condition that *requires* illusions and deceptions is not new: it is a theme found throughout the work of Spinoza, Marx, Nietzsche, and Sartre, as well as in the literary and dramatic works of Dostoyevsky, Ibsen, and O'Neill. Mystifying interpretations of human experience serve the function of interpreting otherwise unintelligible sufferings, unexplained natural forces, and puzzling behaviors, thereby making them more tolerable than they would otherwise be, and supplying for them a schema of putative remedies or coherent responses. This is most clearly seen in shamanistic and religio-magical healing rites, which interpret human powerlessness against a mysterious and threatening natural world, and which supply remedies that give a semblance of power over alien and destructive forces (Torrey 1986; Frank and Frank 1991). Explanatory fictions fulfilling the same basic needs may be at work in contemporary psychotherapeutic settings. The cultivation of the illusion of gaining special insight into the forces that govern the human mind and human behavior, and of having risen above the condition of powerlessness that comes from pain or suffering, is psychologically palliative, even if the insight is widely off the mark.

Taken together, these three guiding assumptions provide a framework for understanding the hypothesis that some therapeutic changes in the psychodynamic psychotherapies are functions of powerful placebos that rally the mind's native healing powers in much the same way that placebo pills and placebo surgeries rally the body's native healing powers; and that the psychodynamic psychotherapies may, at least in *some* instances, trade in placebos while claiming to be truth-tracking. This is not to suggest that veridical insight and self-knowledge are unachievable; they are (Jopling 2000). Pursuing exploratory psychotherapy may simply not be the most reliable and consistent way to achieve it.

Suppose that this alternative hypothesis proves to be both conceptually coherent and empirically valid: suppose, that is, that psychodynamic placebos are at work in a certain percentage of the client population (with certain specific target problems). An important question concerning the *ethics* of giving placebos follows upon this hypothesis.

In medicine, the ethical consequences of giving placebos to patients are weighty, because of the potential for patient deception. Placebos are commonly given to patients without their full knowledge or awareness: they believe they are receiving, or are likely to receive, medically active treatments, when they are in fact receiving lactose pills or placebo surgeries. This typically involves practices of intentional ignorance (Kaptchuk 1986): that is, either deceiving patients, or withholding crucial information from them, or keeping them in the dark. But each of these ways of treating patients violates the fundamental medical principle of respect for patient autonomy. Does the same hold for psychodynamic placebos? Are there any weighty ethical prohibitions against the use of placebos in psychodynamic psychotherapy? If some psychodynamic insights and interpretations are placebos, and if clients are unaware that they are receiving placebos as part of their treatment, then are they the victims of deception, or intentional ignorance? Is giving a client a psychodynamic placebo a violation of his or her autonomy? Are clinical psychologists and psychotherapists who use psychodynamic placebos without first fully informing their clients and gaining their full educated consent violating the Hippocratic oath 'First do no harm'? Could insight and interpretation placebos be as harmful and ethically impermissible as those psychotherapeutically-induced false memories that sometimes result in psychological and interpersonal harm? Finally, are misleading claims about the truth status of psychotherapeutic insights and interpretations tantamount to false advertising?

The position that will be defended in Chapter 7 is that psychodynamic placebos—if they do in fact occur in psychodynamic psychotherapy—should not be regarded as sham treatments or quackery, as placebos have generally been regarded in medical history; rather, they should be regarded as creative attempts to unlock the body's self-healing powers. At the same time, however, the intentional ignorance that is involved in giving psychodynamic placebos is ethically impermissible. As a general rule, clients should not be deceived or kept in the dark by psychotherapists, even if the consequences of intentional ignorance are therapeutically beneficial. If clients believe and have been informed that psychodynamic insights and interpretations are authentic and true, when in fact they are explanatory fictions that operate by means of the placebo effect, then they are the victims of psychotherapist-induced intentional ignorance, the strongest version of which is deception. This is a case of harm, and it falls under the broader class of acts in which the principle of respect for client autonomy has been violated. If, however, clients are fully informed about, and consent to, the use of psychodynamic placebos—that is, if they are informed that psychodynamic insights and interpretations are, or are likely to be, explanatory fictions that help to unlock the body's self-healing powers, *and* that these insights and interpretations do not constitute *bona fide* self-knowledge—then no deception has occurred.

The Principle of Differentialness

As this work offers an alternative explanation of a phenomenon that has been widely studied and debated in the last one hundred years—namely, therapeutic change—it can be considered a contribution to the ongoing debate in the philosophy of social and medical science about the nature of scientific explanation. In particular, it can be considered a contribution to the debate about the possibility of establishing objective and nonrelativistic standards for the evaluation of alternative scientific theories.

The principle of differentialness (Erwin 1985, 1993, 1996a, 1997) that is located near the centre of this debate in the philosophy of science holds that all plausible rival hypotheses purporting to explain some phenomenon P (e.g. therapeutic change) need to be ruled out, before accepting an hypothesis H about P as confirmed. This is one of the basic requirements for any complex scientific investigation that generates a robust body of data about a clearly demarcated phenomenon, along with an hypothesis about that data. 'For any body of data D and hypothesis H, D confirms H only if D provides some reason for believing that H is true, and does not provide equal (or better) reason for believing some incompatible rival that is just as plausible' (Erwin 1997: 75). Take a simple, if strained, example: sustained prayer over a period of three weeks has the power to cure the common cold (Erwin 1997: 75). Suppose this prediction is true: after three weeks of sustained prayer, a common cold clears up. What follows from this? Very little, if anything. It does not follow that prayer was the causal agent responsible for the alleviation of the cold: to assume this is to commit the fallacy of *post hoc ergo propter hoc* ('after this therefore because of this'). Other equally plausible accounts could explain the result just as well, or perhaps even better. It could, for example, be a matter of the self-limiting nature of common colds; or some other causal agent or set of causal agents that have not yet been identified.

The principle of differentialness is not without critics. It has been argued, for example, that: i) there is no need to rule out *all* rival plausible hypotheses, as science goes on without the differentialness condition ever being fully satisfied (Fine and Forbes 1986: 238); ii) scientific hypotheses win support even when there are plausible rivals (Wilkes 1990); iii) there is no need to consider empirical findings from other hypotheses as long as the hypothesis being tested has heuristic value, makes sense out of a wide variety of phenomena, and generates correct predictions (Hall 1963); and iv) the differentialness standard demands too much, because there is an infinite number of alternative (but not always equi-plausible) explanations. But the principle of differentialness does not require that *all* alternative hypotheses to any given hypothesis be ruled out. This would be an endless task (Fine and Forbes 1986: 238). Nor does it require that *any* alternative hypothesis to any given hypothesis be ruled out—since an ingenious mind can always dream up an alternative of some sort (Wilkes 1990: 248–249). The differential standard for evaluating the explanations of the phenomena of therapeutic change in psychotherapy holds the more moderate view that rival explanations of equal plausibility and robustness must be ruled out before accepting as true the explanations supplied by a theory of psychotherapy.[2]

The validity of the differential principle, whether or not it is conclusively established by its proponents by means of formal arguments, is most clearly tested in its *application* to particular areas of controversy. Putting the principle to work in concrete cases is a way of bootstrapping it to a level of legitimacy that formal argument alone may not adequately achieve. The work that follows is an example of how the principle of differentialness can be applied to the puzzling phenomena of therapeutic change in the psychodynamic psychotherapies.

One well-known example of how the principle of differentialness has been applied is Grünbaum's (1984) argument that the suggestion hypothesis serves as a credible rival to a number of central Freudian hypotheses about therapeutic change in classical Freudian psychoanalysis. The clinical data of classical Freudian psychoanalysis are, he argued, hopelessly contaminated by suggestion and expectancy effects, and cannot therefore be taken to support Freudian explanations of therapeutic change.

Wollheim countered by arguing that the absence of a full-blown theory of how suggestion works disqualifies the suggestibility hypothesis as a credible alternative to Freudian explanation. 'He [Grünbaum] never proposes, nor feels the need for, any infilling when he invokes the possibility, indeed the likelihood, of suggestion as the real explanation of what the patient does. In the absence of such infilling, the situation is envisaged in the following way: i) the analyst makes his wishes known; ii) the patient complies' (Wollheim 1993: 111). Wollheim's term 'infilling' is unclear. Perhaps it refers to a robust psychological theory of suggestion that explains the causes, mechanisms, and functions of suggestion. Perhaps his argument is that without such a theory in place, appealing to suggestion as an alternative explanation of the phenomena of therapeutic change in psychoanalysis is unconvincing. Is this a valid criticism?

There is no doubt that more is needed in the way of clear and empirically viable explanations of the phenomenon of suggestion, particularly in the context of psychological healing. More is also needed in the way of clear and empirically viable explanations of the placebo effect, the expectancy effect, and self-limiting disorders. But Wollheim's criticism—that without such 'infilling', any appeal to the suggestion hypothesis reduces to a simple two-stage procedure—simply misses the mark. First, there *is* an *experimental* literature in cognitive and behavioral psychology on the phenomenon of suggestion (Gheorghiu *et al.* 1989; Gheorghiu 1989; Schumaker 1991), self-fulfilling predictions (Jones 1977), and expectancy effects (Kirsch 1999, 2005). This literature can be traced back to the extensive *clinical* work on suggestion done by Bernheim, Delboeuf, Baudouin and others in the Nancy School (Baudouin 1920; Ellenberger 1970), as well as by the French psychiatrist Pierre Janet (1925). There is also a growing literature on placebo effects (Harrington 1997; Peters 2001; Guess *et al.* 2002; Moerman 2002a; Gorski and Spier 2004). Perhaps this literature does not meet Wollheim's demand for theoretical adequacy; or perhaps its relevance to psychotherapy has not been worked out sufficiently clearly. These are different claims, and ones that Wollheim does not substantiate. The so-called 'infilling' that is required to support the theory of suggestion is not as absent as Wollheim makes it out to be.

Second, while it is true that there is still more empirical research to be done on suggestion, placebo effects, and expectancy effects, and the role they play in psychotherapy, it is unrealistic to hold that having such a fully worked out theory is the *only* way to protect Grünbaum's suggestion hypothesis from outright rejection. This argumentative strategy, as Erwin (1996a: 104) notes, sets the standard too high for taking a rival credible explanation seriously. While Grünbaum does not defend a detailed theory of suggestion, what he does offer is neither as primitive nor as incomplete as the two-step mechanism described by Wollheim. Grünbaum's critique of psychoanalysis moves forward on the basis of ongoing research that has identified specific suggestibility factors, ranging from verbal conditioning to subverbal influencing behaviors.

The following work can be considered a contribution to the so-called 'infilling' called for by Wollheim. It offers an account of the varieties of suggestion, placebo effects, feedback effects and other therapeutic interference that occur in the exploratory psychotherapies, particularly as these factors influence psychodynamic interpretations and insights. The following account does not claim to be comprehensive. There are many other causes of therapeutic change than those identified here. Nor is it based on the reductionist assumption that the entire range of therapeutic changes can be reduced to suggestion, expectancy effects, and placebo effects.

Some Preliminary Objections

The alternative hypothesis of therapeutic change that is developed here is bound to meet with considerable skepticism. Three predictable objections are:

a) placebo effects are in fact quite rare in psychodynamic psychotherapy;

b) methodologically scrupulous psychodynamic methods help to screen out placebo effects;

c) rigorous training methods combined with psychotherapist expertise help to minimize placebo effects.

These objections are not convincing without empirical data. Anecdotal evidence and clinical experience do not provide sufficient grounds of support for them. More basically, however, the objections miss the target. The hypothesis that is developed here is not presented primarily as an *empirical hypothesis* about the *actual* presence and *actual* frequency of placebo effects in psychodynamic psychotherapy. It is not claimed here, for instance, that psychodynamic placebos are present in approximately 30–40% of psychodynamic treatments (to use Beecher's 'vintage numbers'); or (say) that approximately 30–40% of all patients suffering from mild to moderate depression respond to psychodynamic placebo; or that 30–40% of all psychodynamic interpretations and insights are in fact placebos. In other words, empirical data are not called upon to confirm or disconfirm the hypothesis—*because it is not, at this stage, an empirical hypothesis.*

Moreover, no use is made of clinical case histories for the purposes of confirming or disconfirming the hypothesis, although on occasion they are called upon for purposes of illustration. Relying upon clinical case histories as a strategy to confirm or disconfirm psychotherapeutic theories is fraught with manifold problems (Meehl 1978, 1990, 1995). First, clinical case histories tend to be presented and interpreted through the filters of a particular psychotherapeutic theory, in such a way that the presentation of the salient psychological, historical, and behavioral facts of the case is theory-mediated. Second, just as null results in the experimental natural sciences tend not to get published, so treatment failures in clinical psychology and psychotherapy tend not to get published. By implication, treatment successes that might be cogently and plausibly explained in terms of placebo effects may not to be published, since they might be considered as impugning the therapeutic efficacy of a treatment. Third, the evidentiary relevance of clinical case histories to questions about the validity of psychotherapeutic theories, or the effectiveness of a particular psychotherapy, is far from clear. Kazdin (1981), for example, identifies five main problems that undermine the evidential support that clinical case studies putatively provide in demonstrating the effectiveness of a therapy: i) case studies often rely on the use of anecdotal reports, such as the client's or psychotherapist's uncorroborated subjective report that some form of therapeutic improvement has taken place; ii) the psychotherapist's use of one-shot or two-shot assessments of clients' improvement to generate case studies has the potential to increase the risk that therapeutic change was a function of the testing itself, rather than the unique ingredients of the therapy; iii) in some clinical cases, the psychological problem that is subject to treatment is acute or episodic, making long-term follow-up difficult; iv) case studies are complicated by the presence of gradual or weak-outcome effects, in contrast to so-called 'slam bang' effects; v) case studies involve only one individual, which is a weak empirical base from which to generalize about therapeutic effectiveness.

If the hypothesis that is developed here is not primarily an empirical one, then what is it? It is a *conceptual hypothesis* about the validity of the *concept* of placebo effects in the psychodynamic psychotherapies. Until psychodynamic placebos can be shown to be conceptually possible—that is, neither logical nor conceptual contradictions—any discussion of the empirical evidence that might support or undermine objections a–c is premature. The logical architecture of concepts guides and constrains the accumulation of clinical and experimental evidence.

But while the main hypothesis that is explored here is conceptual, the study does not take on a purely *a priori* form: it does not follow the high road of armchair psychology. Support for the conceptual possibility of placebo effects in the psychodynamic psychotherapies will come from a variety of directions, both empirical and theoretical: from the philosophical evaluation and logical analysis of core theoretical concepts of psychodynamic psychotherapy (such as the concept of insight); and from recent work in the cognitive, behavioral, and medical sciences on placebo effects. At various points along the way, the philosophical analysis of the concept of insight and the concept of placebo will be tested in light of empirical findings from the cognitive and medical sciences, as well as in light of claims from clinical examples from psychodynamic psychotherapy; at other points philosophical methods will be brought to bear on clinical examples and psychological theories.

Chapter 2

Kinds of Insight

In sooth, I know not why I am so sad:
It wearies me; you say it wearies you;
But how I caught it, found it, or came by it,
What stuff 'tis made of, whereof it is born,
I am to learn;
And such a want-wit sadness makes of me,
That I have much ado to know myself.
Shakespeare, *Merchant of Venice*, I,I,1

Insights True and False

What precisely *is* insight? Why is it considered to be so important in the psycho-dynamic psychotherapies? What does psychodynamic insight target and refer to? And do insights have to be true in order to be therapeutically beneficial? To help explore these questions, three case histories will be presented, one from analytical (Jungian) psychotherapy, one from psychoanalysis, and one from brief psychodynamic psychotherapy. Why turn first to case histories, given the difficulties cited earlier by Kazdin (1981)? First, case histories help to illustrate the hypothesized significance of insight for psychological well-being: that is, they help to illustrate hypotheses about how insights are acquired, hypotheses about how insights stand vis à vis the interpretations supplied by psychotherapists, and hypotheses about how the truth-valuable status of insights functions in the course of treatment. Second, and just as importantly, case histories are notable for what they omit. Many published case histories, for instance, are silent on the question of the truth-value of insights and interpretations. The prevailing uncritical assumption is that they are true. Similarly, many case histories are silent on the question of the truth *criteria* that are considered to be relevant in assessing the truth or falsity of insights and interpretations. These are character-istically bracketed as second-order theoretical issues that have little clinical bear-ing. By the same token, then, case histories do not furnish the relevant kinds of empirical evidence that would to help to address the epistemic problems of psychotherapy. At best, they serve to illustrate these problems, but they cannot directly solve them. Finally, case histories are not unbiased reports of unalloyed fact. Theory typically creeps in to the framing, editing and presentation of case histories. Before being rendered as a case history, for example, some parts of the large mass of clinical case material assembled during the treatment must be foregrounded, and others parts backgrounded. Not every gesture, sigh, association, dream fragment, reported feeling, or comment that makes it into the case notes is equally significant; nor do these bits and pieces of case histories come with labels attached, indicating their level of clinical significance. Whatever the choices about foregrounding and backgrounding, they are made according to prior theoretical commitments about what is psychologically salient and causally relevant (Spence 1982). Typically, case histories do not call these prior commitments to attention. Moreover, discrepant or fragmentary portions of the case material may be subjected to a kind of narrative 'filling in' and streamlining, in the interests of continuity and coherence (Spence 1982). But editorial decisions such as these are not themselves highlighted in case histories, or called into question. What is presented in a case history is never a faithful mirror of what actually transpired moment to moment in the psychotherapist's office.

Case History 1

The first case history illustrates the role of insight in Jungian analytic psychotherapy. It shows the central role of transference and countertransference in the acquisition of insight. More specifically, it shows how insight is not acquired *by* oneself and *for* oneself, but *with* and *for another*. Insight is interpersonally constituted. The case history is described by the Jungian analyst Barbara Sullivan, who worked with her client Christina for five years (Sullivan 2001). Sullivan describes Christina as an intelligent, talented, professionally well-functioning woman, who was suffocating in an unhappy marriage. Nine months before seeking psychotherapy, she abruptly left her two pre-adolescent children and husband, and started to live alone. She 'had reached a point at which she felt she had to choose between her life and her children, and she and I both needed to appreciate how that impossible choice had led to a dreadful wounding of herself' (Sullivan 2001: 52). While imprecise, Sullivan's diagnosis is that Christina suffered from severe narcissistic difficulties and despair. She describes Christina as feeling lost, fragmented, emotionally disconnected, and full of self-loathing and destructive rage. Christina displayed an 'impenetrable coldness' toward others, which protected them from being hurt. Sullivan also describes Christina as suffering from a deep sense of futility and chaos about the meaning and direction of her life. Some of these symptoms showed up in Christina's artworks and dreams, which Sullivan interpreted in terms of Jungian symbol and archetype motifs as revealing an unconscious despair of ever achieving a sense of personal unity.

Sullivan inferred from the relatively fragmentary clinical material that many of Christina's problems must have originated in her childhood. Sullivan does not identify a specific pathogenic event that caused a specific type of repression and a specific chain of symptoms, but rather a pervasively pathogenic family atmosphere. Childhood was a time when Christina 'received every privilege that money could buy and no empathy for any of her emotional experiences' (Sullivan 2001: 52). Sullivan describes Christina as having been emotionally wounded in childhood by a lack of parental affection and empathy. The effect, years later, is that Christina has a 'cold dead part' inside herself.

Psychotherapy was painful, slow, and incomplete. Throughout the early stages of the therapy, Sullivan struggled with her own negative feelings towards Christina, especially her feelings of horror toward a woman who had abandoned her young children. Sullivan also had to cope with Christina's self-loathing, which she described as contagious. The ultimate goal of the treatment, according to Sullivan, was to help Christina become whole again, to accept all aspects of herself, and to develop a new understanding of her life and its meaning. The primary engine of therapeutic change, according to Sullivan, was the intense transference. This allowed Christina to 'develop a different attitude toward herself', one that was more accepting and more understanding. In her ongoing relationship with Sullivan, Christina learned to 'hold herself' as a unified person. Much of this emerged, according to Sullivan, through Christina's rebuffing, contesting, introjecting, and growing from the constant empathy Sullivan felt towards her. 'In our last year of work, Chris realized that these depreciations [of Sullivan] reflected primarily the ways she depreciated herself. But while this insight was useful, the main value of her criticism lay in the experience itself. She turned her human nastiness in my direction and I survived... I was able to maintain my affection for her, pretty much unbroken, through her assaults, and that was crucial in helping her develop and maintain some affection for all of herself, including her darker side' (Sullivan 2001: 53).

According to Sullivan, Christina emerged from dynamic psychotherapy more integrated, whole, and insightful than before. Psychotherapy had allowed her to explore her inner world, and to overcome her inner dividedness. 'In her relationship with me, Chris *developed the capacity to know and hold her whole self* by introjecting my capacity to see and hold her, to unite with her without being injured by her fearful impulses. In the container of our relationship, she *explored* more and more of her inner world, expanding her *familiarity with herself* and her ability to be the whole person she naturally should be' (Sullivan 2001: 55 italics added).

Sullivan's case history illustrates some of the central characteristics of psychodynamic insight. It shows: i) how one of the goals of dynamic psychotherapy is a new and deeper self-understanding, which goes hand in hand with self-growth and self-acceptance; ii) how the acquisition of insight seems to mark a turning point in psychodynamic psychotherapy; iii) how the acquisition of insight can be emotionally catalytic; and iv) the centrality of the psychotherapist–client relationship in the acquisition, validation, and content of insight.

Like most case histories, however, Sullivan's case history is heavily edited, vague on certain concrete details (e.g. the content, depth and durability of Christina's new self-understanding), and weighted down with robust but unexplored theoretical assumptions (e.g. about the unity of the self, the nature of introjection, and the nature of transference). The case history also reveals some of the weighty epistemic and causal assumptions Sullivan makes about the relation between insight, self-growth, and healing. Sullivan assumes uncritically that: a) the transference relation was one the causes of Christina's therapeutic progress; b) Christina's new self-understanding (her 'capacity to know her whole self') was for the most part accurate or truth-tracking; and c) Christina's new self-understanding was one of the causes of her therapeutic improvement. But there is little to recommend taking these assumptions at face value, given that there are a number of alternative explanations of Christina's therapeutic improvement that carry similar levels of plausibility: explanations that appeal, for example, to the natural history of the disorder, placebo effects, suggestion, and the random fluctuation of symptoms over time. These would first have to be ruled out before taking epistemic assumptions a–c as valid.

Case History 2

...he merely told
The unhappy Present to recite the past
Like a poetry lesson till sooner
Or later it faltered at the line where
Long ago the accusations had begun,
And suddenly knew by whom it had been judged,
How rich life had been and how silly,
And was life-forgiven and more humble.
W.H. Auden, *In memory of Sigmund Freud* (1939)

In a revealing but confusing metaphor, Malcolm (1980) likens psychoanalytic treatment to surgery. An extremely powerful intervention is performed by the analyst on the troubled psyche of the analysand, in much the same way that surgery is performed on the diseased body of a patient. The result of this temporary loss of autonomy, however, is something as profoundly transformative and elusive as insight: 'the achieving of insight is as deep and radical

and complex a procedure as the cutting out of a tumor. Insight isn't superficial—it isn't simply learning something mildly interesting about yourself. It is
becoming yourself. It's finding your way to the child in yourself, it is a profound
recognition' (Malcolm 1980: 160). Malcolm's metaphor brings together two
images whose compatibility is not entirely obvious: an anesthetized patient
lying docile on the table, subjected to alien cutting instruments wielded by an
alien hand, and an analysand actively and consciously gaining insight by his or
her own exploratory efforts.

Something like this transformation is seen in Meehl's (1983) case history of
a patient whose physician phobia was lifted shortly after her recollection of a
traumatic childhood event and her acquisition of some insight into its meaning. The case history is more a brief sketch than a full-blown description, and
it excludes details of the early and late stages of treatment, as well as the transference. Still, it is useful insofar as it is focused on the role of insight and
recollection, and insofar as it is situated within an extended and epistemically
informed discussion of the role of suggestion in psychoanalysis.

According to Meehl, the patient's phobia was so severe that she had not had
a physical examination in several years. Despite many efforts of trying to overcome it through sheer will power and self-motivation, she could not manage
to complete dialing the phone number of a physician without collapsing into a
state of high anxiety. She was fully aware that the phobia was 'silly', and that it
jeopardized her health. Her own explanation, which did little to release her
from the grip of the phobia, was that it was caused by the psychological
trauma of a hysterectomy that she had undergone years ago. After seventy
sessions of analysis with Meehl, and a marked reduction in her anxiety, the
phobia remained untouched. Meehl inferred from recurrent themes in his
patient's free associations that there were deeper causes of the phobia, with the
case material pointing to a traumatic encounter the patient 'must have' had
with a physician when she was a child. The physician, Meehl inferred, must
have questioned her about masturbating—and this was a question that would
have caused enormous conflict and guilt in the young patient because of her
puritanical religious upbringing. Since then, the memory was repressed, and it
became the pathogenic cause of the phobia.

In one memorable session, during which Meehl claims to have offered only
'minimal assistance', the patient was able to bring up fragments of intense
visual and auditory memories of the doctor's examining table, and memories
of the physician's probing questions; and then piece together these fragments
into a coherent understanding of how that long-lost event must have been the
cause of her phobia. Near the end of the session the patient expressed doubts
about whether her memories were implanted by the analyst, or whether they

were freely recalled, but these doubts were soon laid to rest. 'She recalled clearly enough, in enough sense modalities, to have a concrete certainty that it was, if imperfectly recalled, essentially accurate' (1983: 358). The next day the physician phobia had lifted, and the patient was able to make an appointment for a general examination with only the slightest level of anxiety. Meehl was confident that there was no suggestion and no placebo effect involved. 'I think most fairminded persons would agree that it takes an unusual skeptical resistance for us to say that this step-function in clinical status was 'purely a suggestive effect', or a 'reassurance effect', or due to some other transference leverage or whatever (75th hour!) rather than that the remote memory was truly repressed and the lifting of repression efficacious' (Meehl 1983: 358).

Despite the fact that Meehl's description of his role in the patient's remembering as 'minimal' considerably oversimplifies the complex interpersonal dynamics and cognitive pressures that must have occurred during treatment, the case history is unusual because of its relative degree of epistemic sophistication. It arises in the context of a discussion of Fliess's so-called Achensee question to Freud, and the epistemic problems surrounding psychoanalytic inferences of past events for which there is no direct evidence. It illustrates clearly how some psychoanalysts conceptualize the role of insight, showing: i) how insight into the putatively hidden or repressed pathogens of a disorder is one of the goals of psychoanalysis; ii) how the acquisition of insight can seem to occasion therapeutic change; and iii) how the acquisition of insight is often emotionally charged and catalytic.

The case history also reveals a number of problematic epistemic assumptions. First, despite Meehl's misgivings about 'unusual skeptical resistance' of skeptics, neither the multi-modal intensity of the patient's remembering nor her feelings of 'concrete certainty' are by themselves sufficient to underwrite the truth of the patient's insight. Some vivid multimodal memories may be false (and implanted or suggested), and some weak multimodal memories may be true. Mnemonic vividness is no more a *criterion* of the truth of memories than mnemonic haziness is a criterion of the falsity of memories; nor do they count as reliable *signs* of the presence of truth and falsity. Moreover, subjective feelings of conviction or uncertainty about memories do not serve as the criteria of truth or falsity, or as reliable signs of the presence of truth or falsity; they are too variable, fleeting, and uncertain. Something else besides vividness and feelings of conviction is required to serve as a criterion for the truth or falsity of insights and memories.

Second, the mere fact that therapeutic change followed the patient's acquisition of insight does not prove that her insight was psychologically and historically true. To assume that it does—that is, without ruling out a number of plausible alternative explanations—is to commit the logical fallacy of *post hoc ergo propter hoc*. There are other explanations of therapeutic change that first have to be ruled out: the change may have simply been a coincidence, or the natural history of the phobia, or the random fluctuation of symptoms, or the effects of some other therapeutic technique, or the effects of other therapeutic factors that were not part of the specific components of the treatment methods of psychoanalysis.

The concept of insight plays a central role in classical Freudian psychoanalysis, as well as in the many divergent branches of psychoanalysis and psychoanalytic psychotherapy (as represented, for example, in the work of Rank, Horney, Ferenczi, Adler, Klein, Kohut, Reik, Winnicott, Wallerstein, Meehl, and Erikson, among others [Wallerstein 1995]). Psychoanalytic definitions of insight are as divergent as they are prolific, and they tend to embody substantive theoretical positions. Consider the following examples. Strachey (1934) defines emotional insight as the culmination of a successful intervention that leads to structural and symptomatic change. Intellectual insight by contrast is a rationalization that does not result in lasting change. Wallerstein and Robbins (1956) define insight as the conscious awareness of intrapsychic changes in defensive operations, traits, wishes and behaviors. Insight is an 'ideational representation' of a change in ego function that does not always correlate with evaluations of structural or behavioral change. Moore and Fine (1968) define insight the following way: 'Analytic insight differs from other cognitive understanding in that it cannot occur without being preceded by dynamic changes leading to the release of energies'. Crits-Christoph and Luborsky (1990) supply a broader definition: 'Rather than perceiving insight as constituting the patient's sudden discovery of hidden or disavowed knowledge, analysts more often perceive the coming of insight as constituting a complex process inextricably associated with the subsequent working through of crucial affects and thoughts in the context of the transference relationship'. Freud conspicuously avoided the term insight, or *Einsicht*. The term only became popular with American and English-speaking European psychoanalysts, who 'thought that they had found an elegant and precise word to express something that belongs entirely to Freud. Analysis aims to offer the analysand a better knowledge of himself; what is meant by insight is that privileged moment of awareness' (Etchegoyen 1991). But while the term *Einsicht* does not appear in Freud's work, a number of cognate terms carry a similar explanatory load: self-knowledge and recognition, amongst others. In the *New Introductory Lectures*, for example, Freud characterized psychoanalysis as aiming to 'strengthen the ego, widen its field of vision, and so to extend its organization that it can take over new portions of the id. Where id was, there ego shall be' (Freud SE 22: 80). Elsewhere, Freud claimed that 'the method by which we strengthen the patient's weakened ego has as its starting point an increase in the ego's self-knowledge' (Freud 1963a: 70).

But what is it to 'widen' the ego's field of vision, and to increase its self-knowledge? And why should the mere acquisition of self-knowledge make any significant difference to the analysand's handling of his or her disorders?

Analysands such as Meehl's patient are regarded as suffering from a deep-rooted cognitive and emotional passivity that interferes with thought and action. Their target disorders are thought to be powerful fantasies, debilitating repressions, phobias, neurotic obsessions, and sexual complexes. Despite the common sense explanations and introspectively-generated reports that neurotic patients initially supply of their behaviors, and that give them the illusion of knowing what they are up to, they are not in possession of any *genuine* knowledge of why their behaviors are self-defeating, repetitive, or life-denying. The explanation given by Meehl's patient for her physician phobia, for instance, only scratches the surface; it is a kind of psychic camouflage for painful and deeply repressed problems. Dissemblance, evasion, and denial, in other words, are typical of patients suffering from neurosis. They are not able to give coherent and accurate accounts of why their behaviors take the particular shape that they do; nor are they able to accurately identify the real external and internal influences operating upon their behaviors. Thus when their analysis begins, they typically offer bowdlerized accounts of their life histories, with gaps left unfilled, sequences of events incoherent, and, as in Meehl's case history, important periods obscured. Freud characterized the life stories of neurotics as resembling 'an unnavigable river whose stream is at one moment choked by masses of rock and at another divided and lost among shallows and sandbanks' (Freud 1963b: 30). Borrowing a Platonic metaphor to illustrate the delicate balance between self-awareness and self-control on the one hand, and self-ignorance and neurotic disorder on the other, Freud likened the relation between the conscious self and the unconscious part of the mind to the relation between rider and horse. 'The horse provides the locomotive energy, and the rider has the prerogative of determining the goal and of guiding the movements of his powerful mount toward it. But all too often we find a picture of the less ideal situation in which the rider is obliged to guide his horse in the direction in which it itself wants to go' (Freud 1933: 108). Prior to psychoanalytic intervention, the deliverances of the conscious self which neurotic patients take as representing their genuine desires and intentions are considered to be little more than *ex post facto* rationalizations for the unruly forces of the unconscious, which operate stealthily but with surprisingly effective purpose behind the scenes. Meehl's patient, for instance, was psychologically minded and self-aware; despite this, she was a victim of powerful and potentially dangerous forces beyond her awareness. Such is the insidious nature of neurosis: its capacity to exist depends on lack of recognition.

It is not only neurotics who are not masters of their own house. A central tenet of the theory of classical Freudian psychoanalysis is that a baseline level of self-ignorance is a given of human psychology, featuring prominently in the everyday lives of normals as well as neurotics.[1] What then is the difference between neurotics before and after psychoanalytic intervention, in terms of the effects of insight into the causes of their target disorders? What possible difference could 'looking into their own depths' make to well-being?

While self-ignorance cannot be fully eradicated with psychoanalytic treatment, it can be modulated in an adaptive direction, and its negative effects on behavior can be weakened significantly. The Meehl case history, for example, seems to shows how analysis was largely an educative process: the analysand acquired a certain level of self-knowledge about the etiology of her disorders, through such mechanisms as memory retrieval and psychoanalytic interpretation. Analysis seemed to allow her the opportunity for a more objective and deeper self-observation and self-criticism than she would have had without any treatment, or with some other form of treatment.[2]

As analysands do not naturally gravitate toward the truth about themselves, it is thought that the interpretive input of the analyst is required to guide their self-explorations in the right direction, and to insure that only the clinical material that is relevant for the purposes of interpretation and insight is focused on. Meehl, for instance, considered his input to be minimal and mostly non-suggestive: only a skeptic, he claimed, would regard his patient's therapeutic progress as a function of analyst suggestion or reassurance. But even Freud acknowledged (with considerable qualification) that in practice this is rarely the case: even innocently-framed questions to elicit clinical material exert some degree of suggestive influence over the analysand's productions. One of the more explicit forms of analyst intervention, which is omitted from Meehl's description of the case history, is the psychoanalytic interpretation, offered to analysands at critical stages in the analysis as an explanation of the disorders from which they suffer. The interpretation is not a simple record of past events and psychological occurrences in the analysand's life; nor is it a fanciful literary construction that floats free of the psychological and historical facts; nor does it force-fit the clinical material into convenient shape, or overinterpret it in order to find psychoanalytic meaning where there is none. The interpretation is claimed to be a work of art, a penetrating account of psychological and historical fact, and a powerful therapeutic tool. It serves to tie together diverse patterns, themes, and clues—many of which are not noticed by the analysand—from the massive bulk of clinical material generated over the course of treatment. Freud (at least at one stage in his career) considered interpretations to be true if they 'tallied' with what is real in the analysand—that is, tallied with the facts of the client's psychology, life-history, and behavior (Freud SE 16: 452; see also Grünbaum 1984; Cioffi 1998). Other psychoanalysts consider interpretations to be true only if they are coherent and meaningful narratives (Schafer 1981, 1992; Spence 1982).

In clinical practice, interpretations are typically offered to analysands as tentative hypotheses to be explored, tested, and revised over the course of the treatment, rather than as finalized and authoritative statements. But how do analyst and analysand finally *know* that an interpretation has tallied with what is real? Tallying is neither self-evident nor immediately obvious; nor is the absence of tallying self-evident or immediately obvious. Moreover, the analyst is in no position to claim to 'know' intuitively, or solely on the basis of clinical experience, that an interpretation tallies with what is real. To make these sorts of claims would be to renounce the scientific method that ostensibly guides psychoanalytic inquiry. Similarly, the analysand is not in a position to claim to 'know' intuitively that an interpretation tallies with the facts. *Ex hypothesi*, the analysand's reflective judgment and introspective acumen are impugned by the presence of the very neurotic disorder that is the object of the interpretation and the target of treatment.

In actual psychoanalytic practice, a number of mutually supportive criteria are called upon to establish the interpretation's accuracy. An interpretation is considered to be accurate: i) if it is followed by significant change in the analysand's conduct; ii) if the analysand accepts it as accurate; iii) if it moves the process of analytic exploration forward, by triggering new discoveries and opening up new topics;[3] iv) if it is analogous to and consistent with a sufficient number of other interpretations in broadly similar case histories; and v) if it makes previously unintelligible experiences in the analysand's life intelligible. None of these criteria counts as a sufficient condition of the accuracy of an interpretation; and no criterion is singly necessary.

If presented at the right time in the treatment, interpretations can—it is claimed—teach analysands a great deal about themselves. New facts may come into view for the first time, and pre-treatment forms of self-understanding may be seen as incomplete, misleading, or as rationalizations motivated by unconscious forces. But the treatment method of psychoanalysis is not limited exclusively to educative processes; nor are the mechanisms of alleviation exclusively cognitive in orientation. It is well known in clinical practice that the mere possession of a veridical interpretation is not equivalent to insight; and it is not enough to have therapeutic efficacy. An accurate but merely abstract knowledge about the unconscious causes of the neuroses is ineffective in changing the neuroses or providing symptomatic relief (Richfield 1954; Rangell 1981, 1992); in some cases, moreover, such knowledge can even interfere with therapeutic progress as part of a 'premature flight into health'.

Had Meehl's patient, for instance, been presented with an interpretation of the causes of her physician phobia well before she so vividly remembered the events in the seventy-fifth hour of analysis, it would have had little effect on her. Freud noticed this phenomenon: 'if we communicate to a patient some idea which he has at one time repressed but which we have discovered in him, our telling him makes at first no change in his mental condition' (Freud SE 14: 175). One of the elements lacking in such cases is a sense that the knowledge of the etiology of a neurotic disorder justifiably *belongs* to the analysand: that is, that it is his or her *own* hard-won knowledge, rather than knowledge picked up adventitiously, or second-hand. It does not, in other words, have the marks of being emotionally charged and strongly identified-with self-knowledge; it is, rather, an abstract knowledge *about* the self. Freud put the point succinctly: 'If knowledge about the unconscious were as important for the patient as people inexperienced in psychoanalysis imagine, listening to lectures or reading books would be enough to cure him. Such measures, however, have as much influence on the symptoms of nervous illness as a distribution of menu cards in a time of famine has on hunger' (Freud SE 11: 225).

Something more is therefore required for genuine insight than mere knowledge about the etiology of neurotic disorders: but what is it? Therapeutically effective insight—what Freud called recollection—must be pitched at the right level of understanding, accompanied by the right kind of emotional attunement and affect (in 'enough sense modalities', as Meehl suggests), acquired at the right stage during the analysis, guided by the right transferential conditions, and propelled forward by the right kind of emotional labor (or 'working through').

Why is the analysand's intellectual understanding of the analyst's interpretations insufficient to bring about insight? Why are repressions and other unconscious forces that are the cause of neuroses so resistant to change when their unconscious meaning is first brought to light through interpretation? Before interpretations could be therapeutically effective and conducive to the acquisition of insight, it is thought that the treatment must somehow break through a well-fortified barrier of emotional and cognitive resistances that is erected by the unconscious to block access to those parts of it that are dangerously sensitive to identification (e.g. Meehl's patient's memories of her traumatic encounter with the physician). During the analysis, unconscious mechanisms of resistance are pressed into service to repress or deflect attention from the pathogenic conflicts that have been excavated and identified in the analyst's interpretations. These mechanisms are canny and insidious: their sole aim is to subvert the analysand's attempts to understand the role of the repressed experiences in the pathogenic conflicts.

The step between interpretation and insight is considered to be a delicate one fraught with the risk of relapse and premature improvement, with analysands struggling against the inertia of repression to keep the interpreted material in full view of conscious awareness. For instance, the doubts that Meehl's patient expressed about the authenticity of her memories of the traumatic event may have been unconsciously motivated rationalizations to keep the painful material at bay. There is always the risk that analytic progress will be derailed if the analysand were to 'allow what had been brought up into consciousness to slip back again into repression' (Freud SE 1916-17: 445). Freud's view is that in these difficult moments, when incipient insight is balanced precariously against the forces of resistance and repression, 'what turns the scale in his [the analysand's] struggle is not his intellectual insight—which is neither strong enough nor free enough for such an achievement—but simply and solely his relation to the doctor' (Freud SE 1916-17: 445). Meehl's case history does not document the transference in any significant detail, but it can be assumed that it was the emotional dynamics of the transference relation, and not an abstract knowledge of the relevant etiology, that provided his patient with the extra psychic momentum that she needed to break through the layers of resistances to consolidate her understanding. Insight and transference, in other words, are thought to be mutually supportive and co-evolving forces. The energy supplied by the emotionally charged relation to the analyst helps to keep the dawning of insight on track.

The transference relation, a central component of the psychoanalytic treatment method, is claimed to be the crucial setting in which the move from interpretation to insight, and insight to lasting therapeutic change, is possible. In the transference relation, the analyst becomes identified (in the mind of the analysand) with the primary figures in the analysand's early childhood experiences, and thus becomes the object upon which highly charged archaic emotions are projected. Because it is in the transference relation that the primary driving conflicts of the neurosis become foregrounded, the analyst is placed in the special position of being able to control the analysand's regression to critical childhood and infantile events—the very events that are thought to be at the crux of the neurosis. With the evidence of the transference clearly at hand—virtually staring the analysand in the face—the analyst can vividly demonstrate how the interpretation *must* fit the relevant facts of the past. This is a highly emotional stage of the analysis, with the analyst often forcefully repeating the interpretation to the analysand—'browbeating' according to Grünbaum (1984)—to help with his or her 'working through' the barrier of unconscious defenses.

The Meehl case history might give the impression that the acquisition of insight in psychoanalysis is sudden and dramatic (Meehl 1983: 355–356):

a kind of 'eureka' experience, or a startling, global realization.[4] Eureka insights, however, are relatively uncommon. In actual clinical practice, insight is commonly a drawn-out and slowly consolidated series of realizations, one building upon another with increasingly synergistic effect. 'The sudden tidal wave of illumination or enlightenment is rare compared to the numerous small ripples of insights which are experienced and intellectually assimilated over a long period of time. Moreover, the therapeutic insights tend to be circumscribed and more specific to certain problem areas than the profound and general eureka experiences, such as those described to occur during religious conversion or revelations in which the 'whole truth' suddenly is revealed' (Ludwig 1966: 315). Eureka insights are not only relatively uncommon, but they may even be counter-therapeutic. The psychoanalyst Ernst Kris (1956: 452) characterizes as 'deceptively good' those analytic hours in which there are sudden revelations and hasty movements. By contrast, the 'good hour' involves a slow and hesitant advance (Kris 1956: 452):

> It concerns the degree to which insight reaches awareness. Interpretation naturally need not lead to insight; much or most of analytic therapy is carried out in darkness, with here and there a flash of insight to lighten the path. A connexion has been established, but before insight has reached awareness (or, if it does, only for flickering moments), new areas of anxiety and conflict emerge, new material comes, and the process drives on: thus far-reaching changes may and must be achieved, without the pathway by which they have come about becoming part of the patient's awareness... As analytic work proceeds, the short-circuit type of reaction to interpretation decreases, so that more and more the flickering light stays on for a while; some continuity from one insightful experience to the other is maintained, though naturally what was comprehension and insight at one point may be obliterated at another. But by and large, even those phases seem to become shorter, and the areas of insight may expand.

Under *ideal* treatment conditions, and with an ideally successful analysis, analysands such as Meehl's patient would finally be able to recognize desires *as desires* of such and such a type, tracing them back to their causes, and separating from them the elements of fantasy and unconsciously driven instinctual need that threaten to interfere with their satisfaction. Thus armed, analysands would be able to distinguish real desires from irrational wishes and infantile wish-fulfillment schemas. They would also be able to discriminate genuine memories from unconsciously distorted memories; and identify their present situation with a certain adaptive degree of objectivity, without the overlay of unconscious memories of the past that are characteristically projected upon the present in the form of restrictive templates of thought, emotion, and action. Whatever control analysands would be able to exert in changing their behaviors through an increased self-understanding would first be based on the recognition of archaic motives and instincts, and the tracing of their causal history back to the sexual conflicts of infancy and early childhood.

Obviously, the analysis of unconscious motives and instincts would not cause them to disappear; but they would be tamed in such a way that the psychologically healthy analysand would be able to choose to express or sublimate his or her appetites without being driven irrationally by them. Hence Freud's characterization of psychoanalysis as a form of self-exploration that leads to self-knowledge, with analysis putting the analysand in a position 'to extend, by the information we give him, his ego's knowledge of his unconscious' (Freud 1963a: 65).

This is what might be achieved under ideal conditions, with an ideally successful treatment. But such things do not exist. No one fully achieves this state of self-transparency; it is at best a therapeutic ideal to which analysands aspire. Nor would its full realization be entirely desirable: psychoanalytic self-transparency would be painfully burdensome. But even in degrees, psychoanalytic insight is supposed to afford a measure of freedom and self-control that would not be available to those who have not undergone psychoanalysis. Aware that the ideal of rational self-transparency and self-control was *only* an ideal, Freud's actual expectations for therapeutic improvement were in fact quite moderate: 'Much will be gained if we succeed in transforming your hysterical misery into common unhappiness. With a mental life that has been restored to health you will be better armed against that unhappiness' (Freud SE 2: 305).

Case History 3

The third case history illustrates the role of insight in brief psychodynamic psychotherapy. It is described by the well-known psychiatrist Jerome Frank, and is based on his treatment of a client who suffered from episodes of severe depression, preoccupation, and irritability (Frank and Frank 1991: 205–210).[5] Frank notes that the client's presenting symptoms had recurred at one to two-week intervals from shortly before the client had married. With the birth of her daughter, the client was determined to be a perfect mother, a decision that only exacerbated her irritability and led to frequent violent outbursts. The client feared that she would fail her child just as her mother had failed her, and the intensity of these feelings contributed to her growing fear of impending insanity.

Frank learned in the first interview that the client's mother had been absent during much of her infancy, and then had vanished from her life when she was three years old. The client's father remarried and soon went overseas on military service for a year and a half, an absence which generated in the young child considerable emotional distress. At the age of fourteen the client discovered some of her mother's letters, which contained information suggesting that she had suffered a serious mental illness and had committed suicide.

This precipitated a lengthy downturn in the client's state of mind, character-ized by irritability, withdrawal from social interaction, fantasies about her own suicide, and brooding over her father's involvement in and responsibility for her mother's death. The client's unhappiness lasted for eighteen months, after which time she returned to her 'normal self'. This period of psychological stability lasted until late in her courtship, which was marked by conflict and opposition from both families. The client, Frank notes, was reluctant to confide in her psychotherapist.

At a relatively early stage in the psychotherapy Frank presented to the client a broadly psychodynamic interpretation of the cause of her symptoms. The gist of the interpretation was that abandonment by her mother and father at such an early age had led the client to fear putting trust in other people, including her husband. This, Frank told her, explained her earlier depressive episodes, as well as the manifest distrust she displayed during the therapeutic hour. Despite the relative simplicity of Frank's reconstruction, it triggered in his client a series of insights that were followed by positive therapeutic changes: 'As the patient said in the next interview, my interpretation 'went off like a gong'. She confirmed her acceptance of it by spontaneously attributing the recurrence of her depression and irritability during her courtship to her fiancé's periodic threats to terminate the engagement because of family opposition. She recognized that these threats had reactivated the feelings that followed her desertion by her mother and father' (Frank and Frank 1991: 206).

For the three months she was seen by Frank following the initial interpreta-tion and insight, the client remained free of symptoms. During this time she came to accept that her mother had committed suicide; she felt more recon-ciled toward her father; she abandoned her aspirations of trying to be a perfect homemaker and mother; and she began to share her feelings more openly with her husband. Looking back over her past, she came to realize that she had failed to communicate with her husband, and had confused speaking her feel-ings aloud with reciting them to herself. The psychotherapy had enabled her to acquire a number of insights into her behaviors, feelings, upbringing, and present situation that she would not otherwise have acquired; and it led—or so it seemed—to positive behavioral changes and a marked decrease in the presenting symptoms.

As with Sullivan's case history, Frank's case history illustrates how psychotherapists think about the central characteristics of insight. It shows: i) how the acquisition of insight is considered to mark a turning point in psychodynamic psychotherapy, and how it is considered to have prophylactic effects with respect to presenting symptoms; ii) how the acquisition of insight can be emotionally catalytic; iii) how congruence between the psychotherapist's interpretations and the client's insights can be therapeutically effective; and iv) how interpretations can appear to stimulate the flow of insights without any overt signs of suggestion or emotional manipulation.

The case history also hints at the puzzling epistemic questions about interpretations and insights. An epistemically uncritical construal of this case history would hold the following: a) Frank's interpretation was one of the causes of his client's therapeutic progress; b) the interpretation was true, or truth-tracking, and therefore therapeutically effective; c) the client's insights were one of the causes of her therapeutic improvement; and d) the client's insights were true, or truth-tracking, and therefore therapeutically effective. The same epistemically uncritical construal would hold that false or incomplete interpretations and insights would not have had the same level of therapeutic effectiveness; or perhaps none at all. Clearly, other causes of therapeutic change were at play, including the all-important interpersonal dynamics arising from the increasingly trusting relationship Frank was establishing with the client.

Is the epistemically uncritical construal of the case history plausible? On what grounds could the interpretations and insights in this case history be assessed as veridical? Is it possible that the client's improvement was caused by false interpretations and insights—that is, explanatory fictions with robust instrumental value and a high degree of subjective plausibility? Frank conspicuously does not commit himself to the veridicality of his interpretation, or to the veridicality of the client's subsequent insights. He suggests, cautiously, that his interpretation was 'plausible' and 'reassuring'; that it enabled her to acquire insights through 'relabeling' her feelings as normal; and that it allowed her 'to construct a more optimistic apologia and enhanced her sense of mastery' (Frank and Frank 1991: 207). 'The healing power of my interpretations seemed to lie more in the general attitude they conveyed than in their precise content' (210). Elsewhere Frank writes: 'An effectively reassuring explanation simultaneously promotes patients' feelings of mastery and offers hopes of recovery' (128).

Interpretations and insights that to clients seem 'plausible', 'reassuring', and 'mastery enhancing' may also be false, inaccurate, or incomplete. Plausibility is not equivalent to truth; nor is it a sufficient condition for truth. Outside of psychotherapeutic contexts, for example, it is not uncommon for people to hold beliefs about the behavior, psychology, and personality of others (or themselves) that seem to be plausible, but are in fact false, incoherent, or vacuous. Similarly, it is not uncommon for people to reject beliefs that seem implausible, and yet are in fact true. Astrological explanations of personality, for example, appear to many to be plausible, and to have a high degree of explanatory power; but they are pseudo-explanations, because they are compatible with any state of affairs in the world. Not only is plausibility commonly confused with truth; it is also common for people to be influenced by beliefs they regard as plausible, that are in fact false: that is, to deliberate over them, make decisions on their basis, and act upon them.

Plausibility is often confused with truth in psychodynamic psychotherapy. Interpretations and insights are the prime candidates for confusion here. Frank's interpretation may have been plausible but false, just as the insights the client experienced after his interpretation went off 'like a gong' may have been plausible and reassuring, but also false, inaccurate, or incomplete. Frank does not explicitly rule out these possibilities. The common factors approach that he defends (see Chapter 3) holds that what matters for therapeutic effectiveness is (among other factors) that clients are provided with a rationale, conceptual scheme, or myth that supplies a *believable* explanation for the client's symptoms, and prescribed a manageable but progressively difficult procedure for resolving them. But the rationale or conceptual scheme need not be psychologically or historically true (or truth-tracking) in order to be believable; nor does it need to be true to be therapeutically effective. False, inaccurate, or incomplete insights and interpretations may still be credible.

Obviously, interpretations and insights must satisfy certain minimal levels of psychological coherence in order to count as plausible and credible: they cannot display glaring cognitive vices, such as being wildly off the mark, irrelevant, obscure, vague, self-contradictory, or plain bizarre. But once these minimal cognitive criteria are satisfied, false interpretations and insights may be just as plausible and credible as veridical interpretations and insights; perhaps even more so. Frank hints at this: 'Therapists... who believe that only 'correct' interpretations will lead patients to change, find it hard to accept that the attitude their words convey may contribute more to therapy than the words' precise content' (Frank and Frank 1991: 210).

Frank's interpretation satisfied these minimal levels of psychological coherence. It was not arbitrary; it was not a fanciful story made up on the spot, without any attention to the clinical material and the facts of the case. At the same time, however, it was not a detailed and comprehensive explanation of the facts of the case, since many of these facts were simply not available to Frank. The interpretation was offered early in the course of the therapy, at a point when the clinical material was still quite thin, and Frank's knowledge of the client's background, psychological problems, and personality still limited. Other interpretations might just as well have gone off 'like a gong'. There was nothing stopping Frank from constructing different interpretations of the client's problems, with different levels of plausibility: foregrounding themes that were backgrounded in the actual interpretation, backgrounding themes that were foregrounded, emphasizing certain causal connections over others, and so on. Alternative interpretations may also have been therapeutically effective. Some may have been much more psychologically speculative, with more tenuous connections to the facts than the one he presented; others may have been more empirically robust. Similarly, it is reasonable to suppose that a number of alternative insights might have been as therapeutically effective as the insights the client actually acquired, as long as they met minimal standards of plausibility. Does this mean that truth in the psychodynamic psychotherapies is therapeutically dispensable?

Insight Research

This question about insight and truth takes on new meaning in light of the following sampling of passages about insight, all culled from psychodynamic psychotherapy literature, including textbooks, literature reviews, and research papers. The sampling is neither complete nor rounded: it is a selective, scattered, and partial glimpse of a huge and multifaceted field (Castonguay and Hill 2007). Still, it is useful for illustrating some common themes. One of these, as will become clear, is that insight is one of the central goals of psychodynamic psychotherapy, and one of the essential components of psychological well-being. Another common theme is that the insights clients acquire in psychodynamic psychotherapy are authentic and true. As will be evident from this sampling, however, there is little discussion of the possibility that these insights may be fictional, false, over-simplified, incomplete, or tainted by self-deception or illusion. It should also be evident that there is no significant discussion of the possibility that insights may need to be graded on an epistemic scale of better to worse, or more truth-tracking and less truth-tracking.

- [P]sychoanalysis is the best method available to achieve the more ambitious goal of fundamental alteration of character structure, with eradication or reduction to a minimum of neurotic mechanisms... Psychoanalysis attempts the ultimate in exploration, with a goal of the maximum in self-knowledge and structural alteration of the personality... The greatest field, and often the most rewarding one for exploratory psychotherapy which does not involve the more ambitious goals of psychoanalysis, lies in those clinical conditions which are appraised as relatively recent decompensations arising out of upsetting life experiences... The psychotherapist's capacity to detect the nature of the event and the reasons for the patient's excessive reaction to it enables him to penetrate the neurotic conflict, actively conduct the exploration, and finally expose the whole sequence of predisposition, overtaxing event, and neurotic response. (Knight 1952: 121)

• Interpretations, as meaningful explanatory interventions, appeal to an ego which is actively experiential in the sense of emotional participation in, and acquaintanceship with, current and past events; as well as to an ego which is introspective, self-observant and responsive in terms of intellectual recognition and explanation... With proper timing and appropriate blending of the intellectual and emotional, the material which is brought to consciousness is dynamically accessible to interpretations, and the insights which follow feel authentic and immediately applicable to inner and outer life. (Valenstein 1962: 332)

• In a successful analysis, the patient eventually becomes aware of the previously unconscious elements in his neurosis: he can fully feel and experience how his neurotic symptoms grew out of the conflicts of which he is now conscious; and he can fully feel and experience how facing up to these conflicts dispels the symptoms and, as Freud put it, 'transforms neurotic suffering into everyday misery'; and how flinching will bring back the symptoms again. (Waelder 1962: 629)

• 'Insight', psychoanalytically oriented or depth psychotherapy is based on Freud's recognition that psychological problems are developmental, and that only by obtaining insight into the process that gives rise to them can a resolution based on cause be reached. (Basch 1980: 171)

• The ultimate goal of psychoanalytic intervention is the removal of debilitating neurotic problems. Not much new in that. But the unswerving credo of the traditional psychoanalytic therapist is that, ultimately, the only final and effective way of doing this is to help the patient achieve insight. What does insight mean? It means total understanding of the unconscious determinants of one's irrational feelings, thoughts, or behaviors that are producing so much misery. Once these unconscious reasons are fully confronted and understood, the need for neurotic defenses and symptoms will disappear... The true meaning of this insight is then burned into the patient's consciousness by the working-through process. This refers to a careful and repeated examination of how one's conflicts and defenses have operated in many different areas of life. Little may be accomplished by a simple interpretation that one's passivity and helplessness are really an unconscious form of aggression. Once the basis for the interpretation is firmly laid, it must be repeated time and time again. The patient must be confronted with the insight as it applies to relations with a spouse, a friend, or a supervisor, and, yes, even as it affects reactions to the therapist. Patients must be helped to work through all corners of their lives with this insight. (Phares 1980: 342–343)

◆ [Insight is] the affective experiencing and cognitive understanding of current maladaptive patterns of behavior that repeat childhood patterns of interpersonal conflict. (Strupp and Binder 1984: 24–25)

◆ The primary goal of psychodynamic psychotherapy is insight. When the therapist intervenes, the ultimate purpose would always be to foster understanding. [The therapist] tunnels through the darkness of ignorance bringing meaning and purpose where none existed. (Nichols and Paolino 1986: 13–14)

◆ From the beginning, of course, I had known that the pure forcefulness of my argument would not penetrate deep enough to effect any change. It almost never does. It's never worked for me when I've been in therapy. Only when one feels an insight *in one's bones* does one own it. Only then can one act on it and change. Pop psychologists forever talk about 'responsibility assumption', but it's all words: it is extraordinarily hard, even terrifying, to own the insight that you and only you construct your own life design. Thus, the problem in therapy is always how to move from an ineffectual intellectual appreciation of a truth about oneself to some emotional *experience* of it. It is only when therapy enlists deep emotions that it becomes a powerful force for change. (Yalom 1989: 35)

◆ Let us turn to the idea of insight in depth and nuclear complex insight that is supposed to be the essence of psychoanalytic theory, or other exploratory psychotherapies. I wonder at the whole complex procedure of working through a patient's problems, so that all sorts of emotional and intellectual processes and experiences go on side by side with establishing connections and relations [sic]. The achieving of insight and the effect of acquiring insight as a therapeutic phenomenon is a reciprocal, and almost a feedback mechanism. For example, we cannot make certain interpretations until the patient is ready. This means that a great deal more must go on in a patient before he is able to see the connections. If he is ready, then the seeing of connections will be meaningful and helpful. This being made ready is a complex procedure consisting of many phenomena, among which are even preliminary insight experiences. I would therefore say that insight is the acquiring by the patient of an understanding of connections and relations. This may take place at many levels, and is an integral part of the reciprocal manner in which the deeper forms of psychotherapy develop. (Frosch 1990: 720)

- Through gaining insight, which is an education process, it can be discerned how old patterns were created—and how unconscious forces shaped unwanted behavior. As a result of greater insight into these unconscious processes (making the unconscious conscious), the number of choices is increased. It should be emphasized, however, that insight *per se* does not bring about change. (Hollender and Ford 1990: 6)

- Kris (1956) stated what most therapists have experienced, namely, the discovery that insight, either cognitive or emotional, is often insufficient to bring about real change in our patients. Fried (1982) suggested 'that what matters clinically is that insight into most conflicts, be they preoedipal or oedipal, does not rectify deficits and malformations. They have to be corrected through the very repetitive experiences and challenges that groups offer in abundance.' (Rutan and Stone 1993: 139)

- The ultimate goals of psychoanalysis and those treatments weighted toward the expressive end of the continuum involve the acquisition of insight, which may be defined as the capacity to understand the unconscious meanings and origins of one's symptoms and behavior. Although Freud never used the term insight, he did define the goal of analysis as making conscious what is unconscious, which is certainly a significant aspect of insight. (Gabbard 1994: 91)

- Essentially, psychoanalysis continues the rationalist spirit of Greek philosophy, to 'know thyself'. Knowing one's self, however, is understood in quite a different way. It is not to be found in the pursuit of formal, logical analysis of thinking. As far as the individual is concerned, the sources of his neurotic suffering are by their very nature 'unknowable'. They reside outside the realm of consciousness, barred from awareness by virtue of their painful, unacceptable quality. By enabling the patient to understand how neurotic symptoms and behavior represent derivatives of unconscious conflicts, psychoanalysis permits the patient to make rational choices instead of responding automatically. Self-knowledge of a very special kind strengthens the individual's ability to make choices and seek fulfillment. For the successfully analyzed individual, freedom from neurotic inhibition is often experienced as a liberating, self-fulfilling transformation, which promotes not only self-actualization but also the ability to contribute to the advancement and happiness of others. Knowing oneself may have far-reaching social implications... Although there are many ways to treat neuroses, there is but one way to understand them—psychoanalysis. (Arlow 1995: 16–17)

- The power of insight ultimately rests on the ability of human beings to use their intelligence to understand themselves and alter their behavior, given the new information developed in the course of psychotherapy. Allen Wheelis (1956) adds that insight also 'implies the belief that no inner danger is so bad that not knowing about it will be better than knowing'. (Kotin 1995: 172)

◆ The simplest and most frequent answer given to the question of what brings about change is the patient's acquisition of insight, aided largely by the therapist's interventions, especially their interpretations and clarifications. The expansion of patients' self-understanding and awareness allows them to break out of their neurotic mode, to resolve their conflicts, and to resume growth and maturation... [B]y becoming more fully aware of one's defenses, wishes, needs, resistances, character traits, and conflicts, one is in a much better position to exercise control over them. Otherwise, they continue to exert an insidious influence beyond one's ken or control. If one has been anxious, inhibited, unproductive, or depressed, the route to overcome such dysfunctional states, according to psychoanalytic therapy, is by becoming conscious of the conflicts underlying these symptoms. (Messer and Warren 1995: 93)

◆ More practically, insight is the first clear awareness of an implicit general tendency, control mechanism, or habit, and working through consists of breaking the habit by becoming increasingly aware of its subtle intrusion into our behavior again. (Jacob 1996: 157)

◆ Successful psychotherapy fosters the capacity for self-analysis, a direct reinvestment that allows you to end psychotherapy yet continue to progress, to apply self-understanding gained through working with your therapist to new life situations as they arise. (Vaughan 1997: 182)

◆ For the current investigation [a study about the reliability and validity of measures of self-understanding of interpersonal patterns], self-understanding was defined as the understanding of maladaptive interpersonal patterns described in modern theories of short-term dynamic psychotherapy... Self-understanding was further defined across a continuum from mere recognition of a problem area to a deeper understanding of the historical origins of the pattern. Using this definition, the client can gain self-understanding by coming to recognize his or her own wishes, responses of self, and responses of others. The next level of understanding involves the recognition that these interpersonal patterns are replicated across different relationships. Deeper understanding occurs when the client comes to understand the interpersonal origins of these wishes and responses. (Connolly *et al.* 1999: 473)

◆ [T]he central belief of the psychodynamic approach [is] that our emotional problems have their origins in childhood experiences. As long as the troubling thoughts, feelings and memories of these experiences are repressed by the unconscious processes, they are inaccessible and therefore cannot be understood or resolved. Psychodynamic therapy aims to bring the unconscious into conscious awareness so that the individual may gain insight and understanding. Freud once said 'One cannot fight an enemy one cannot see'. (Dryden and Mytton 1999: 17)

♦ It is important, for instance, that the client responds well to the basic techniques—that the client takes some initiative for speaking, and does not rely on the counselor for advice or solutions. To make good use of the psychodynamic approach, the client needs to show some insight (understanding) of her or himself, and also to respond thoughtfully (although not compliantly) to linking responses and interpretations. (Jacobs 1999: 44)

♦ [I]t is through the process of self-awareness, self-understanding, and self-revelation that true growth occurs... Insight into one's problems is a necessary prerequisite before any real and lasting change can occur. (Kottler and Brown 1999: 28)

♦ The dynamic concept of insight supposes an awareness of the interaction between external and internal reality, that is, between objective and subjective experience... All psychodynamic schools of thought agree that partial failure of insight results from the operation of defenses: for example, denial of an external fact such as a painful bereavement, or the projection of an unwanted internal impulse. Just as understanding between people can lead to reconciliation, so can self-understanding and insight lead to reconciliation with disowned aspects of oneself... Repressed and split-off parts can be restored to the self in the new climate of experimentation and growth, if the therapeutic relationship provides the necessary security and flexibility. The person is enabled to discover the extent of his internal world, perhaps even to discover for the first time that he has one. (Bateman et al. 2000: 74–75)

♦ Knowledge alone does not inform conduct. Insight is rarely a transforming event. Still, insight is a useful, perhaps necessary, ingredient for change. Whatever it may be called—self-knowledge, self-awareness, insight—it is still central to most schools of psychotherapy. (Gaylin 2000: 147)

A great many theoretical variations of psychodynamic psychotherapy are represented in this sample: divergent conceptions of the contents of insights, divergent ideas about the ways in which insights are acquired, and divergent views about the relative therapeutic weight assigned to the emotional dynamics of the psychotherapist–client dyad. Despite these differences, however, three dominant themes emerge: i) insight is essential to psychological well-being;

ii) insight into the causes of maladaptive behaviors and psychological problems is, minimally, a necessary (but not sufficient) condition for therapeutic progress; and iii) insights refer to real psychological, behavioral, or historical forces, entities, objects, or situations.

Other themes emerge as well. Many of the passages suggest that the *causes* of psychological disorders are found in the past, particularly in early childhood experiences, and in the defense mechanisms that were erected during childhood to keep painful feelings, wishes, and conflicts out of conscious awareness. Defense mechanisms work silently, efficiently, and behind the scenes: hence the repeated references to the importance of making conscious what is unconscious, and the repeated references to the sheer difficulties of this process, because of the manifold unconscious forces (or resistances) opposing the work of exploratory therapy (e.g. erotic or hate-dominated relations with the psychotherapist, acting out, and resistance to recovery). Also hindering the work of therapeutic exploration are: repression (i.e. the client's active attempts to push out of awareness painful memories and feelings), denial (i.e. the client's attempts to divert attention from painful feelings and ideas), and regression (i.e. the client's tendency to return to earlier ways of experiencing in order to avoid conflicts). The psychodynamic psychotherapies tend to share a number of other key theoretical (and experience-distant) concepts, which diverge markedly from common sense psychological explanations: transference, repression, reaction formation, displacement, reversal, sublimation, and splitting, among others. These are among the basic building blocks of psychodynamic explanations.

Another theme that emerges from these passages is the tension between insight and the transference relation. The question of which one is more important for therapeutic improvement has divided researchers in psychodynamic psychotherapy for years (Crits-Christoph and Luborsky 1990; Wallerstein 1995). A number of theoreticians and clinicians contend that the real engine of therapeutic change is the transference relation, and not the acquisition of insight (Eagle 1993). Others contend that a careful and well-timed balance between insight and transference is required for therapeutic progress. However this issue comes to be resolved, it is generally agreed that insight alone is not a sufficient condition for therapeutic change—a view that can be traced at least as far back as Spinoza's philosophical psychology (1677/1992). Once insights are acquired, they must be emotionally, behaviorally and psychologically consolidated by means of a 'working through' process. In Phares' (1980) terms, they must be 'burned into the consciousness' of the client: that is, repeated, reiterated, identified with, deeply felt—without running the risk of suggestion, coercion, or brainwashing (see also Valenstein 1962).

Much of the impetus for this working-through process comes from the client–therapist dyad, considered by some clinicians to be a re-enactment of the parent–child relationship, by others to be an ideally supportive and nurturing relationship, and by others to be a corrective emotional experience (Alexander and French 1946).

These are just some of the more noticeable common themes running throughout these passages. There are also many noticeable oversights and omissions. What is striking about *all* of the passages (and the works in which they are imbedded) is the relatively scant attention that is paid to the *epistemic* complexities and liabilities surrounding insight. The prevailing assumption is that the insights clients achieve in exploratory psychotherapy are authentic and true (or minimally, truth-tracking); and that insights refer to, or are about, something real. There is almost no discussion of the issue of whether the insights acquired in psychodynamic psychotherapy might be epistemically problematic: for example, false, incomplete, overly simplistic, trivial, driven by psychotherapist suggestion, empirically impoverished, contaminated with self-deception or illusion, or the vehicles of the placebo effect. There is almost no discussion of how the basic epistemic distinction between appearance and reality might affect psychodynamic insights. (None of the passages approaches the level of methodological sophistication displayed by Freud, who, as Grünbaum (1984, 1993) showed, was driven by a concern to address the epistemic challenges of the suggestion hypothesis (Freud 1954; Meehl 1983)).

Another common omission is the absence of any discussion of the question of the *truth criteria* that are called upon when insights are evaluated as true or false. None of these passages addresses the epistemic question of *what it is* that makes one insight true and another false, or the question of what it *means* to say that an insight is true or false. Each is silent on the question of whether the truth of insights consists (for example) in their correspondence with psychological facts (the correspondence theory of truth), or their internal coherence and consistency (the coherence theory of truth), or their pragmatic value (the pragmatic theory of truth)—three of the more well-known theories of truth. Closely related to this is a general absence of discussion of the evidentiary criteria that are called upon to evaluate and validate insights: that is, criteria specifying what *counts* as good and bad evidence in the validation of the truth or falsity of an insight, and *what it is* in virtue of which something is good or bad evidence.

It would be tempting to extrapolate beyond the confines of this relatively small sampling of psychodynamic theorizing, and conclude with the broad generalization that the concept of insight in psychodynamic psychotherapy is *both* a core concept that is accorded enormous explanatory leverage, and a concept that is, at least from the point of view of logic and epistemology, poorly defined, ambiguous, and even muddled. Such an extrapolation would not be far from the truth, but with the exception of a handful of philosophers and psychodynamic theorists, few have ventured this far. Kubie is one of the few who have. He writes that 'unfortunately, this most fundamental of all elements in psychoanalytic therapy [namely, insight] has never been adequately tested and verified... [I]ndeed, it is fair to say that this cornerstone of the modern conception of a dynamic psychotherapeutic process confronts us with many complex and unsolved problems' (Kubie 1975: 59–60). Marmor is another: 'But what is insight? To a Freudian it means one thing, to a Jungian another, and to a Rankian, a Horneyite, an Adlerian or a Sullivanian, still another. Each school gives its own particular brand of insight. Whose are the correct insights? The fact is that patients treated by analysts of all these schools may not only respond favorably, but also believe strongly in the insights which they have been given' (Marmor 1962: 289). But these critical comments from within the field of psychodynamic psychotherapy have mostly gone unaddressed.

Clinical Psychology's Quicksilver

Perhaps as compensation for conceptual sloppiness, criteriological vagueness, and epistemic oversights, there have been several attempts within psychodynamic psychotherapy research to bring some rigor to the study of insight, with a view, among other things, to making the concept of insight more scientifically respectable.

If the concept of insight could be operationalized satisfactorily, and *if* client insight could somehow be made to yield to measurement that is not arbitrary or force-fitted, then it might be possible to determine with some degree of precision how insight interacts with other client and treatment variables. A number of deep theoretical and clinical issues could then be addressed with some degree of scientific rigor: for instance, the relation between insight acquisition and treatment outcome, the therapeutic interventions most effective in stimulating insight, the relative contributions of emotional versus intellectual insight to overall therapeutic progress, and the relation between psychological mindedness (or, more broadly, client suitability) and insight acquisition.

But is the *very idea* of a science of insight a coherent idea? Insight is the quicksilver of psychodynamic psychology research: elusive, private, and highly individual, it seems to be the one phenomenon that is least likely to yield to scientific scrutiny. Insights are not observable like behaviors. Nor are they measurable like behaviors. No two clients' insights are the same, or mean the same thing. No two clients arrive at insights in the same way. No two clients experience their insights in the same way. Few if any clients naturally quantify or grade their insights in ways that are relevant to the psychologists who seek to measure insights. To further complicate matters, the theoretical and psychometric principles that govern the measurement of insight—principles of psychological salience, psychological causality, and insight prototypicality, among others—are not independent of changing cultural and historical norms. No *a priori* limit could be set to the variety of new types of insight measures that may be generated at any one time across the changing history of clinical psychology. With changes in the forms of social life, in the historically embedded vocabularies of sentiment, memory, personality, and character, and in the explanatory goals of clinical psychologists, will come changes in the types of relevant insight measures. Any measurement of insight is therefore necessarily incomplete: there will always be something that is left out of any ostensibly objective measurement instrument.

How then could something so intensely subjective, individual, and multifaceted be captured with standardized measurement instruments? How could insight measures be designed to range across diverse subject populations, when the contents, depth, and force of insights are mediated by variables such as age, gender, education, mental health, psychological mindedness, and cultural background? Are insight measures destined to measure only some thin and lifeless slice of the actual phenomenon—or, worse, some artifact that bears little significant relation to it?

Despite its quicksilverish appearance, insight has not proven to be scientifically invisible. Beginning in the 1950s, a research program has gradually emerged dedicated to investigating the nature, conditions, frequency, and relevance of insight in psychodynamic psychotherapy. The basic assumption shared by all researchers in this program is that there is *something* that is open to *some* form of psychological measurement, even if it is only what clients *report* about their insights (rather than the insights themselves), or what they *say* about their insights in structured questionnaires, scales, or inventories, or what is displayed in their *behaviors* that might plausibly be correlated with insight or its lack. This assumption is neither implausible nor speculative. Even very crude measures of insight could be conducted in the homespun terms of folk psychology, far from the clinic or laboratory. This might involve, for example, asking a group of people who share roughly similar psychological problems to answer a series of simple 'Yes' or 'No' questions: 'Do you know what your feelings about X are?' 'Do you know why you have these feelings about X?' 'Do you see a pattern in your feelings about X and other X-like situations?' and so on. The questions could be fine-tuned by asking respondents to rank their answers on a simple Likert-type scale. Emerging from this would be a crude data base, from which a number of rough generalizations about insight could be made—although the results would not have significant explanatory or predictive power. While still in its infancy, the scientific study of insight has advanced considerably further than random folk psychological samplings (Messer and McWilliams 2007).

A simplified skeletal model of the scientific measurement of insight would take the following form. First, stimulus materials would be administered to carefully selected groups of psychodynamic psychotherapy clients at different time intervals, with the first set of measurements serving as a baseline against which subsequent measurements are compared. The instruments pressed into service for this task would be varied, reflecting the theoretical orientations, hypotheses, and subject populations of the insight researchers. But however varied the instruments might be, they would include some of the following: standardized insight scales, insight questionnaires, self-reports, hypothetical situations, psychological inventories, and comparative self-ratings.

Second, respondents would be constrained to respond to the stimulus materials with one of a limited number of structured choices: for example, 'Yes' or 'No', or numeric gradations on a Likert-type scale. This would serve to rule out the messy excess information that comes with free-response methods. Next, scoring procedures would be applied to the uninterpreted data, with a view to minimizing the role of experimenter interpretation and bias. Then the data would be subjected to scale indices that would have been subjected to experimental fine-tuning and replication studies. The point of administering these materials would be to define the content of clients' self-understanding with more precision than is available to folk psychological methods and first-person methods. With increasing refinements in the design of these measurement instruments would come increases in predictive and explanatory rigor, not to be found in common sense psychology. At the same time, insight measures would have to be designed that control for such things as Hawthorne effects, expectancy effects, compliance effects, experimental subordination effects, and other effects that could contaminate the data.

The history of insight research from the 1950s onwards is a messy but more or less true-to-form instantiation of this skeletal model. In the 1950s psychotherapy researchers thought, not implausibly, that client insight could be measured objectively by looking at the degree of congruence between client self-descriptions and the descriptions supplied by others (Dymond 1948; Feldman and Bullock 1955; Kelman and Parloff 1957; Mann and Mann 1959).

The guiding hypothesis was that clients whose insight-based self-descriptions were more congruent with the psychological descriptions provided by others—presumably, experienced psychotherapists and psychological experts—were more likely to have accurate insights than those whose self-descriptions diverged sharply from the descriptions of others. This particular branch of the insight research program encountered a number of methodological and design flaws, including halo effects, rating accuracy problems, and lack of information to rate the behaviors of others (Gage and Cronbach 1955). Even if it had not foundered on these grounds, however, it would have run up against a number of difficult logical and epistemic problems. Congruence of first and third-person descriptions is a measure of simple intersubjective agreement, but not—without further measures—a measure of the depth, accuracy, or truth value of the relevant descriptions. Congruent first-person and third-person descriptions might be false, simplistic, or implausible; and self-descriptions that are incongruent with the descriptions of experts may be true or truth-tracking. The mere fact that there is congruence does not guarantee descriptive accuracy and truth, but simply pushes the question of accuracy and truth one step back. There is another epistemic issue at stake too. Third-person descriptions vary as much from first-person descriptions as biographical descriptions vary from autobiographical descriptions: they have different influences, serve different ends, and mean different things. Failure to bring first-person descriptions (and the insights they convey) into line with third-person descriptions may simply show that what clients consider relevant to their lives is what observers consider irrelevant (Jopling 2000); or it may simply show that observers lack much of the relevant information.

The difficulties of the congruence approach spurred the development of other approaches—but these too encountered logical, epistemic, and methodological problems. Some insight researchers, for example, thought that the measurement of insight should be placed squarely in the hands of psychological experts, rather than in the hands of clients reporting on their own insights; and that the measurement instruments should be designed for and deployed by experts, rather than the people measured by the instruments. There are good reasons for this. First, the data collected on self-report measures do not rule out the possibility that the clients filling out the measures suffer from self-deception, self-misunderstanding, and misestimation (Jopling 2000). Second, when filling out self-reports, questionnaires, or inventories, clients are vulnerable to mistakes, self-deception, context effects, and experimenter influence; or worse, they are vulnerable to hidden systematic errors in judgment and inference that can lead to experimental artifacts that contaminate the data. Self-reports of behaviors and attitudes, for instance, have been found to be strongly influenced by features of the research instrument, such as the wording of the question, format, and context (Schwartz and Sudman 1992, 1994, 1996; Schwartz 1999; see also Jones 1977, Greenberg 2007). Researchers who rely on these instruments often overlook these factors: 'as researchers, we tend to view our questionnaires as 'measurement devices' that elicit information from respondents. What we frequently overlook is that our questionnaires are also a source of information that respondents draw on in order to determine their task and to arrive at a useful and informative answer. [W]e are often not fully aware of the information that our questionnaires—or our experimental procedures—provide, and hence miss the extent to which the questions we ask determine the answers we receive' (Schwartz 1999: 103). The lesson to be learned here is simple: it is one thing for respondents to achieve high scores on a self-report about insight, another to actually have accurate and valid insights.

The strategy of the so-called third-person approach was to avoid these difficulties by leaving the measurement of insight to experts. Variations in this approach have been defended by Morgan *et al.* (1982) and Tolor and Reznikoff (1960), among others. Tolor and Reznikoff (1960), for instance, developed an insight scale consisting of twenty-seven hypothetical situations measuring insight. Each hypothetical situation was designed to invoke one or more of thirteen defense mechanisms, and for each situation there were four interpretations. Only one of these interpretations was counted as more insightful than the others, with insight being defined as the ability to understand the causal factors underlying attitudes and behaviors. Even with the help of a more precise definition of insight, however, the study shows little about the epistemic conditions of insight. A correct understanding of the motivations of other people (or oneself) in hypothetical situations is no guarantee that insights into one's own behaviors are accurate or truth-tracking (Roback 1974).

In the 1980s, Morgan *et al.* (1982) designed a nine-item rating scale for measuring client insight in moderate-length psychodynamic psychotherapy, with experienced psychologists serving as raters. The scale was applied to two early-in-treatment sessions and two late-in-treatment sessions, and the scale items (below) were rated on a ten-point Likert-type scale that was designed to measure degree of emotional insight. Clients themselves were not asked to fill out the scale, for all the obvious and not-so-obvious reasons: this was the business of the experts.

1. Patient recognizes specific phenomena (ideation, affect, behavior) relevant to the problems being discussed.
2. Patient recognizes habitual patterns of behavior.

3. Patient recognizes that he or she plays an active rather than a passive role in producing his or her symptoms and experiences. He or she becomes increasingly conscious of provoking behaviors that are related to production of symptoms and experiences.

4. Patient recognizes particular behaviors as indications of defensiveness or resistance.

5. Patient connects two problems which were previously unconnected, or sees their immediate relevance.

6. Patient becomes increasingly aware of previously unconscious (repressed) thoughts, feelings, or impulses.

7. Patient is able to relate present events to past events.

8. Patient is able to relate present experiences to childhood experiences.

9. Patient's awareness of psychological experience appears to be cumulative.

The findings of the Morgan *et al.* study were mixed. While the scale correlated strongly with operationalized measures of the therapeutic alliance, the interaction between treatment phase and outcome was not significant. That is, the most improved patients were not those who gained insight from early to late in the treatment. This was a disappointing result for those who hold that insight is a necessary condition for improvement. The validity of this result, however, is weakened by methodological and epistemic problems similar to those that hampered the congruence approach. First, the study assumes a high degree of theoretical congruence between judges using the rating scales. In this study, the judges were experienced psychoanalysts who were given training in using the scales and in coding procedures. But it is doubtful if the results would be the same if judges with different theoretical backgrounds were called upon; or if judges had different levels of clinical experience and training; or if the ratings of judges with different psychoanalytic approaches were combined. Second, the ratings do not measure the *accuracy* or *truth-value* of the patients' insight; they simply measure the *presence* of insight (or 'recognition'), and its level of intensity. What the study design does not rule out, in other words, is the condition in which patients receive high scores on all nine measures, while still having insights that are false, incomplete, irrelevant, or superficial. Question 2, for example, measures the extent to which the patient recognizes habitual patterns of behavior. Suppose a patient is scored highly on this measure by all judges. From this, it does not follow that the patient actually is insightful. Patients may come recognize patterns which are not psychologically salient, and overlook patterns which are; or they might see patterns where none exist; or their insights may be decontextualized. The rating scale does not rule out these possibilities.

Moreover, a patient who receives a low score on the scale may in fact have an accurate and truth-tracking recognition of a real pattern of habitual behavior, but may not display the expected level of confidence. But these difficulties did not spell the end of the third-person approach to the measurement of insight.

Yet another variation of the third-person approach to insight research focused on the relationship of individual differences in insight to treatment outcome, with the goal of determining whether clients who are successful in acquiring insight are more likely to get better as a result of psychotherapy than clients who are not successful. Suh, O'Malley, and Strupp (1989), for example, used the Vanderbilt Psychotherapy Process Scale to predict therapeutic outcome. Included in the scale is a seven-item subscale that measures the extent to which patients engaged in self-exploration during therapy sessions. The drawback with the subscale is that it did not measure the validity, depth, or accuracy of insight, but simply the *prevalence* of self-exploration. High scores on these scales are no guarantee of accuracy or validity, because clients who are actively engaged in self-exploration may be off-track in their explorations.

In more recent studies, Crits-Christoph (1984) and Crits-Christoph and Luborsky (1990) developed measures of self-understanding using guided (as opposed to unguided) clinical judgment. The goal of these measures was to determine the relation between the *level* of self-understanding displayed by clients during exploratory therapy, and the treatment outcome. The self-understanding scale that was designed to measure level of insight was narrowly defined, and reflected a theoretical orientation that would not likely be found in other insight measures. It focused mainly on clients' understanding of 'core conflicts' in different 'object-related domains': that is, clients' insight into different types of interpersonal relationships and their conflicts, which the experimenters called the Core Conflictual Relationship Theme (CCRT). The empirical data for the study were supplied by clients' narratives about their interpersonal relationships, as these were developed during a number of psychotherapy sessions. The narratives were coded so as to capture the clients' main wishes, as well as the clients' views of responses from others and responses from self. Judges—not clients—then evaluated the extent to which clients demonstrated degrees of self-understanding relative to an independent operationalized criterion. Clients' self-understanding was evaluated with respect to CCRT in general, CCRT in relation to the psychotherapist, CCRT in relation to parents, and CCRT in relation to two significant others.

There are at least two basic but unstated conditions that must be met in the administering of a scale such as this. First, respondents must be honest in reporting their feelings. The data supplied by those respondents who are dishonest, self-deceived, or frivolous would skew the data supplied by those who are not, and would give an imbalanced picture of respondents' insight. Second, respondents must be psychologically-minded. If they have little interest in or experience of psychological matters, their responses could be superficial and unhelpful.

Two significant findings emerged from the study: i) self-understanding with respect to core conflictual relationships with the psychotherapist was associated with therapeutic improvement; and ii) self-understanding with respect to core conflictual relationships with significant others was correlated with higher scores on global adjustment measures. The study did not measure acquisition or gain in insight–something that would require testing over longer periods of time—but only level of insight. Nor did it address whether clients' self-understandings were true or truth-tracking.

In a related study that focused on the self-understanding of interpersonal relationships and their conflicts, Connolly *et al.* (1999) developed the Self-Understanding of Interpersonal Patterns Scale, a first-person approach to the measurement of insight. In the standard version of the SUIP, clients in psychodynamic psychotherapy are instructed to read each item and then circle 'Yes' or 'No' to indicate whether the pattern is 'relevant to their current life' (Connolly *et al.* 1999: 482). They are then instructed to fill out the four-point self-understanding scale for each item that they have circled as 'yes'.

Self-Understanding Rating Scale

a) I recognize that I feel and act this way with a significant person in my life, but I don't know why.

b) I can see that this experience has become a pattern with multiple people in my life, but I don't know why.

c) I'm beginning to see a link between these experiences and past relationship experiences, but the connection is not yet clear.

d) I can clearly see that I feel and act this way because of past relationship experiences.

Interpersonal Patterns

1. I feel the need to save others when I see them having a tough time and therefore try to solve their problems for them.

2. I feel the need to guide others when I see them about to make a mistake and wind up telling them what to do.

3. I feel the need to please others and let them push me to do something I don't want to do.

4. I need someone to truly understand me, and feel hurt when he/she cannot relate to my feelings.

5. I feel the need to keep someone close, and do whatever is necessary to keep him/her with me even when they need to leave me.

6. I feel the need to change someone, and wind up helping him/her to think more like me even when he/she has beliefs or values different from mine.

7. I feel the need to be understood by others, and get defensive or angry when others are not able to see things as I see them.

8. I feel the need to be close to someone and have difficulty letting them have the space they need.

9. I am very dependent on others for approval, and feel hurt when they reject me.

10. I need to be trusted by someone, and feel rejected when they do not trust me.

11. I need to trust someone, yet I distance myself from that person when they do not trust me.

12. I feel the need to be accepted by someone, and feel bad about myself when he/she doesn't like me.

13. I need someone to take care of me, and I feel abandoned when he/she is not helpful.

14. I need someone to be reliable, and I feel disappointed when he/she lets me down.

15. I need to feel accepted by others, and I feel bad when they oppose what I want to do.

16. I need to feel free of responsibility, and I distance myself from someone I care about because they are too dependent on me.

17. I need to be respected by someone else, but I am forced to distance myself when they do not live up to my expectations.

18. I want to accept someone else, but I am forced to distance myself when they do not live up to my expectations.

19. I feel the need to avoid conflict, and keep quiet even when someone else mistreats me.

While the SUIP illustrates some of the psychometric strengths of insight measures, it also illustrates some of the epistemic weaknesses and oversights. What does this insight scale *really* measure—the actual content of respondents' insights about their interpersonal patterns, as it claims to do, or something else? Is it possible for instance, that their responses reveal more about the experimental strategies and theoretical extrapolations of the insight psychologists who designed the scale, than about the respondents' actual insights? Is it possible that the scale reveals more about how respondents *think* they should answer the questions about their interpersonal patterns, than it does about their actual insights into those patterns? Again, is it possible that the data yielded by the scales reflect (to a certain extent) a degree of interference that is caused by the testing procedures themselves?

One argument in support of a moderate skepticism regarding the psychology of insight measurement is the following: insight measurement is intrinsically Procrustean, and displays questionable ecological validity. Measurement instruments such as the SUIP scale are inexact and poorly fitted to the contours of the actual insights that they putatively measure. The very choice and framing of the questions in the scale assures this. Questions are structured in such a way as to i) systematically factor out from the participants' responses all extraneous information about background context and complicating idiographic factors; ii) target insights in highly generalized or typical contexts; and iii) constrain respondents to characterize themselves in terms that may be more relevant to the experimental purposes of the insight psychologist than to their own purposes. Because of the standardized format of the questions, the data they yield contain few personal narrative elaborations, fine-grained details, individual differences, and qualifications—the very things that are normally the stuff of insight. The stimulus materials capture only a thin slice of a multifaceted and diachronic reality, like a standardized psychological cookie-cutter that is force-fitted upon the phenomenon.

In defense of insight measurement, however, it could be argued that the Procrustean character of the insight measures is simply the nature of the case. To demand exacting representational accuracy and individual specificity where none can be had is a non-starter, so the failure of insight psychology to measure individual insights is not a lamentable flaw but simply the price paid for any scientific study that seeks generalizability across large populations.

To determine if this is a cogent defense against the charge of Procrusteanism, take as an example the statement in SUIP item 4, to which respondents are asked to answer with a 'Yes' or 'No' (Connolly et al. 1999: 482): 'I need someone to truly understand me, and feel hurt when he/she cannot relate to my feelings'. The question is framed in standardized terms: that is, it is broad enough to range over and be answered by diverse people in diverse interpersonal situations, with different understandings of the terms involved. But the crucial terms in the statement are deliberately left undefined. Epistemically complex terms such as 'truly understand', and psychologically complex terms such as 'I need' and 'I feel hurt', are presented in the statement without examples, clear behavioral referents, operational definitions, or prototypes that might supply a stabilized common meaning. This forces respondents to rely on their own interpretations of the terms, or to guess at the meanings intended by the psychologists administering the scale. The problem with this, however, is that respondents and insight psychologists might diverge widely in their under-standings of the relevant terms, and this could result in a skewed data set, or a data set that is more reflective of the categories of the experimental tasks of insight psychology than of the respondents' actual insights.

For example, the statement 'I need someone to truly understand me, and feel hurt when he/she cannot relate to my feelings' is vague on a number of fronts. First, the nature of this need to be understood by another is not speci-fied. It is left up to the respondent to fill in the meaning of the relevant terms, and to determine the depth and pervasiveness of the need, and its place in the economy of personal needs. It is also left up to the respondent to guess at the meaning of the term 'other person'. The question does not specify the degree of closeness to the other, nor does it instruct the respondent on the decision criteria that should be used in cases where a number of other people concur-rently serve this role, but do so in different ways (e.g. partners, family members, friends, professional counselors). Again, the question is silent on what it means to be 'truly understood' by the other. It is left up to the respon-dent to decide whether this means a comprehensive understanding, a psycho-logically deep understanding, a professional understanding, an accurate understanding, or a heartfelt understanding.

Suppose, again for the sake of illustration, that the respondent answers SUIP item 4 with a 'Yes'. He or she is then instructed to rate this self-understanding according to the four-point scale. Suppose the respondent rates it as 'd', indi-cating the highest comparative degree of insight into the matter: 'I can clearly see that I feel and act this way [namely, 'I need someone to truly understand me, and feel hurt when he/she cannot relate to my feelings'] because of past relationship experiences'. As with SUIP item 4, this statement is silent on a number of issues. First, the phrase 'because of past relationship experiences' is silent on the nature of the relevant causal connections, and the specific kind of forces or entities that are putatively at work in causing his or her current feel-ings and actions (e.g. unconscious forces, personality factors, libidinal forces, cognitive forces). It is left up to the respondent to determine the meanings of these terms. Respondents who are in one kind of psychodynamic treatment setting may (for example) assume that these terms refer to traumatic child-hood events of a sexual nature, whereas respondents in another psychody-namic setting may assume that they refer to traumatic events of a non-sexual nature. Second, it is left up to the respondent to fill in the meaning of the term 'clearly see'. Given the many varieties of knowledge, belief, and opinion that might be plausibly covered by this term, it is not clear what precise epistemic claim is being made when d) is chosen. The phrase 'I can clearly see that x' could be construed as 'I know that x', 'I believe that x', or 'I am of the firm opinion that x'. Failure to spell out these differences in the instructions accompanying the scale could mean that respondents conflate knowledge with belief or opinion; and that different respondents will interpret this vague term in different ways. Moreover, as the self-rating does not contain any second-order epistemic measures that could serve to rule out common failures of knowledge or belief, a respondent might claim that he or she 'clearly sees' the interpersonal situation, when in fact he or she is self-deceived, confused, or mistaken about it. Nothing in the scale rules out this possibility.

Efforts to make insight yield to precise measurement continue. The overall goal is to determine precisely how insight interacts with other variables in psychotherapy, and thereby to put psychodynamic psychotherapy research on a more solid scientific footing *vis à vis* other modalities of psychotherapy. With new measurement instruments devised to detect the presence, level, and therapeutic effectiveness of insight, comes new empirical data, which in turn can be used to validate or falsify theoretical hypotheses. Crits-Christoph and Luborsky (1990: 419–20) take an optimistic view of the future of this tradition:

> Assuming advances in the clinical and theoretical literature on insight, empirical research can begin to move forward. Because of the primitive status of research in this area, progress is needed in all phases of research, beginning with scale development. More work on the reliability and particularly the validity of instruments designed to assess the various types of insight is needed... Specifically, it will be of interest to further examine the overlap between emotional insight and experiencing so that the nature of the constructs being measured is further clarified. With clinical rating instruments for assessing insight, it will be critical to determine the necessary level of clinical expertise, skill, and training of judges, as well as the optimal size of the rated unit of measurement (whole sessions or brief segments) and optimal time frame (within treatment) for sampling... Research is needed on the overlap and separate contributions of emotional insight and content-based insight... [T]he relationship of these variables to treatment outcome could be assessed using advanced statistical methods such as causal modeling. This would help test alternative explanations such as whether the insight is only concomitant to, or a result of, behavior change, rather than a cause.

Of the many challenges facing the insight research tradition, however, it is fair to say that just as many are epistemic in nature as methodological. For every effort to operationalize and measure insight, there are nagging questions about the truth-value and accuracy of insight, as well as questions about truth criteria and evidentiary criteria. Until the measurement instruments rule out inaccurate, incomplete, self-deceptive, trivial, or empirically impoverished insights, the data they yield cannot be considered entirely reliable or valid.

A Formal Definition of Insight

Where lists of definitions of insight tend to err on the side of confusion, and operational definitions tend to err on the side of artificiality, formal definitions tend to err on the side of abstractness. Formal definitions overlook content, detail, and context in favor of shared general structures. Moreover, the very idea of supplying a formal definition of insight may seem hopeless, given the fractionated field of psychodynamic psychotherapy. There is little congruence between different psychotherapeutic schools on the theoretical terms used to identify the changes experienced by clients during the course of therapy: e.g. insight, recognition, recollection, self-knowledge, understanding. To a Freudian, insight means one thing; to a Jungian, it means another; to a Kleinian it means another; and so on (Marmor 1962). Moreover, there is little congruence between the different psychodynamic schools on the issue of the *contents* of clients' insights. Simply saying that insights are about the salient facts of a client's psychology, developmental history, behavior, emotions, interpersonal relations, and personality is unhelpful, because the precise content of these concepts is in dispute. The insights clients acquire in short-term psychodynamic psychotherapy about their behaviors, personality, and psychological make-up, for instance, pick out issues, and highlight clinical material, very differently from the insights clients acquire in classical Freudian psychoanalysis, which in turn are different from the insights clients acquire in Jungian analysis; and so on. This lack of congruence is even found between psychotherapies representing different branches of one particular school. There is also little congruence on the relative importance of insight *vis à vis* the interpersonal dynamics of the psychotherapist-client dyad in exploratory psychotherapy.

Despite these challenges, however, certain common elements stand out as linking together the concept of insight across the psychodynamic psychotherapies (Hill *et al.* 2007). Insight can be defined formally as the condition that occurs when clients acquire an emotionally charged and action-guiding understanding of:

i) the kinds of disorders from which they are suffering, and the symptoms with which the disorders are associated;

ii) the causes and/or meanings of their disorders;

iii) the relation between the causes and/or meanings of their disorders, and their overall life processes, including their behaviors, emotions, and personality.

A further condition applies once conditions i–iii have been satisfied. Insight is the condition that occurs when:

iv) clients *believe* that their understanding of i–iii is valid, and when they *believe* that the validity of their understanding is measured against and confirmed by the relevant psychological, behavioral, and historical facts.

Condition iv stipulates a notional or belief-indexed state. It is satisfied even if in fact the client's understanding has little or no such validity.

This formal definition of insight can be rendered even more schematic. Insight involves:

A.i) the client's recognition and understanding of the target disorders D, and symptoms S;

A.ii) the recognition and understanding of the specific causes C and/or meaning M of target disorder D;

A.iii) an understanding of the relation of symptoms S, causes C and/or meaning M to the client's life processes L (e.g. life history, behaviors, interpersonal situation, emotions, and personality).

Each of these components identifies a necessary condition of insight; and each one is dependent on the others, with the order in which they are identified serving as the order of their dependence. The recognition and understanding of the target disorders D is required for the recognition and understanding of symptoms S, which is required for the recognition and understanding of causes C. These are required for the understanding of the relation of S and C to life processes L.

Chapter 3

The Standard View

The Standard View: A Model

As the sampling of case histories, theoretical positions, and research methods in Chapter 2 has revealed, there are important theoretical differences between the major schools of psychodynamic psychotherapy on the nature, function, and content of insight and interpretation. Along with these come important clinical differences, particularly on the comparative therapeutic efficacy of insight and transference. The specific psychological content of insights and interpretations acquired during the course of classical Freudian psychoanalysis diverges—sometimes dramatically—from the psychological content of insights and interpretations acquired during the course of Kohutian psychotherapy, which in turn diverges from the psychological content of insights and interpretations acquired during the course of Kleinian analysis. As Marmor (1962) suggests, clients 'discover' different facts about their psychology, behavior, emotions, and personality depending on the different treatment methods to which they are exposed; they identify certain themes as salient and others as unimportant, depending on the different therapeutic approaches into which they are socialized; and they assimilate and embody their discoveries in different ways.

Despite these theoretical and clinical differences, however, the psychodynamic psychotherapies are not so distant from one another that there is no possible ground for broad theoretical and clinical agreement, particularly on a number of basic *epistemic* issues that are relevant to the goals and core defining features of psychodynamic psychotherapy. For instance, most would agree that psychodynamic exploration does not follow an arbitrary or haphazard course, but is authentic and truth-tracking; and most would agree that the targets picked out for psychodynamic exploration are genuine, rather than made-up or therapy-dependent fictions, or artifacts of the very treatment methods used to get at them. Moreover, most would agree that the insights acquired by clients during the course of their explorations are effective instruments of therapeutic change.

For the sake of precision, these broad points of agreement about the epistemic character of insight and interpretation can be formalized as a set of explicit principles: the principle of exploratory validity, the principle of therapeutic specificity, the principle of interpretive agency, the principle of therapeutically effective insight, and the principle of intraclinical confirmation. These principles, which will be called the Standard View of insight and interpretation in psychodynamic psychotherapy, serve as a kind of epistemic skeleton upon which the many different approaches to psychodynamic psychotherapy are built, and from which the many differentiating features stand out. It is important to bear in mind that the Standard View is a standardized model not of psychodynamic psychotherapy *per se*, but only of the main *epistemic* characteristics of psychodynamic psychotherapy.

Exploratory Validity

According to the principle of exploratory validity, psychodynamic psychotherapy provides clients with a valid method of psychological exploration that leads ultimately to veridical self-knowledge (Farrell 1981). Whatever the particular theoretical orientation—Freudian, Jungian, Kleinian, psychoanalytic, Kohutian, brief—the practice of psychodynamic psychotherapy affords clients the opportunity for discovering certain salient facts about themselves: viz. facts about their personality, behaviors, emotions, interpersonal relations, motives, and developmental history, as well as facts about the etiology of their target disorders. These facts exist prior to therapeutic exploration in the same way that the facts of geography exist prior to exploration. The facts are logically independent of the specific theoretical framework by means of which they are discriminated, identified, and described; and they are logically independent of the treatment methods and exploratory procedures brought to bear upon them.

Given the logical independence of theory and fact, the psychodynamic psychotherapist can be regarded as a catalyst who expedites the flow of antecedently existing material, or promotes the excavation of latent thoughts and desires. The facts speak, as long as the right treatment method and the right therapeutic approach are brought to bear upon them. If the exploratory work of psychodynamic psychotherapy is conducted in a methodologically scrupulous manner, then there is little risk of contamination of the clinical material by the treatment method: that is, little risk of creating psychological artifacts.

Clearly, what *counts* as a psychologically relevant fact is a highly contested issue, varying from one psychodynamic theory to another. In psychoanalysis, for example, the facts that are the object of therapeutic exploration, interpretation, and insight include such things as neuroses, complexes, infantile traumas, and unconscious drives. These are said to exist antecedently to and independently of the psychoanalytic theoretical apparatus, in the same way that physiological processes like digestion exist independently of theories of the physiology of digestion. In Adlerian psychotherapy, the facts that are the object of therapeutic exploration and insight are different: they include such things as a client's deep-lying feelings of inferiority. These too are also claimed to exist antecedently to and independently of the Adlerian theoretical apparatus. Despite differences concerning the precise nature and content of the factual, however, the psychodynamic psychotherapies converge on the idea that there is something factual rather than fictional or artifactual that it is the object of psychotherapy to explore, and that it is the goal of insight to capture: that is, something given, and prior to psychotherapeutic intervention. Exploratory psychotherapy, in other words, does not make up its own facts in the process of exploration.

Freud's archaeology metaphor illustrates clearly the principle of exploratory validity. The analyst's task of reconstruction, Freud claims,

> resembles to a great extent an archaeologist's excavation of some dwelling place that has been destroyed and buried, or of some ancient edifice. The two processes are in fact identical, except that the analyst works under better conditions and has more material at his command to assist him, since what he is dealing with is not something destroyed but something that is still alive—and perhaps for another reason as well... [I]t must be borne in mind that the excavator is dealing with destroyed objects of which large and important portions have quite certainly been lost... No amount of effort can result in their discovery and lead to their being united with the surviving remains. The one and only course open is that of reconstruction, which for this reason can often reach only a certain degree of probability. But it is different with the psychical object whose early history the analyst is seeking to recover... All of the essentials are preserved; even things that seem completely forgotten are present somehow and somewhere, and have been merely buried and made inaccessible to the subject. Indeed, it may, as we know, be doubted whether any psychical structure can really be the victim of total destruction. It depends only upon analytic technique whether we shall succeed in bringing what is concealed completely to light. (SE 23: 259–260)

Against the principle of exploratory validity, it might be argued that "since real life is too complicated to be fully explained, all interpretation by a therapist, and all insights of a patient... are incomplete and inexact" (Shapiro 1971: 461–2). This is a version of the epistemically moderate view that reality is always richer and more complex than our knowledge of it. There are at least three ways that the principle of exploratory validity can respond to Shapiro's claim. The strong construal of the principle would hold that psychodynamic insights and interpretations are *essentially* valid and accurate: that is, they capture *all* of the most salient and most relevant psychological, historical, and behavioral facts in a client's life, even if they do not capture all of these facts in exacting and complete detail. The moderate construal of the principle of exploratory validity would hold that psychodynamic insights and interpretations capture a *core cluster* of the most salient psychological, historical, and behavioral facts in a client's life—but not all of the relevant facts, nor all of the relevant facts in exacting detail. The weak construal of the principle of exploratory validity would hold that psychodynamic insights and interpretations are oriented to the truth, or truth-tracking. A corollary to this would hold that with further investigation, reflection, and corroboration, they would eventually reach the truth. The principle of exploratory validity would lose much of its force if it is held that psychodynamic insights and interpretations are no more than useful tools or heuristic devices that allow clients and psychologists to structure inquiry and make sense out of the phenomena. This is the instrumentalist approach, and it is incompatible with psychodynamic claims to exclusivity. *Qua* tools, insights and interpretations come in many different sizes and shapes: psychodynamic tools just happen to be one such shape, but they are not the only one. Tools, moreover, can only be evaluated one against the other in terms of their usefulness and function (and sometimes in terms of other criteria, such as aesthetic appeal, parsimony, and coherence), rather than in terms of their relation to the facts.

Therapeutic Specificity

The principle of therapeutic specificity holds that the precise application of a psychotherapeutic treatment method M has exact, clearly delineated, and non-suggestive effects on the target disorders D (either on the symptoms or causes of D). The treatment methods of the psychodynamic psychotherapies, in other words, are not a hodge-podge of various techniques that work by hit and miss; nor are they amorphous or fuzzy techniques; nor do they operate by means of placebo effect or suggestion. Rather, they deal precisely and effectively with specific problems that cannot be accessed by any more suitable means. The treatment methods of the psychodynamic psychotherapies are defined by a finite and precisely specifiable set of mechanisms or characteristic factors, and these engage the target disorders as a key engages a lock. Just as a properly cut key fits precisely onto the tumblers of a lock, so the uniquely contoured mechanisms of the characteristic factors of the treatment method fit precisely onto the contours of the target disorders, and exert upon them a precise countervailing force. And just as the tumblers of a lock resist the efforts of inadequately cut keys, or keys cut to open different locks, so target disorders resist the efforts of treatment methods that do not contain the right characteristic factors. Again, just as locks do not mold themselves like silly putty around the keys inserted into them, so target disorders can not be shaped or molded to fit the treatment methods that are applied to them: they yield only to precisely fitted characteristic factors.

The principle of therapeutic specificity can be formalized as follows: psychotherapy T1 is differentiated from psychotherapies T2, T3, T4...Tn by virtue of the precise and controlled application of its characteristic treatment factors, which generate specific, non-placebo, and non-suggestive effects in remedying the target disorders D. For example, if a client A is diagnosed as suffering from disorder D1 (e.g. a neurotic obsession), according to therapeutic theory T1 (e.g. psychoanalytic psychotherapy), with symptoms S1, and is treated with method M1 (e.g. with characteristic factors such as analysis and free association), for time t1–t2, then disorder D1 will be ameliorated *because* of the precise application of the characteristic components of the treatment M1. By comparison, the non-characteristic factors of the treatment method—for instance, the cost of psychoanalytic psychotherapy, or the physical setting in which it occurs—will have no clinically significant effect on the disorders.

Fromm, for example, captures the spirit of the principle of therapeutic specificity as it applies to classical psychoanalysis: 'many patients have experienced a new sense of vitality and capacity for joy, and *no other method than psychoanalysis* could have produced these changes' (Fromm 1970: 15, italics added). So too does Kris (1956: 445–6): 'the analytic situation with its requirements and rules, including the reclining position and the 'anonymity' of the analyst, is no conglomeration of random procedures, of accidental survivals of Freud's early steps in therapy or of his personal idiosyncrasies, but a set-up designed for the double purpose of cure and quasi-experimental exploration.'

Interpretive Agency

The principle of interpretive agency is a sub-principle of the principle of therapeutic specificity. It holds that the interpretations (and clarifications or explanations) formulated by psychodynamic psychotherapists about their clients are valid and intrinsically effective instruments of therapeutic change. Interpretations move the process of exploration forward in new ways by helping to make otherwise puzzling experiences intelligible for clients. The agency of therapeutic interpretations is not derivative: that is, it is not derived from some more powerful set of factors that operates through or behind them, such as suggestion, persuasion, the cognitive dissonance of the therapeutic encounter, placebo effects, or expectancy effects. Because interpretations reframe clients' explorations in a manner that is putatively non-suggestive, they are instrumental in guiding clients to a position from which they will eventually acquire their own insights.

A corollary to the principle of interpretive agency that is shared by most psychodynamic psychotherapies is that only veridical interpretations possess genuine therapeutic agency. False, inexact, or incomplete interpretations, by contrast, lack this special agency. As false interpretations run up against a refractory psychological, historical, and behavioral reality, they will unavoidably fail to generate significant and lasting therapeutic changes; or they will result in misdirected or transient therapeutic improvement. Glover (1931), for example, argues that in the context of psychoanalysis, inexact interpretations may be temporarily useful to analysands, but in the long run they will be counterproductive. While they are plausible enough to yield some degree of emotional and cognitive gratification, they are also inaccurate enough to interfere with the real movement of analytic exploration, by playing into the hands of unconscious defenses. The partial gratification yielded by inexact interpretations serves to alleviate the anxiety and cognitive dissonance caused by analysis as it penetrates into deeper parts of the psyche, but the analysand reaches an exploratory plateau, and his or her ego is lulled into thinking that it can relax its attention.

Waelder succinctly captures the principle of interpretive agency insofar as it functions in psychoanalysis: 'Whenever a psychoanalyst is satisfied that he has untied the Gordian knot of a neurosis and has correctly understood its dynamics and its psychogenesis, his confidence is based on two kinds of data, one of outside observation of events, the other of the patient's self-observation. The first is the experience, repeated countless times during the working-through period of the analysis and again countless times during the person's later life, that this particular interpretation, or set of interpretations, and no other, can dispel the symptoms when they reappear, that they alone are the key that opens the lock' (Waelder 1962: 629–30).

Freud's friend Fleiss argued that psychoanalytic interpretations operate principally by suggestive influence and other non-truth-valuable factors (Meehl 1983). Freud adamantly rejected this criticism. His response illustrates the central importance attributed to the principle of interpretive agency in psychoanalysis:

> But you will now tell me that, no matter whether we call the motive force of our analysis transference or suggestion, there is a risk that the influencing of our patient may make the objective certainty of our findings doubtful. What is advantageous to our therapy is damaging to our researches. This is the objection that is most often raised against psychoanalysis, and it must be admitted that, though it is groundless, it cannot be rejected as unreasonable. If it were justified, psychoanalysis would be nothing more than a particularly well-disguised and particularly effective form of suggestive treatment and we should have to attach little weight to all that it tells us about what influences our lives, the dynamics of the mind or the unconscious. That is

what our opponents believe; and in especial they think that we have 'talked' the patients into everything relating to the importance of sexual experiences—or even into those consequences themselves—after such notions have grown up in our own depraved imagination. These accusations are contradicted more easily by an appeal to experience than by the help of theory. Anyone who has himself carried out psychoanalyses will have been able to convince himself on countless occasions that it is impossible to make suggestions to a patient in that way. The doctor has no difficulty, of course, in making him a supporter of some particular theory and in thus making him share some possible error of his own. In this respect the patient is behaving like anyone else—like a pupil—but this only affects his intelligence, not his illness. After all, his conflicts will only be successfully solved and his resistances overcome if the anticipatory ideas he is given tally with what is real in him. Whatever in the doctor's conjectures is inaccurate drops out in the course of the analysis; it has been withdrawn and replaced by something more concrete. (Freud SE 16: 452)

Freud was confident that truth would eventually emerge in the conflict of interpretations, because of the self-correcting character of analytic exploration, and the inherent recalcitrance of neuroses to the misdirected causal agency of false, inexact, or suggestion-based interpretations. A properly applied psychoanalytic method, separating those clinical data that have genuine evidential value from those that are contaminated by suggestive influence, would eventually sift out false interpretations. 'Any danger of falsifying the products of the patient's memory by suggestion can be avoided by prudent handling of the technique' (Freud SE 18: 251).[1]

Therapeutically Effective Insight

The fourth core principle that is shared by the psychodynamic psychotherapies is the principle of therapeutically effective insight: the insights acquired by clients during the course of their explorations are valid and intrinsically effective instruments of therapeutic change. As with therapeutically effective interpretations, the agency that accrues from clients' insights is not derived from some more powerful set of factors that operates *through* or *behind* the mechanism of insight acquisition, such as suggestion, persuasion, or expectancy effects; nor is it something that merely *happens* to accompany the acquisition of insight; it is rather an intrinsic property of insights, and it serves to mobilize other therapeutically beneficial factors that are not directly related to insight-acquisition. Those clients who have acquired insight are considered to be well on the way to achieving a significantly higher degree of self-acceptance, emotional maturity, and self-responsibility than before they began psychotherapy.

Basch (1980: 171) captures the principle of therapeutically effective insight: 'Insight', 'psychoanalytically oriented', or 'depth' psychotherapy... is based on

Freud's recognition that psychological problems are developmental, and that only by obtaining insight into the process that gives rise to them can a resolution based on cause be reached'.

The corollary to this principle holds that only veridical insights are therapeutically effective. As the brief review of psychodynamic literature shows (above), it is usually assumed uncritically that the insights clients acquire during psychotherapy are true or truth-tracking. It is by virtue of their truth-value, and not by virtue of any non-truth-valuable factors (such as their pragmatic value, cognitive availability, or aesthetic appeal), that they function like a key opening a lock: that is, they correspond precisely to the contours of the actual psychological, behavioral, and experiential reality they describe. False, inexact, or fictitious insights, by contrast, lack this special agency; they are ineffective (or they generate only transient therapeutic improvements) because they founder against the facts. Truth-tracking insight, in other words, is a necessary condition for therapeutic improvement. This corollary is defended, for instance, by the psychoanalyst Segal (1962), who claims that insight must be 'correct' in order to be therapeutic. Insight 'must reach the deep layers of the unconscious and illuminate those early processes in which the pattern of internal and external relationships is laid down, and in which the ego is structured. The deeper the layers of the unconscious reached, the richer and the more stable will be the therapeutic result' (Segal 1962: 212).

Intraclinical Confirmation

The fifth core principle that is shared by the psychodynamic psychotherapies is the principle of intraclinical confirmation: the agreement of clients' insights with psychotherapists' interpretations counts as partial intraclinical confirmation of the explanatory hypotheses postulated by the relevant therapeutic theories; and the failure of agreement counts as partial intraclinical disconfirmation (Grünbaum 1984, 1993). At a certain stage near the end of exploratory therapy, clients are considered to be in a strong position to confirm or disconfirm—through introspection, self-observation, memory, or inference to the best explanation—their psychotherapists' interpretations. This in turn comes to count as partial confirmation or disconfirmation of the explanatory entities postulated by the psychodynamic theory's etiology. Other forms of confirmation may come from experimental and extra-clinical means.

Intraclinical confirmation is particularly important for interpretations about traumatic events in childhood, considered by many psychodynamic theories to be a primary cause of subsequent psychological disorders. Confirmation is secured if clients agree with their psychotherapists' reconstructions of traumatic childhood events, and if their insights agree with the constructions. Agreement is based upon a number of factors: by direct memory of the relevant events, by finding the psychotherapist's reconstructions cognitively and emotionally compelling, by inferring the existence of the relevant events through the impartial evaluation of compelling contemporary evidence, and so on.

In psychoanalysis, for example, the analysand's acquisition of insight into the etiology of his or her disorders serves as clinical validation of the theoretical claims that: i) previously repressed material is one of the primary causes of the client's disorders; and ii) the analyst's interpretations are therapeutically effective, and not the result of placebo effect. This corroboration in turn lends valuable clinical support to psychoanalytic theories of personality and development, and to the general psychoanalytic theory of the unconscious dynamics of the mind. Thus, one of the ways that the causal linkages between the analysand's ostensibly pathogenic infantile experiences and his or her adult psychology are clinically validated is through the analysand's memory of those experiences (Grünbaum 1984, 1993).

The Standard View: Criticisms

The Standard View of the role of interpretation and insight in psychodynamic psychotherapy can be summarized as follows:

i) The psychodynamic psychotherapies provide a valid method of personal discovery that allows clients to acquire *bona fide* insights, and to acquire veridical self-knowledge.

ii) The methods of the psychodynamic psychotherapies have specific, non-suggestive, and non-placebogenic effects.

iii) One of the primary agents of therapeutic improvement in the psychodynamic psychotherapies is therapeutic interpretation.

iv) One of the primary agents of therapeutic improvement in the psychodynamic psychotherapies is the acquisition of insight.

v) Client insights count as valid means of confirmation of the interpretations and explanatory theories of the psychodynamic psychotherapies.

These five principles are singly necessary and mutually dependent. Together they constitute a formal model of the role of insight and interpretation in psychodynamic psychotherapy, around which are generated stronger and weaker versions.

The Standard View is a bare-bones formal model, not of psychodynamic psychotherapy and psychoanalysis per se, but of the epistemic status of insight and interpretation *within* psychodynamic psychotherapy and psychoanalysis.

Most *theories* of psychodynamic psychotherapy instantiate this model, but all do so in different ways, and with different emphases accorded to the role of insight and interpretation. Most clinical *practices* of psychodynamic psychotherapy aim to instantiate this model, but again all do so in different ways, and with different emphases. If a psychotherapy did not contain some variation of these five interlinked principles, it would be hard to see how it could be considered an exploratory or insight-oriented psychotherapy.

As it has been noted, across the various theoretical and clinical instantiations of the Standard View, little attention is paid to the logical and epistemological questions surrounding insight and interpretation. Perhaps this would not be so problematic if the Standard View were intended to serve only as a *normative epistemic ideal*: that is, if it depicted only the role of insight and interpretation under ideal epistemic conditions. As such, it could be considered as a model that sets an epistemic norm for the day-to-day practices of exploratory psychotherapy to emulate, rather than as a model that is in fact instantiated in the general features of existing clinical practice. Any logical or epistemological defects encountered at the level of clinical practice could then be regarded as remediable flaws in the individual implementation of the normative ideal, rather than as flaws in the ideal itself. But it is doubtful if such a weak version of the Standard View would be acceptable to most systems of psychodynamic psychotherapy.

Psychodynamic psychotherapy and psychoanalysis have met with many different criticisms from a number of disciplinary angles. These include the common factors criticism, the efficacy or outcome criticism, the placebo comparator criticism, the clinical judgment criticism, the limits of cognition criticism, and the skeptical criticism.

The common factors criticism holds that the psychodynamic psychotherapies are therapeutically effective not because of any set of factors that are unique to their treatment methods, but because of factors that they share with all other psychotherapeutic and healing modalities (Calestro 1972; Strupp 1972a, 1972b; Torrey 1986; Robinson *et al.* 1990; Frank and Frank, 1991; Piper *et al.* 1998; Lambert and Barley 2001). What this means for the Standard View is that the particular content and theoretical slant of psychodynamic interpretations and insights is less therapeutically important than the fact that *some* form of interpretation and insight occurs at all.

The efficacy criticism holds that when the treatment outcomes of psychodynamic psychotherapy are compared with those of other psychotherapeutic modalities using a number of common measures for therapeutic effectiveness, there is little empirical evidence to show that they demonstrate clear therapeutic superiority. In other words, they are no more effective than other forms of psychotherapy that place little emphasis on interpretation and insight (Eysenck 1960; Bergin and Garfield 1971; Luborsky *et al.* 1975; Svartberg and Stiles 1991). What this means for the Standard View, then, is that the therapeutic efficacy assigned to insights and interpretations may be overstated; they may be just as—or less—therapeutically effective as behavior modifications and corrective emotional experiences that do not involve interpretation and insight.

The placebo comparator criticism holds that there is empirical evidence that suggests that the psychodynamic psychotherapies are no more (and in some cases less) therapeutically effective than credible placebos such as wait lists, pill placebos and minimal psychotherapist contact (Eysenck 1960, 1965, 1969, 1985, 1994; Prioleau *et al.* 1983; Erwin 1997). What this means for the Standard View is that the therapeutic agency attributed to insights and interpretations may not outperform the therapeutic agency of credible placebos.

The clinical judgment criticism holds that there is empirical evidence to suggest that the clinical methods used by psychotherapists to interpret clinical data, and to make diagnoses, predictions, and clinical judgments, do not generally outperform statistical or actuarial methods (Meehl 1953; Faust 1986; Dawes, Meehl, and Faust 1989; Dawes 1994; Koehler 1996; Garb 1998; Garb and Boyle 2003). This is due in part to the fact that the clinical judgments are vulnerable to a number of systemic cognitive biases (e.g. confirmatory bias, illusory correlations, overconfidence) that are not found in actuarial methods. Moreover, while psychotherapists claim to understand human behavior, there is empirical evidence to suggest that their training, credentials, and years of clinical experience are largely irrelevant to the success of psychotherapy (Dawes 1994). What this means for the Standard View is that psychodynamic interpretations that claim to make sense of an individual *qua* individual, in all of his or her complexity, and on the basis of expert knowledge, clinical intuition, or years of experience, have negligible accuracy, despite the inflated confidence that psychotherapists display in their clinical judgments. Faust (1986: 426) for example applies these findings to psychoanalysis: 'Psychoanalytic theories require judgments about multidetermined behaviors, interacting drives, and inverse or curvilinear relations (e.g. reaction formations). If individuals have difficulties integrating more than small amounts of information or correctly identifying even simple two way interactions, what is the likelihood that therapists can make far more complex judgments accurately? Therapists undoubtedly capture something about their clients, and therapists' interpretations can be convincing and useful, but their judgments almost certainly leave much of the true variance untouched. If the judgments required by specific therapy approaches cannot be made, then one cannot truly exercise the specific therapy approaches; this inability would thereby preclude specific treatment effects and result in similar outcomes across treatment modalities.'

The so-called limits of cognition criticism holds that the psychodynamic psychotherapies operate with a model of insight that is psychologically and cognitively unrealistic given the architecture and design constraints of human cognition and the cognitive unconscious. A great deal of experimental research in cognitive and social psychology shows that human beings are particularly prone to confabulation, error, and systemic bias in thinking about the causes of their behaviors (Nisbett and Wilson 1977; Nisbett and Ross 1980; Piatelli-Palmerini 1994), in identifying their contemporary states of mind (Wilson 1985, 2004), in the recall of past events (Loftus 1993; Loftus and Ketchum 1994; Neisser 1994b; Neisser and Fivush 1994), and in accurately assessing their personality traits (Sundberg 1966; Snyder *et al.* 1977; Dickson and Kelly 1985). What this means is that insight, at least as it is modeled in the Standard View, with its emphasis on veridical insight, is unachievable.

The skeptical criticism of the Standard View holds that the theories of the psychodynamic psychotherapies rest on implausible or inconsistent epistemological foundations, which collapse under analysis. What this means is that client insights may be contaminated with suggestion, and may have no credible value as supplying intraclinical confirmation of the theories of the psychodynamic psychotherapies.

For the sake of economy, only some of these criticisms will be addressed in any detail.

A Common Factors Criticism

The common factors criticism of the Standard View holds that psychodynamic psychotherapies are therapeutically effective not because of any set of factors that are unique to their treatment methods (e.g. depth exploration, interpretations, insights), but because of factors they share with *all* other healing modalities, from religio–magical healing to contemporary psychiatric healing, including modalities that make no use of exploration, interpretation, and insight. If this is a valid critique, then whatever therapeutic benefits psychodynamic interpretations and insights might appear to occasion are in fact derived from some more powerful set of factors that operate *through* or *behind* them. Psychodynamic exploration, interpretation, and insight might seem to be the uniquely configured keys that open the lock to a client's psyche and disorders, but this agency is an appearance only. The real engine of therapeutic change lies elsewhere, and functions independently of the putatively unique factors of psychodynamic psychotherapy. This means that the interpretations and insights that are regarded by psychodynamic psychotherapists as instrumental in triggering therapeutic change might in fact be false, irrelevant, or fictitious—and yet this does not affect the continued operation of the common therapeutic factors. The idea that interpretations and insights have merely a borrowed or epiphenomenal therapeutic agency contrasts sharply with the Standard View's principle of therapeutic specificity and the principle of therapeutically effective insight.

The common factors approach tends to deflate the exaggerated claims to therapeutic uniqueness and therapeutic expertise sometimes made by psychodynamic psychotherapies. It is not uncommon to find competing psychotherapeutic schools trying to differentiate themselves one from another in the therapeutic marketplace by claiming to offer unique approaches to healing, with uniquely configured etiologies, symptomatologies, and treatment methods that are tailored specifically to certain disorders.[2] Classical Freudian psychoanalysis, for example, is presented as an approach constituting a species all its own: it is not derived from, nor dependent upon, any more fundamental approach. Arlow, for example, claims that 'although there are many ways to treat neuroses, there is but one way to understand them—psychoanalysis.' (1995: 17; see also Kris 1956: 446; and Fromm 1970: 15). Similar claims for uniqueness or unique therapeutic outcomes are sometimes made by other psychodynamic psychotherapies.

What are some of the common factors that psychodynamic psychotherapies share with one another, with all other modalities of psychotherapy, and with all modalities of healing? There are a number of different models of the common factors (Calestro 1972; Strupp 1972a, 1972b; Bergin and Lambert 1978; Parloff 1986; Torrey 1986). Frank's model (1983, 1989; Frank and Frank 1991), perhaps the most well-known in this research tradition, identifies four basic factors:

1) an emotionally charged and trusting relationship with someone who is recognized by the community as a healer;

2) a specially configured healing environment which reflects the healer's prestige and authority, and which provides the appearance of safety;

3) a rationale, conceptual scheme, or myth that supplies a believable explanation for the client's symptoms, and prescribes a manageable but progressively difficult procedure for resolving them;

4) a set of procedures or rituals that call for the active participation of both client and psychotherapist, and that is believed by both to be the primary means of restoring the client to health.

These, according to Frank, are the four basic building blocks of all forms of psychological healing—the psychological equivalent of the primary chemical elements of matter. Together they constitute a prototherapeutic *infrastructure* that maps out in advance all possible permutations that can occur in any modality of psychotherapy, psychodynamic or otherwise. Every form of psychotherapy engages these elements in varying combinations, and with varying surface features that express their effects. Neither the most benignly non-directive nor the most aggressively directive psychotherapeutic approaches can suspend or neutralize the operation of these elements.

These are not the only factors common to all healing modalities. On the basis of this infrastructure, a number of narrower common factors are also pressed into service. Together, these constitute a prototherapeutic *superstructure*. These factors include:

- The client's level of suggestibility.
- The client's adoption of interpretations that are self-validating within the healing context.
- Placebo effects.
- The client's desire to reduce the cognitive dissonance generated by the encounter with the psychotherapist (Festinger 1957).
- The pressures of social consensus about the authority of the psychotherapist.
- The psychotherapist's personal qualities of charisma, conviction, and supportiveness.
- The power of therapeutic rhetoric and persuasion (Glaser 1979).
- The naming of symptoms.[3]
- Expectancy effects.
- The anxiety-reducing use of repetitive reminders (e.g. the ritual of taking medicine, or of repeating pithy maxims and rules, or doing homework).
- The client's modeling of his or her behavior after the psychotherapist's behavior.
- The client's tendency to relate unrealistically to the psychotherapist, and to react with more hope and optimism than is warranted by the situation.

How do these factors influence interpretations and insights in the psychodynamic psychotherapies? Does their presence mean that interpretations and insights are mainly epiphenomenal: that is, intellectualized surface phenomena that trail behind the real engine of therapeutic change, and that have no real causal influence? Does it mean that the specific content of interpretations and insights is irrelevant for therapeutic progress, as long as a placeholder insight—that is, *some* minimally satisfactory form of insight—is in place? Does it mean that placeholder insights that are inexact, false, irrelevant, or fictitious are as good as veridical insights, as long as the clients *believe* they are

true, and as long as their presence is upheld by the operation of the infrastructural and superstructural factors?

A number of common factors stories could be told about psychodynamic
interpretations and insights. All of them, however, would concur with some
version of the following minimalist story. Clients engaged in psychodynamic
therapy are exposed to a number of powerful forces that render them more
suggestible to certain kinds of interpretations and insights than they would
otherwise be. These forces, which include expectancy effects, cognitive dissonance, therapeutic rhetoric, and psychotherapist authority, begin with the
socialization of clients *as clients of such and such a therapeutic modality*; that is,
as clients of (for example) Kleinian psychoanalysis, or short-term psychodynamic psychotherapy. These forces are also pressed into service in the socialization of clients *as self-interpreters* within such and such a therapeutic
modality: that is, as clients who are learning to view themselves in terms of a
particular therapeutic rationale, conceptual scheme, or myth. Client socialization
moves forward with the help of leading questions from the psychotherapist,
nonverbal cues, behavioral reinforcement, and other forms of therapeutic
influence which have the effect of selecting and cultivating psychological
themes that clients would not have otherwise construed as significant.

One way therapeutic influence is transmitted to the client is through exposure to the therapeutic theory (including symptomatology, nosology, and
etiology) that guides the day-to-day progress of the therapy. Aware of the
kinds of symptoms and causal issues their psychotherapists are attending to,
clients are guided in their own explorations to look in certain directions rather
than others, and to look for certain kinds of evidence rather than others. This
prepares clients in advance for accepting certain kinds of psychodynamic
interpretations and insights that they would not otherwise have considered as
explanatorily plausible. What clients learn is expected of them as outlined in
the overarching theory that governs their psychotherapy—that is, the kinds of
discoveries they can be expected to make, and the kinds of insights they can be
expected to acquire—tends to reinforce the very symptoms that are ostensibly
uncovered and solved by the therapy's treatment method.

The fact that powerful non-modality-specific factors are operating through
or behind psychodynamic interpretations and insights does not mean that
they are empty or trivial; nor does it mean that they are eliminable on the
grounds that they are surface phenomena, and that in their absence a
psychotherapy can be constructed that relies exclusively on the operation of
common factors. Just as interpretations and insights are held in place by the
covert operation of infrastructural and superstructural factors, so these
common factors require something to be held in place as a receptive vehicle

for their operation. Interpretations and insights serve as a deflective and unifying focus for clients' attention and efforts.

Much of this happens below the surface. From the client's point of view, the naïve realism of the Standard View goes without question. It is crucial for the success of the psychodynamic psychotherapies that clients believe that they are engaged in a collaborative project that offers them a valid method of self-exploration; and it is crucial that they conduct themselves *as if* this is in fact what is occurring. The fact that clients need to believe that their explorations are valid, and are converging upon some significant truth about their psychological make-up, personality, and behavior, is an essential component of the experience of being a client. It is unlikely that clients can successfully engage in an activity as emotionally demanding as exploratory psychotherapy in the specific awareness that it 'works'—yields insight and therapeutic progress—for reasons significantly different from those supplied by psychotherapists (in other words, by the operation of common factors), and for reasons other than those that are suggested by their own experiences. A critical and philosophically detached approach to the progress of exploratory psychotherapy, which would entail a meta-clinical awareness of the contingency of any one particular therapeutic practice—viz. that it is one of many alternative therapeutic interventions that work by virtue of the agency of common factors rather than characteristic factors of the psychotherapy—would undermine the valuable life-sustaining momentum of clinical practice. The illusion of real exploratory agency is an essential part of psychodynamic psychotherapy, even if the principles of therapeutic specificity and therapeutically effective insight are epistemically flawed.

A Cognitive–Psychological Criticism

A great many experimental findings in cognitive and social psychology call into question our naïve confidence about the reliability of introspection, memory, causal self-attributions, and human judgment. These findings are part of a broad skeptical trend about traditional philosophical and folk psychological assumptions about the unity of consciousness, first-person privileged access, introspective accuracy, and human rationality. If the human mind is much more unsystematic, modular, and self-opaque than was once thought by philosophers and psychologists, and if human thought is driven by myopic reasoning strategies, cognitive biases and blind spots, availability and representativeness heuristics, opportunistic oversimplification, and massive perceptual and cognitive compartmentalization (Piatelli-Palmerini 1994), then human beings are much more like strangers to themselves than privileged authorities concerning themselves (Wilson 1985, 2004).

If these experimental findings are applicable beyond the experimental domain of cognitive psychology to the clinical domain of the psychodynamic psychotherapies, then there may be grounds for regarding psychodynamic exploration, interpretations, and insights as assuming cognitively unrealizable competencies. Human beings may lack the fine-tuned cognitive resources—perhaps even the basic cognitive architecture—that is required to realize the ideal of veridical insight that is so highly prized in exploratory psychotherapy. This is not for lack of will-power, or sufficiently rigorous exploration, or the right treatment methods. Underprivileged access to mental states and their causes may simply be an evolutionarily fixed design constraint of the cognitive architecture of human beings, in much the same way that fixed design constraints in the human perceptual apparatus support the experience of some colors and sounds, but are not designed for the reception of other wavelengths of light and other sound frequencies.

If this, or some emerging story that resembles this, is the case, then it would be reasonable to assume that more relaxed therapeutic ideals than those defended in the Standard View ought to be encouraged, in order to accommodate the design constraints that account for the manifold biases that govern how human beings think, introspect, remember, and perceive: that is, something less than the veridical interpretations and insights assumed by the Standard View, and something more consistent with causal opacity and the compensatory fictional explanatory strategies it evokes. It is, after all, not an unfair theoretical demand to require that psychodynamic psychotherapy be guided by commitment to a minimal form of psychological realism, and that it take seriously the design constraints of human cognition and perception. Such a commitment would mean that psychodynamic theory construction and clinical practice consider: i) the question of the realizability of the psychological and motivational structures that are presupposed by a particular psychodynamic theory and treatment method; ii) the question of whether the kinds of persons required for the realization of a particular therapeutic ideal of psychological health, including the goal of insight, are psychologically possible; and iii) the question of whether a particular therapeutic ideal presupposes too much plasticity on the part of creatures with such and such cognitive endowment and affective capacities (Flanagan 1991).

The philosophical ideal of self-knowledge as one of the goods of human life, and as an important component of human rationality, has come under attack from several directions in recent work in cognitive and social psychology. One branch of research in social psychology, for example, has adduced evidence that seems to show that self-knowledge may be more psychologically maladaptive—and even conducive to unhappiness and depression—than creative self-deceptions and positive illusions; and, contrary to a well-established tradition in cognitive theories of depression, that 'depressives' are more realistic than 'normals' in their perception of themselves and the world (Taylor and Brown 1988; Taylor 1989; Jopling 1996b). Positively biased 'creative' illusions about the self—including unrealistically positive self-evaluations, exaggerated perceptions of personal control, and unrealistic optimism about the future—are thought to play a more significant role in the maintenance of mental health, as well as in the maintenance of caring interpersonal relations and a sense of well-being, than accurate self-perceptions and self-knowledge. One of the primary goals of psychodynamic exploration, however, is the removal of self-deception and unrealistic self-evaluation.

Another branch of research in social psychology has adduced evidence that appears to show that people are generally mistaken in their self-reports and self-descriptions, when these purport to supply causal explanations of their own behaviors, motives, or thoughts; and, that people generally tend to rationalize or confabulate in their causal self-attributions according to empirically underdetermined schemas picked up from the immediate social and cultural environment (Nisbett and Wilson 1977; Nisbett and Ross 1980; Wilson 1985, 2004). Despite the fact that a great deal of human behavior is caused by subpersonal mental states located far below the experiential surface, people are unusually prone to proposing *ex post facto* explanations of why they engage in certain behaviors, why they make certain decisions, and why they experience certain emotions. The assumption that makes these explanatory efforts intelligible is an essentially philosophical one: viz. that most thought and action can be traced back to conscious thoughts and decisions. This optimistic assumption may be false.

Echoing a theory also defended by Spinoza ('all men are born ignorant of the causes of things', and 'men are conscious of their desire and unaware of the causes by which they are determined' (Spinoza, 1677/1992: 57)), Nisbett, Wilson, and Ross defend a strong version of the causal opacity of behavior and thought. To do so, they adduce a large body of experimental evidence that appears to show that people are not especially skillful at picking out the real causes of their behaviors; and that people are less adept at identifying accurately the mental processes that explain their behaviors than they are at engaging in causal confabulation. This undermines two longstanding beliefs about the first-person point of view and its relation to human agency: viz. that people shape their behaviors in such a way that their actions are the result of conscious choices made between carefully considered alternatives; and that people do not engage in actions and behaviors without adequate justification. The experimental literature suggests, on the contrary, that people demonstrate a pronounced willingness to confabulate or deceive themselves in order to protect the belief that they always act rationally. Counter-attitudinal advocacy experiments, for example, consistently show that when people are asked about their actions after the fact, they typically reconstruct their perceptions, memories, and stories of their conduct to fit the conception of how they believe they *should* act, based on what they have previously learned is a socially appropriate story for such action.

Yet another area of research in social psychology that has damaging consequences for the Standard View concerns the so-called 'Barnum effect' in personality psychology:[4] viz. that people generally tend to accept bogus personality profiles (based on descriptions of hypothetical persons) as containing accurate and revealing insights about themselves just as readily as they accept *bona fide* personality profiles (Ulrich *et al.* 1963; Dmitruk *et al.* 1973; Snyder *et al.* 1977). The descriptions that the experimental participants identify as true of themselves consist of 'one-size-fits-all' statements that could be true of almost anyone, but nonetheless display some degree of psychological plausibility. In some circumstances the participants even tended to accept *bogus* personality descriptions as more accurate than the *bona fide* personality descriptions (Sundberg 1966; Snyder *et al.* 1977; Dickson and Kelly 1985). If the Barnum effect is observable in social psychology experiments, and also in real world contexts, then it is possible that it is at work in exploratory psychotherapy, especially when the interpretations offered to clients are highly schematic and thin on detail. 'Research evidence has consistently indicated that a patient's belief in interpretations and his consequent anxiety reduction do not depend on the accuracy of the interpretations. Investigators have found that individuals will enthusiastically accept bogus interpretations as accurate descriptions of their own personalities' (Fisher and Greenberg 1977: 364).

This is by no means an exhaustive list of the experimental work in cognitive and social psychology on introspective accuracy, causal self-attribution, and self-knowledge (see Neisser 1994a; Neisser and Fivush 1994; Neisser and Jopling 1997); nor is the attack on introspective accuracy and causal self-attribution an historically recent phenomenon unique only to cognitive and social psychology. Spinoza and Nietzsche, among others, placed a great deal of emphasis on the causal opacity of human behavior.[5] But the list is indicative of the broad skepticism in the cognitive sciences about 'autophenomenology' (Dennett 1991; Jopling 1996a), and the explanatory relevance of knowledge claims and causal self-attributions that are made from the first-person point of view. If the experimental findings are valid, then there is a *prima facie* case against *veridical* insight as an attainable goal in the psychodynamic psychotherapies.

Introspection, Causal Self-Attribution, and Insight

Nisbett, Wilson, and Ross's well-known findings about the nature of human inference, and the systematic failures of introspective self-reports to identify accurately the causal circumstances of mental states and behaviors (Nisbett and Wilson 1977; Nisbett and Ross 1980; Wilson 1985, 2004), lend a degree of credibility to the epistemological critique of the psychodynamic psychotherapies. Watters and Ofshe (1999: 203) summarize the critique succinctly: 'That our thoughts cannot trace their own course can be an odd notion at first, but it is one that has widening importance for the idea of psychotherapy. The basic work of psychodynamic therapy is to do exactly what the research shows we have little capacity to do: trace our thoughts and behaviors to their mental origins. If the patient and psychotherapist have no ability to trace the course of thoughts, and if the patient has no internal sensitivity to when such cause and effect stories are wrong, what is really going on in therapy? Is there any reason to believe that the patient and therapist are any more accurate in identifying strings of causation than the subjects and observers in Nisbett's studies?'

The experimental evidence adduced by Nisbett, Wilson, and Ross suggests that people do not have privileged access to the inner goings-on of their minds; and that the introspective mechanisms people *claim* to use when furnishing explanations of their inner goings-on do not afford reliable knowledge about the real causes of processes such as memory, perception, and thinking. The real causal action occurs at a sub-experiential level, in what has been called the cognitive unconscious. Despite this, causal self-attributions are commonplace. Low-level experience-near causal self-attributions are an accepted part of common sense psychological discourse. Experience-distant versions are an accepted part of the psychodynamic psychotherapies. Clients are typically encouraged to explore their less than fully conscious motives, and to excavate the hidden causes of their behaviors and feelings. The assumption that makes such self-attributive practices intelligible seems to be that the mere fact of authorship of the relevant actions, decisions, or judgments guarantees some form of introspective access to the causal processes that explain them. But the experimental evidence seems to show otherwise. In appealing to introspective self-observation to explain their behaviors, people characteristically tell more than they in fact know: they go beyond the given experiential and psychological evidence. More significantly, people characteristically 'tell more than they *can* know' (Nisbett and Wilson 1977).

Nisbett, Wilson, and Ross are careful not to make the eliminativist claim that introspection is epistemically bankrupt in first-person explanations of mental states and causal self-attributions. They do not claim that introspection ought to be eliminated in favor of non-introspective methods. Nor do they embrace epistemic skepticism, and deny outright the possibility of all forms of self-knowledge: 'each of us is privy to a wealth of data pertinent to the generation of such accounts' (Nisbett and Wilson 1977: 203). This access *sometimes* places first-person introspectors in a better position than external observers to generate accurate causal self-attributions. But mere *proximity* to the workings of the mind is not a sufficient condition for introspective accuracy; and the mere usage of introspective idioms, and the display of introspective behaviors, is not sufficient evidence that introspection is in fact taking place. Nisbett, Wilson, and Ross suggest that accurate causal self-attributions are less likely to be the result of some special mechanism of introspective access than they are to be a function of the subject's awareness of the causal generalizations that have been established to be objectively correct by culturally-accepted theories of causation. 'When trying to decide why they performed a certain action, people call upon reasons that are available in memory and representative of (or similar to) the response, and use their culturally-learned and idiosyncratic theories about 'why I performed behavior X'. Similarly, if access to internal states is sometimes limited, people may call upon the explanatory system to infer how they feel. These conscious inferences are influenced by theories about oneself and about what feelings seem like plausible reactions to a stimulus.' (Wilson 1985: 17). The verbal explanatory system used in self-description and self-attribution relies heavily on representativeness and availability heuristics (Tversky and Kahneman 1974; Kahneman *et al.* 1982).

Nisbett and Wilson claim that first-person introspective reports alleging to discriminate between the causes of mental states and behaviors are just as vulnerable to theory-induced errors as causal inferences about external events (Nisbett and Wilson 1977: 248; Wilson 1985). In some experiments, for example, participants were unaware of the existence of external stimuli that exerted a decisive influence on their higher-order actions. One series of experiments showed that as the number of bystanders increased, participants were less likely to help others who were in situations of distress. Despite this, participants consistently denied that this variable had any effect on their own helping behavior. In other experiments, participants were unaware that their behaviors were responses to external stimuli. 'Even when subjects [were] thoroughly cognizant of the existence of the relevant stimuli, and of their responses, they [were] unable to report accurately about the influence of the stimuli on the responses' (Nisbett and Wilson 1977: 242).

In those experiments where participants produced subjective reports about causal connections that happened to be correct, it was not because the participants enjoyed direct introspective access to how their higher mental processes were in fact influenced by external causal forces. The accuracy of their causal self-attributions was a function of the 'incidentally correct employment of *a priori* causal theories' (Nisbett and Wilson 1977: 233). That is, accurate causal self-attributions linking a particular response to a particular stimulus were more likely to have been drawn from extant theories and psychological generalizations that enjoyed broad cultural support, than to have been the result of accurate introspection of the relevant causes. 'We propose that when people are asked to report how a particular response is influenced by a particular stimulus, they do so not by consulting a memory of the mediating process, but by applying or generating causal theories about the effects of that type of stimulus on that type of response. They simply make judgments, in other words, about how plausible it is that the stimulus would have influenced the response' (Nisbett and Ross 1980: 248).

Extrapolating from experimental contexts such as these to the clinical situations of the psychodynamic psychotherapies, these findings appear to cast doubt on the reliability and veridicality of psychodynamic interpretations and insights. By implication, they appear to cast doubt on the Standard View. If introspective self-observation is unreliable for relatively low-level cognitive processes involving simple memory and perceptual judgment, then it is even more likely to be unreliable in exploratory psychotherapy, where the introspective targets include complex cognitive, emotional, and behavioral causes with long causal histories. Moreover, the idea that causal self-attributions are often a function of the 'incidentally correct employment of *a priori* causal theories', rather than the result of accurate introspection, suggests that the real function of the exploratory work of psychodynamic psychotherapy is to teach clients how to employ a new *a priori* causal theory. What clients take to be deep and accurate insights into their psychology and behavior may really be stock psychodynamic causal generalizations and confabulations they have learned during therapy. This learning is then reinforced by the pressures of cognitive dissonance in the therapeutic encounter, and by the drive toward disambiguation. When confronted with the complex and ambiguous social situation that is psychodynamic psychotherapy, clients typically report attitudes and make self-assessments that are most likely to win approval of their psychotherapists, and therefore reduce the level of cognitive dissonance caused by the encounter with the psychotherapist's initially alien theory and explanatory apparatus.

The fact that people rely more on shared cultural agreements, heuristics, and *ad hoc* generalizations about how certain stimuli and certain responses are supposed to connect, than they do on accurate observation, does not mean that the causal theories or narratives supplied by the relevant social context (e.g. psychotherapy) are always false. The important point made by Nisbett, Wilson, and Ross is that people do not generally have the ability *not* to fall back upon the causal generalizations supplied by shared theories or culturally sanctioned narratives, nor the ability to gauge when these generalizations are accurate or inaccurate. What does this mean for the psychodynamic psychotherapies?

Watters and Ofshe (1999) offer one answer. Instead of allowing clients to explore the deeper dimensions of their psyches, the psychodynamic therapies supply them with socially sanctioned causal theories that hook up nonverifiable causes with certain psychological and behavioral effects in the absence of any reliable introspective reports that might validate the causal connections. '[T]he vast number of psychodynamic schools of talk therapy appear as nothing more than a testing and breeding ground for these shared cultural narratives. Psychodynamic therapy offers a new and interesting world of possible narratives by which patients can come to believe they understand the origin of their thoughts and behaviors. These narratives become plausible in the patient's eyes through the process of influence embedded in therapy. Considering that patients have little or no internal capacity to disconfirm such cause-and-effect stories, it is not surprising that each generation of psychodynamic psychotherapists has had patients who have adopted its narratives. To convince patients of the validity of the cause-and-effect narrative, therapists need not offer a true explanation, they need only immerse the patients into a new subculture and overwhelm the patients' previously held narratives.' (204).

Grünbaum offers a similar answer in his critique of classical Freudian psychoanalysis. 'The upshot of the work of Nisbett, Wilson, and Ross for our concerns is essentially the following: the purported deliverances of the analyzed patient's introspection, besides not actually being obtained introspectively, are often not even trustworthy, let alone are they the products of the subject's privileged epistemic access to the validation of psychoanalytic interpretations' (Grünbaum 1984: 208-9). The findings of Nisbett, Wilson, and Ross, according to Grünbaum, undermine claims about the validity of the analysand's insight—and, by implication, claims about insight in the other forms of psychodynamic psychotherapy—in a number of ways. First, they undermine appeals to introspection as a potential source of intraclinical validation of the explanatory hypotheses postulated by the psychoanalytic theory of personality and psychogenesis. Second, they undermine appeals to introspection as a potential source of evidence that would block the alternative hypothesis that therapeutic change is due to suggestion, placebo effects, and expectancy effects. Third, they undermine appeals to the analysand's introspective confirmation to underwrite claims about the therapeutic efficacy of the acquisition of insight. Finally, they undermine appeals to introspective self-observation as the source of the analysand's conviction of the veridicality of the analyst's interpretations.

To illustrate this, Grünbaum cites the example of therapeutically elicited memories of traumatic events in infancy and early childhood—one of the more common targets of insight in psychoanalysis. 'Even if a patient can claim veridical recall of an episode as having been emotionally painful, we have no good reason to give credence to any etiologic role the analysand may assign to the trauma on purportedly introspective grounds' (Grünbaum 1984: 217). Why is this? In cases of 'reawakened' memories of infantile or early childhood traumas, it is more likely that the analysand has picked up the relevant causal explanation through socialization into the therapeutic culture, and through exposure to the analyst's theory-imbedded interpretations, than through introspective observation of the alleged causal connections. The empirically impoverished character of introspection, Grünbaum claims, also explains the curious phenomenon of analysand assent to bogus interpretations (Grünbaum 1984: 217–18).

One moderate conclusion to be drawn from the findings of Nisbett, Wilson, and Ross is that the tendency in cases of causal self-attribution to rely on culturally-endorsed theories of causation drawn from the surrounding society can always interfere with careful reflective self-inquiry and self-evaluation. Theories of causation serve a double role: as compensatory mechanisms for causal opacity, and as coping mechanisms for dealing with pressing psychological difficulties. If this is the case, then the psychodynamic psychotherapies are good candidates for supplying clients with ready-made causal generalizations, with the corresponding risks this would bring to the empirical component of their therapeutic explorations.

It would be a serious misrepresentation, however, to claim that the findings of Nisbett, Wilson, and Ross mean that insight and self-knowledge are unattainable ideals, and that all claims to self-knowledge are systematically false. At most, the findings support the modest conclusion that what people know about themselves is most often not known by means of *introspective self-observation*. Nisbett and Ross suggest that the knowing practices that lead to self-knowledge are the same as those that lead to knowledge of others. 'Knowledge of the self is produced by the same strategies as knowledge of other social objects... [A]ccurate perception of self and accurate perceptions of others ultimately depend on the successful performance of the same 'scientific' tasks—that is, collecting, coding, and recalling data, assessing covariations, inferring causal relations, and testing hypotheses' (Nisbett and Ross

1980: 195). This is one way self-knowledge is acquired. But there are other ways of self-knowing (Jopling 2000; see also Neisser 1988; Neisser and Jopling 1997), not all of which are based on the knowing strategies that lead to knowledge of other people and social objects; and there are other dimensions of the self (besides the causal–historical dimension) that serve as the target of self-knowledge.

Some Skeptical Criticisms

The more obvious and entrenched an idea is, the more difficult it is to find alternative explanations for what it allegedly explains. As has been seen, a number of claims made on behalf of the psychodynamic psychotherapies seem to have acquired the status of the obvious: for instance, that psychodynamic treatment involves deep self-exploration, that it leads to insight or self-understanding, that psychodynamic insight is true or truth-tracking, and that insight is essential to psychological well-being. A dose of skepticism is useful here in helping to see around what might seem obvious. It is also useful in debunking myths that have hardened into fact, and, as Hume phrased it, undermining 'lofty pretensions'. Hume championed skepticism, or at least a version of it which he characterized as mitigated (as opposed to excessive): the suspension of judgment, the renunciation of idle speculation, the carefully targeted deployment of doubt, and the constant awareness of the dangers of hasty judgment (Hume 1774/1998: 84–5). Skepticism, Hume claimed, is both durable and useful, and is an invaluable antidote to dogmatism, which is the epistemic default condition of most people. 'The greater part of mankind are naturally apt to be affirmative and dogmatical in their opinions; and while they see objects only on one side, and have no idea of counterpoising argument, they throw themselves precipitately into the principles, to which they are inclined; nor have they any indulgence for those who entertain opposite sentiments. To hesitate or balance perplexes their understanding, checks their passion, and suspends their action... But could such dogmatical reasoners become sensible of the strange infirmities of human understanding, even in its most perfect state, and when most accurate and cautious in its determinations; such a reflection would naturally inspire them with more modesty and reserve, and diminish their fond opinion of themselves, and their prejudice against antagonists... [I]f any of the learned be inclined, from their natural temper, to haughtiness and obstinacy, a small tincture of Pyrrhonism might abate their pride, by showing them, that the few advantages which they may have attained over their fellows, are but inconsiderable, if compared with the universal perplexity and confusion, which is inherent in human nature. In general, there is a degree of doubt, and caution, and modesty, which, in all kinds of scrutiny and decision, ought forever to accompany a just reasoner' (Hume 1774/1998: 192).

The Standard View invites a number of skeptical inquiries. The skeptical responses to the principle of interpretive agency can be summarized as follows:

i) The plausibility and coherence of psychotherapists' interpretations are neither necessary nor sufficient to underwrite their claims to veridicality.

ii) The thematic agreement between psychotherapists' interpretations and clients' insights is not a guarantee of the veridicality of either the interpretations or the insights.

iii) The occurrence of therapeutic change following psychotherapists' interpretations is not a guarantee of the veridicality of the interpretations, nor a guarantee that the interpretations are the specific causal agent of therapeutic change.

The skeptical responses to the principle of therapeutically effective insight can be summarized as follows:

iv) The mere acquisition of insights by clients is not a guarantee of the veridicality of the insights.

v) Clients' and psychotherapists' convictions, feelings, or intuitions about the validity of insights are not a guarantee of the veridicality of the insights.

vi) The occurrence of therapeutic change following the acquisition of insights is neither a guarantee of the veridicality of the insights, nor a guarantee that the insights are the causes of the change.

i) The principle of interpretive agency holds that psychodynamic interpretations are valid and intrinsically effective instruments of therapeutic change; and that only veridical interpretations possess genuine therapeutic agency. But in virtue of what is an interpretation true? What is the meaning of truth here? Is it the correspondence of the interpretation with the facts of the client's psychology and history, or the internal coherence of the interpretation, or the instrumental value of an interpretation—or what? And what are the signs of truth? Questions like these are seldom addressed in the theoretical and clinical literature of psychodynamic psychotherapy. On the few occasions when they have been addressed, the two criteria of truth most readily called upon are the correspondence criterion and the coherence criterion. According to the former criterion, an interpretation is true if it corresponds with the psychological and historical facts it interprets. Freud's so-called 'tally argument' is a version of this (Grünbaum 1984). According to the latter criterion, an interpretation is true if it is internally coherent and narratively satisfying (Spence 1982). If other theories of truth and evidence are at play in the psychodynamic psychotherapies, they are not explicitly stated and defended, and can only be guessed at.

The principle of interpretive agency is burdened with a number of other unwarranted assumptions. First, unless it is shown that what appears to be a therapeutically effective interpretation is *not* a vehicle of unrelated (i.e. non-interpretive) forces that are operating through or behind it, it cannot be assumed that it has intrinsic therapeutic agency. A number of alternative explanations can be given of the fact that an interpretation seems to be therapeutically effective. It could, for example, be a simple case of the temporal contiguity of the interpretation and the therapeutic improvement: the former happens to precede the latter. But temporal contiguity is not a reliable sign of a causal relation. Something else could have caused therapeutic change at roughly the same time that the interpretation was given to the client. Again, therapeutic improvement could be a function of therapeutic suggestion, or the doctrinal compliance (Ehrenwald 1966) of the client with the psychotherapist's theoretical stance as this is expressed in the interpretation. In such a case, the content and truth value of the interpretation is of less therapeutic importance than its suggestive power, or its capacity to induce agreement. Finally, the timing of the interpretation may be coincident with the natural remission of symptoms if the psychological disorder is self-limiting, and if it follows a natural onset, course, and duration. Each of these factors, in other words, would first need to be ruled out before concluding that an interpretation was effective in bringing about therapeutic change.

Second, as Frank's case history illustrated, the mere fact that an interpretation is internally coherent is neither necessary nor sufficient to underwrite its truth. False, fictitious, or bogus interpretations may display the marks of coherence, and may be narratively satisfying. On this basis they may be regarded as true by client and psychotherapist alike. Moreover, true interpretations may lack the degree of coherence displayed by false but satisfyingly coherent narratives, and on this basis may be regarded as false by clients and psychotherapists. There is no incompatibility between interpretive coherence and falsity.[6]

This should not be surprising. Interpretations are not like mirrors or videotapes. They do not capture every salient detail of the psychological and behavioral make-up of clients with exacting precision; nor are they 'read off' the clinical material. The coherence of an interpretation is often purchased at the expense of veracity. Historical and psychological accuracy may yield to the same kinds of selective and compensatory devices that are deployed in works of fiction: interpretive 'filling in', 'smoothing over', and editorial streamlining, among other devices (Spence 1982). Much of this is unavoidable.

After a certain number of hours of exploratory therapy, psychodynamic psychotherapists find themselves confronted with a mass of heterogeneous clinical material, the boundaries and patterns of which are not immediately obvious. The clinical material includes clients' verbal and nonverbal behaviors, self-reports, memories, dreams, transference behaviors, tics and mannerisms, physical appearance, physical health, and so on. A number of critical decisions thus confront psychotherapists at every stage of the process of interpreting the clinical material. Before the development of an interpretation can even proceed, psychotherapists must decide about what to count as a sufficient amount of clinical material. That is, they must decide about how much longer to allow the production of clinical material to continue, taking into consideration the overall progress of the therapy, the needs of the client, and the psychological capacity of the client to deal with an interpretation. This decision must be made without influencing clients positively or negatively about the amount and content of material that is expected from them. Ideally, the flow of clinical material would not be artificially interrupted by this decision. But if clients are somehow influenced, then psychotherapists must decide how best to neutralize the potentially self-validating beliefs that clients hold about the clinical productions expected of them.

Once a sufficient mass of clinical material has been assembled, psychotherapists must then make a number of decisions about the kinds of clinical material that will count as relevant to the development of an interpretation: decisions about what psychological themes to foreground, what early childhood events to focus upon, what patterns of resistance and denial to highlight, and what defense mechanisms to unravel. But none of these are easy to decode. Even if the emotionally charged events and interpersonal relations of early childhood continue to exert powerful influences over a client's thoughts, feelings, and behaviors, in the form of defense mechanisms and neurotic complexes, the evidence of the relevant causal connections between past pathogenic events and contemporary symptoms is highly fragmentary and diffuse. First, there is rarely any objective historical evidence of the putatively pathogenic emotionally charged events of childhood: few if any photographic records, documents, diaries, or journals exist, and there are rarely credible eyewitnesses. Moreover, first-person memories of the relevant events, especially as these are reported in therapy sessions, are often blurred, contradictory, or malleable (Loftus *et al.* 1989a; Loftus *et al.* 1989b; Crews 1990; Loftus 1993; Loftus and Ketchum 1994; Neisser 1994b; Neisser and Fivush 1994). To complicate matters, the clients' present-day psychological disorders are unreliable indicators of the occurrence of specific *types* of pathogenic childhood events; and they are completely unreliable as indicators of specific details of time and place. Eissler, for example, notes that 'it is not difficult... to demonstrate to a patient that he once harbored aggressive feelings against a beloved father; but a true reconstruction goes beyond the mere unearthing of a hidden impulse and includes those specific details of time, place, environment and inner processes that conjoined to produce a trauma. Yet to take hold of these is a formidable task' (Eissler 1969: 462).

Take Frank's case history again. The client suffered from episodes of severe depression, preoccupation, and irritability. Frank's interpretation highlighted the client's abandonment by her parents at an early age, which, he claimed, led the client to fear putting trust in other people. A single-factor causal explanation of this type *might* happen to be correct. The client's symptoms *may* have been caused by this *kind* of sequence of events, specific details of time, place and actual subjective state notwithstanding. But any moderate fallibilist approach to differential diagnosis must also allow that the symptoms are complex enough to be compatible with a number of other *kinds* of traumatic events in the client's past, or *kinds* of dysfunctional interpersonal relations. Moreover, the symptoms are complex and diffuse enough to be compatible with much more recent biological, neurobiological, and environmental causes in the client's history that have little causal relevance to her childhood experiences. The true explanation of the client's disorders might take a multifactorial rather than monofactorial form, pinpointing multiple concurrent paths of causation operating at many different nonreducible explanatory levels.

In the absence of direct historical and psychological evidence, then, psychodynamic psychotherapists intent on constructing interpretations must *infer* the existence of emotionally charged events in early childhood from the mass of clinical material; and they must *infer* the existence of the causal relations between these putatively pathogenic events and the presenting disorders. But there is an unavoidable degree of slack between the mass of clinical material and the psychological inferences that are made on its basis: that is, there is a kind of empirical underdetermination of psychodynamic inference. This means that psychodynamic interpretations based upon inferences are less likely to be faithful reconstructions of the historical past and the psychological facts, than they are to be inference-rich psychological generalizations that have been generated inductively on the basis of prior clinical experience with similar cases within a broad theoretical framework (such as Freudian psychoanalysis or Kleinian psychoanalysis).

The epistemic obstacles facing the attempts to fill out the connection between the interpretation and the psychological and historical facts might seem more surmountable if clients' confirmations of interpretations were relatively unproblematic. Psychodynamic interpretations, after all, are not self-evidently true. Nor are they true because the psychotherapists who develop them *say* they are true. Nor are they true because they make sense to psychotherapist and client alike. Interpretations must be confirmed or disconfirmed. According to the Standard View's principle of intraclinical confirmation, this must proceed within the clinical setting, using the responses of clients as a guide: that is, clients' memories, assent or dissent, nonverbal behaviors, therapeutic progress, and insights. To an uncritical eye, it might seem that if clients have memories of the *specific* childhood events and feelings described in the interpretation, then the interpretation is true, and the inferences upon which it rests are valid. Similarly, it might seem that if clients claim to have memories of the *types* of childhood events and feelings described in the interpretation, then this would count as moderate empirical confirmation for the inferences upon which the interpretation rest. Again, it might seem that if clients have no memories of the *types* of childhood events and feelings described in the interpretation, then this would be considered strong empirical disconfirmation for the inferences upon which the interpretation rests. Assent to an interpretation, in other words, might seem to be a reliable sign of its truth; dissent might seem a reliable sign of its falsity or incompleteness. But client responses to interpretations are epistemically unreliable.

Freud's reflections on the epistemic unreliability of client recollection as a way to authenticate the putative psychological and historical facts identified in interpretations of early childhood events apply equally well to nonpsychoanalytic psychodynamic psychotherapies. Late in his career Freud wrote: 'The path that starts from the analyst's construction ought to end in the patient's recollection; but it does not always lead so far. Quite often we do not succeed in bringing the patient to recollect what has been repressed. Instead of that, if the analysis is carried out correctly, we produce in him an *assured conviction* of the truth of the construction which achieves the same therapeutic result as a recaptured memory' (Freud SE 23: 265–266, emphasis added).

This is a striking concession, given Freud's rejection of suggestion therapeutics, and his earlier adherence to a version of the principle of interpretive agency. It means that psychoanalysts may produce in analysands assured convictions about the truth of alternative constructions that stress different themes and psychological meanings. This applies equally well in the psychodynamic psychotherapies. More than one interpretation of childhood events may be therapeutically effective: that is, more than one key may open the lock to a psychological disorder. But this raises the vexing issue of how conflicts between more or less equally plausible interpretations of early childhood events—say a Freudian interpretation, a Kleinian one, and a Horneyan one—are rationally resolved. All three interpretations cannot be psychologically and historically true. But in the absence of direct historical and psychological evidence, and reliable analysand responses, it is far from clear how conflicts could be decided, except on grounds of parsimony, aesthetic appeal, instrumental value, or plausibility. Even these grounds are open to dispute, however, with no universally agreed-upon criteria available that would help to resolve disputes about competing claims to parsimony or plausibility.

Second, Freud's concession seems to allow the possibility that psychoanalysts may with relative ease produce in analysands assured convictions about the truth of false constructions. That is, psychoanalytic interpretations may result in false but therapeutically effective memories of childhood events, and false but therapeutically effective beliefs in the psychoanalytic explanation of behavior, emotion, and personality. The same is generally true of the many psychodynamic psychotherapies. Freud earlier claimed that false constructions, failing to 'tally' with what is real in the analysand, would fall by the wayside, and would have no lasting therapeutic effect. But his later concession (from 1937) suggests otherwise. The degree of conviction of analysands is neither necessary nor sufficient to establish that the interpretations they are convinced about are true. Because of analyst expectations, the cognitive dissonance of the analytic situation, and other emotional pressures of analysis, analysands may assent to historically and psychologically false constructions of the events and feelings of their childhood; and their assent may be a function of factors that have nothing to do with the truth-value of the constructions presented to them. This undermines the Standard View's principle of interpretive agency.

Another problematic epistemic consequence of the empirical underdetermination of psychodynamic interpretations is what might be called 'interpretive force-fitting'. Interpretations risk acquiring a schematic one-size-fits-all character the less they are like faithful reconstructions of the actual contours of historical and psychological fact, and the more they are like inference-rich psychological generalizations that are generated inductively on the basis of prior clinical experience with similar cases within a broad theoretical framework. Force-fitted interpretations have the following character: given such and such clinical evidence, *types* ABC of childhood events and feelings *must* have happened, *types* LMN of defense mechanism *must* be the cause of these presenting symptoms, and *types* XYZ of resistance *must* be working against the therapy. Rather than conforming to the mass of clinical material, these interpretations are imposed onto it in order to satisfy the theoretical demands of the relevant psychodynamic theory. Such was the gist of Fliess's critique of Freud; and it is a critique that applies beyond psychoanalysis to other exploratory psychotherapies. In formulating his often ingenious psychological interpretations, Freud (claimed Fliess) read his own theoretical biases into the thoughts and feelings of his patients (Freud 1954: 334, 337). He did this by selecting and editing the clinical material in such a way that the material fitted the profile and scope of the kinds of interpretations *demanded* by the theory of psychoanalysis (Meehl 1983).

There is a clinical side to the risk of interpretive force-fitting: namely, the risk of force-fitted eliciting of clinical material. Clients are not indifferent to interpretations. They may respond in such a way that their memories, insights, nonverbal behaviors, dreams and other clinical productions come to fit the interpretations that are force-fitted upon them. The complex mutual interplay between the force-fitted interpretation and the clinical productions that are fitted by the interpretation may generate artifactual clinical material that would not otherwise have occurred during the therapy. Just as alternative selections from the clinical material could have been made, thus yielding different interpretations, so each alternative interpretation in its turn would exert different effects on the clients, and elicit different kinds of clinical material.

Another of the unwanted epistemic consequences of force-fitted interpretations of early childhood events and feelings is the distortion of temporal perspective. Simply put, following Kierkegaard's formulation, life lived forwards is confused with the fact that it is understood and interpreted backwards. More technically, this is the confusion of the retrospective perspective with the prospective perspective. The confusion results in psychodynamic interpretations acquiring an element of temporal artificiality that is more characteristic of psychological fiction than psychological fact.

How does this confusion arise? Psychodynamic interpretations of childhood experience are unavoidably after the fact. The events of the client's childhood have long passed. Interpretations must smooth over or fill in the loose ends of the history of early psychological development, where both well-founded objective evidence and accurate recall are absent. But this gives to the interpreted events of early childhood the appearance of a linear, forward-looking, and fully intelligible development—characteristics which were not present at the time of the events themselves, or were not experienced as such. With such a move, the role of historical randomness and subjective uncertainty in the face of the future is kept to a minimum. With sufficiently robust interpretive filling in, certain temporal determinations are read into events after the fact; that is, temporal distinctions such as beginning, middle, and end, and climax and dénouement, are inserted into the weave of childhood events, when in actuality they were not present at the time the events occurred. In the actual moment of occurrence, the events of early childhood were not experienced in the terms identified under the interpretation: it was not known what they would later be, or what they would later mean. With after-the-fact interpretive filling in, the realized future is read back into the interpretation of the past event, with the achieved outcome of a series of events called upon as the key to their meaning. But this conflates the prospective perspective with the retrospective perspective, with the result that interpretations acquire a fictional character that the series of events they putatively interpret do not actually have (Jopling 2000).

Considerations such as these weaken the principle of interpretive agency, and the corollary to the principle that states that only veridical interpretations possess genuine therapeutic agency.

ii) Clients often concur with their psychotherapists' interpretations. As Frank's client remarked, his interpretation went off 'like a gong', and it triggered a series of important insights which further developed the interpretation. Not all interpretations go off like gongs. But some form of cognitive and emotional agreement is therapeutically significant, and it is considered to serve as a source of intraclinical confirmation. Failures of concurrence, on the other hand, are often taken as signs of resistance to therapy: that is, as signs of intellectualizing, delaying exploration, or holding onto the disorder. But concurrence has little probative value. The mere occurrence of thematic agreement between interpretations and insights is not a guarantee of the veridicality of either. False insights may display substantial thematic agreement with false interpretations; and veridical insights may display poor thematic agreement with veridical interpretations. Even if there is significant thematic agreement between true interpretations and true insights, it is still possible that the agreement has occurred for reasons that have nothing to do with the truth value of the proffered interpretations. Thematic agreement may be a function of the power of therapeutic suggestion, yielding to the cognitive dissonance of the therapeutic situation, the psychotherapist's charisma or authority, or the presence of an unspoken *folie à deux* between psychotherapist and client. These alternative explanations would have to be ruled out before concluding that thematic agreement between interpretation and insight is a sign of the truth of the insight. It does not follow from this, however, that thematic agreement has no epistemically significant role to play in the course of therapy. It may, for example, serve as a reliable indicator that therapeutic exploration is moving ahead satisfactorily according to the norms of the therapeutic theory.

iii) The mere acquisition of insights by clients does not mean that the insights are veridical, even if the insights are compelling, plausible, endorsed by a highly experienced psychotherapist, or followed by therapeutic progress. This is as true within as without the psychotherapeutic context. Outside of the context of psychotherapeutic exploration, for example, it is not uncommon for people to experience blinding realizations, introspective breakthroughs, or moments of surprisingly clear self-awareness following upon reflective self-examination. But it is also not uncommon for people to experience blinding realizations that are false, introspective breakthroughs that are in fact exploratory dead-ends, and moments of self-awareness that are illusory (Farrell 1981, Jopling 2000). That is, the mere acquisition of insight is insufficient to establish its truth. Insights need to be checked and re-evaluated to minimize the possibility of false, self-deceived, or deluded insights that masquerade as true.

There are several other considerations that underline the importance of the distinction between the mere occurrence of insight and the truth-value of insight. The occurrence of insight can be explained by a number of factors unrelated to the truth-value of the insight: for example, expectancy effects; therapeutic suggestion; explanatory compliance; transient insight-mimicking realizations, the spurious nature of which becomes apparent later; or pervasive but undetected strategies of self-deception that find support within the therapeutic setting itself (see Chapter 6).

iv) Just as the mere fact of acquiring insights is not a guarantee that the insights are veridical, so clients' levels of conviction about the validity of their newly-won insights, or their emotionally charged responses to insights, are not a guarantee that the insights are veridical. Feelings of conviction carry no probative weight. They wax and wane for reasons that are often unrelated to the truth-value of the insights. In an appropriately suasory or coercive environment, for instance, clients may become convinced about—even form strong identifications with—psychologically bogus insights; and in the absence of such an environment they may remain indifferent to veridical insights, and unconvinced by the otherwise compelling evidence that supports them. Furthermore, the level of conviction displayed by clients may be a function of temporary lapses of critical judgment occasioned by exposure to the psychotherapy itself. A feeling of conviction may arise, for instance, as a result of systematically weakened epistemic standards that have been brought about by prolonged exposure to the lax epistemic standards and practices of the therapy.

It does not follow from this that the level of conviction and the emotional arousal surrounding insights have no therapeutic significance. Strong feelings of conviction may *happen* to accompany an insight that is true, or close to the truth. But the fact that clients become emotionally aroused at certain key exploratory stages in the therapy, and become convinced they have acquired insights that they would not otherwise have acquired, is not sufficient to underwrite the veridicality of what they have acquired in their aroused state.

v) Just as clients' convictions about their insights are not a guarantee of their veridicality, so psychotherapists' convictions about the authenticity of their clients' explorations, and the truth of their clients' insights, are not a guarantee that the insights are true. Psychotherapists are no more immune than nonexperts to mistaken explanations of the motivational and psychological make-up of their clients, even when their clinical interventions bear all the marks of being conducted correctly according to the standards of the psychotherapeutic theory and the clinical norms of the community of practitioners. Psychotherapists are not impartial observers. They have strong interests in seeing their work succeed; they operate with theoretical orientations that have the potential to blind them to damaging counter-evidence; they have only a finite amount of clinical material with which to work; they have only a finite amount of time within which to bring about therapeutic improvement; and they often have strong feelings towards their clients. Appeals to consistency with previous case histories, or to consensus among similarly trained psychotherapists, do not guarantee the veridicality of insights.

vi) The occurrence of positive therapeutic change in clients following the acquisition of insight is not a guarantee of the veridicality of insights or interpretations. To infer therapeutic efficacy from this is to commit the fallacy of *post hoc ergo propter hoc* (after this therefore because of this). Just as some psychoanalyzed patients may feel better *after* receiving psychoanalytic treatment, so almost all of those people who suffer from colds may get better *after* drinking coffee for a sufficient number of days (Grünbaum 1977: 222). But the fact that cold symptoms happen to remit after drinking coffee does not justify any conclusion about the therapeutic efficacy of coffee. A number of alternative causal explanations first have to be ruled out before such a conclusion would be warranted. Similarly, there are a number of alternative explanations that first have to be ruled out before accepting that therapeutic change was a direct function of the characteristic factors of the treatment method of psychoanalysis. These explanations would include the possibility of: remission of symptoms due to extra-clinical events (e.g. the passage of time); therapeutic improvement that is driven by client compliance and subservience to medical authority; therapeutic change as a function of placebo effects of the treatment method; and therapeutic improvement as a function of the false, deception-engendering, or fictitious character of the insights.

Moreover, positive post-insight therapeutic changes may have occurred because of factors less related to the truth-value of the insights than to their capacity to persuade clients with their *apparent* explanatory power. This would accord with one of the central findings of the common factors approach: one of the functions of psychotherapy is to supply clients with coherent and socially sanctioned rationales that appear to explain psychological problems, and that give otherwise puzzling symptoms a name—but the rationales (and the therapeutic theories which imbed them) may be false or trivial. That is, therapeutic agency in many cases rests on clients' *belief* in the validity and veracity of the rationales they are given—actual truth-value notwithstanding.

At this point, it should be clear that certain claims about the psychodynamic psychotherapies cannot simply be taken at face value: claims, for instance, that what occurs in psychotherapy is *bona fide* exploration and discovery, and claims about the validity of psychodynamic interpretations and insights. The mere fact that clients emerge from psychotherapy *claiming* to have a greater clarity about themselves than they had at the outset of the treatment does not justify any robust conclusion about insight or self-knowledge; and the fact that the insights clients achieve in psychotherapy happen to be followed by improvements in their condition is not sufficient to show that the insights caused these improvements. Naturally, it is hard to imagine what else the psychodynamic psychotherapies could possibly be doing if they were *not* engaged in the exploration of the psyche, and not helping clients to get in touch with a deeper self: such is the power of uncritical assumption. This is precisely the point of developing an alternative explanation. Clients in the psychodynamic psychotherapies may be engaged in something that *looks* like *bona fide* exploration and discovery, but is in fact something else: they might, for example, be responding to the psychological equivalent of a sugar pill. But first, what *is* a placebo?

Chapter 4

Placebos and Placebo Effects

Charms and Fair Words

If a person a) is poorly, b) receives treatment intended to make him better, and c) gets better, then no power of reasoning known to medical science can convince him that it may not have been the treatment that restored his health.

P. Medawar, *The Art of the Soluble*

Placebos suffer a poor reputation in contemporary scientific medicine. They have been regarded by clinicians as fake, imaginary, unscientific, or unreal treatments, given mainly to placate anxious, gullible, or difficult patients. They have been regarded by bioethicists as vehicles for the deception or coercion of patients. And they have been considered by methodologists as no more than the 'noise' that needs to be factored out in randomized controlled trials. To make matters worse, the physicians who give placebos have been criticized as manipulative, uncaring, or unconcerned with the autonomy and dignity of patients—or just plain incompetent; and the use of placebo therapeutics in clinical situations, and placebo controls in trial situations, has been criticized as unethical (Bok 1974, 2002; Simmons 1978; Veatch 1982; Beauchamp and Childress 1983; Rothman and Michels 2002). Even the Latin etymology of the term 'placebo' seems to be damning: 'I shall please'.

From a broad historical point of view, however, these criticisms are newcomers on the scene. The deliberate use of placebos and symbolic treatments has ancient roots. So too does the practice of benevolent paternalism, and the principle of beneficence, once the foundation of the medical relationship (Veatch 1972, 1982; Beauchamp and Childress 1983). By contrast, the principle of respect for patient autonomy, and the emphasis on transparency, informed consent, and truth-telling in medical treatment, are historically recent developments, with origins in the Kantian commitment to the universal duty of veracity (Rawlinson 1985: 404; see also Faden and Beauchamp 1986).

Long before the concept of placebo had made its appearance in medical thinking, Socrates recognized the healing power of rhetoric and persuasion. Observing the soul doctors of the day, he said that 'the cure of the soul has to be effected by the use of certain charms, and these charms are fair words' (Plato 1961; see also Gill 1985; Nussbaum 1994). Hippocrates also recognized the healing power of the symbolic and linguistic elements in the patient–doctor relationship, and acknowledged the importance of protecting patients from knowledge that may be harmful to them (Lain Entralgo 1970). Physicians, he claimed, must use their authority and charisma, and the mystery of their esoteric knowledge, to heal. They must practice their art 'calmly and adroitly, concealing most things from the patient while attending him. Give encouragement to the patient to allow himself to be treated, turning his attention away from what is being done to him; sometimes reprove sharply and emphatically, and sometimes comfort with solicitude and attention, revealing nothing of the patient's future or present condition' (Hippocrates 1979: XVII). It is, he wrote, 'sometimes simply in virtue of the patient's faith in the physician that a cure is effected' (Hippocrates, Regimen, II). The first duty of the Hippocratic physician is not truthfulness and informed consent, but a proper paternalism (Rawlinson 1985).

Medical practices involving benevolent paternalist deception and heightened patient credulity continued unabated throughout the Renaissance period, with Montaigne's descriptions of the placebo-responsive merchant of Toulouse, and the woman who believed she had swallowed a pin, being the most vivid (2003: 117). In *The anatomy of melancholy* of 1628 Robert Burton wrote: 'A third thing to be required in a patient is confidence, to be of good cheer, and have sure hope that his Physician can help him. Damescen the Arabian requires likewise… that (the Physician) be confident he can cure (the Patient) or at least make the patient believe so, otherwise, his Physick will not be effectual… and, as Galen holds, confidence and hope can do more good than Physick. Paracelsus assigned it for an only cause why Hippocrates was so fortunate in his cures, not for any extraordinary skill he had, but because the common people had a most strong conceit of his worth'.

Defenses of the therapeutic role of benevolent deception were fairly common in the eighteenth century. Peter Shaw, for instance, wrote in 1750 that the 'principal Quality of a Physician, as well as of a Poet (for Apollo is the God of Physic and Poetry) is that of fine lying, or flattering the Patient… And it is doubtless as well for the Patient to be cured by the Workings of his Imagination or a Reliance upon the Promise of his Doctor, as by repeated doses of Physic' (cited in Rawlinson 1985). It was also in the eighteenth century that the term placebo came into widespread use. In Quincy's lexicon placebo was defined as 'a commonplace method in medicine'. One medical dictionary in 1785 described the placebo as 'calculated to amuse for a time, rather than for any other purpose'. Another dictionary from 1811 described the placebo as 'given more to please than to benefit the patient' (Shapiro 1968). Thomas Jefferson, characterizing placebo use as a 'pious fraud', wrote that 'one of the most successful physicians I have ever known assured me, that he used more of bread pills, drops of colored water, and powders of hickory ashes, than of all medicines put together' (Brody 1982: 112).

In the nineteenth century the intentional and unintentional use of placebos was widespread. One of the clearest justifications of benevolent paternalistic deception was made by Thomas Percival in 1803. Percival identified two conditions under which it is justified to deceive patients: a) when full disclosure of the patient's condition would be harmful to the patient; b) when some ruse would be necessary to insure the success of the treatment. Oliver Wendell Holmes also defended the use of placebos and benevolent paternalistic deception in medicine in his *Medical Essays*: 'Your patient has not more right to the truth you know than he has to all the medicine in your saddlebags... He should get only as much as is good for him' (Holmes 1883). Holmes was sensitive to the symbolic power of medical language, and deliberately used extravagant and esoteric technical terminology in order to impress patients with his medical authority, allay their anxieties, or supply them with diagnoses when none were available or required. Diagnoses such as 'spinal irritation' and 'congestion of the portal system' were the equivalent of diagnostic fictions.

Placebos were also documented in literature in the nineteenth and early to mid-twentieth centuries. Writers such as Fyodor Dostoevsky (1880/1981: II:3), Mark Twain (Ober 2003), Jerome K. Jerome (1889/1964; see Chapter 5), George Bernard Shaw (1911/1941), Sinclair Lewis (1980), and Patrick O'Brian (1998; see also Marshall 2004) wrote fictional and often highly comical accounts of the use of placebos, nocebos, sham cures, and symbolic healing rituals. In the play *The Doctor's Dilemma* (Shaw 1911/1941), for example, Shaw's colorful character Dr. Sir Ralph Bloomfield Bonnington is portrayed as 'a walking placebo' (Brody 1997: 77). His medical reasoning is muddled and his scientific understanding spotty, but he has a genuine therapeutic touch. 'Cheering, reassuring, healing by the mere incompatibility of disease or anxiety with his welcome presence. Even broken bones, it is said, have been known to unite at the sound of his voice'.

The practices of placebo use and benevolent paternalistic deception flourished well into the 1900s. The Harvard physician Richard Cabot (1903), for instance, wrote that he was 'brought up, as I suppose every physician is, to use placebo, bread pills, water subcutaneously, and other devices... How frequently such methods are used varies a great deal I suppose with individual practitioners, but I doubt if there is a physician in this room who has not used them and used them pretty often... I used to give them by the bushels'.

The Shaman Quesalid

Viewed from an outsider's perspective, benevolent paternalistic deception and other forms of intentional ignorance flourish in the history of many non-Western medical practices, particularly in ritualized healing practices that deploy powerful symbols and metaphors to increase patients' levels of credulity and hope (Hahn and Kleinman 1983). But symbolic healing rituals are not typically considered by their practitioners to be merely imaginary or spurious, in the same way that Holmes, Cabot and others considered their own practices to be merely imaginary or spurious; nor were patients considered to be victims of benevolent deception when they received symbolic treatments. The distinction between placebo and nonplacebo treatments is not as clearly established in some non-Western medical practices as it is in Western medicine. Symbolic healing 'is often quite effective, just as placebos are often effective… because human beings structure and partly create their experiences of illness and recovery through shared symbols and metaphors' (Harrington 1997: 7).

Take for example the 'charms' and 'fair words' of the Vancouver Island Kwakiutl shaman Quesalid, as depicted by Lévi-Strauss (1963) (who based his account on that of the anthropologist Franz Boas [1930]). Quesalid's medical training began for what seem to be all the wrong reasons. Initially skeptical about the validity of shamanistic explanations and treatment methods, and incensed over what he regarded as the exploitation of patients by means of shamanistic trickery, Quesalid trained to become a shaman in order to debunk shamanism. To his astonishment, however, his use of shamanistic treatment methods produced what his peers and patients regarded as cures. Quite inadvertently, Quesalid became the most powerful shaman in his region, and his healing powers at the height of his career were legendary.

The treatment method for which Quesalid became famous was based on an elaborate and esoteric ceremony which embodied many of the common factors identified by Frank (1983, 1989, 1991). The high point of the ceremony involved the shaman extracting a hidden tuft of bloodied down from his mouth, and then reporting to his patient that he had successfully sucked out the pathological body in the form of a bloody worm. Quesalid believed that the technique was bogus: that is, that it had no connection with any known etiology, and that it worked for reasons other than the ones he offered to his patients. He thus knew that he was deceiving his patients with an elaborate explanatory fiction; he also knew that his patients neither shared nor detected his medical skepticism. The procedure nonetheless remained his most potent therapeutic tool (Lévi-Strauss 1963: 175). Quesalid continued to regard other shamans as charlatans, but it is not clear if he regarded himself in the same light. Lévi-Strauss claims that 'we cannot tell, but it is evident that he carries on his craft conscientiously, takes pride in his achievements, and warmly defends the technique of the bloody down against all rival schools. He seems to have completely lost sight of the fallaciousness of the technique which he had so disparaged at the beginning' (Lévi-Strauss 1963: 173).

There are a number of explanations of the effectiveness of Quesalid's treatment that serve as credible alternatives to the shamanistic explanation. One explanation is that therapeutic improvement was due to the self-limiting nature of his patients' illnesses. Quesalid probably knew that most of the symptoms of common illnesses remitted on their own, with time. Shrewd as he was, he may even have concocted for himself rough and ready baseline rates of the onset, duration, course, and remission of the common illnesses in his society. By taking only those patients whose illnesses were in the latter third of their natural progression, he would have been assured of a welcome coincidence of treatment and symptom remission. This points to another alternative (but incomplete) explanation of Quesalid's success: his canny choice of patients. With careful screening, Quesalid may have managed to avoid treating untreatable patients, taking on only those whom he suspected had a high chance of success.

Yet another alternative explanation is the placebo hypothesis. Quesalid's treatments may have succeeded because he supplied his patients with interpretation and insight placebos, thereby giving them a believable rationale, conceptual scheme, or myth that made sense of their unintelligible and frightening symptoms. In doing so, he gave their disorders a name—the Rumplestiltskin effect (Torrey 1986)—thereby increasing his patients' levels of hope and their sense of control. Quesalid also provided patients with procedures or rituals that called for their active involvement, and which they (and others in their community) believed were the primary means of the restoration of health (Frank 1989). From a clinical point of view, it was irrelevant that Quesalid's explanation—the shamanistic etiology, nosology, and pathology—was false, or an elaborate explanatory fiction: it was therapeutically effective as long as his patients (and the surrounding community) *believed* that the explanation was true. Quesalid became famous because he was the therapeutic agent for the placebo effect. Lévi-Strauss writes:

> That the mythology of the shaman does not correspond to an objective reality does not matter. The sick woman believes in the myth and belongs to a society which believes in it. The tutelary spirits and malevolent spirits, the supernatural monsters and magical animals, are all part of a coherent system on which the native conception of the universe is founded. The sick woman accepts these mythical beings or, more accurately, she has never questioned their existence. What she does not accept are the incoherent and arbitrary pains, which are an alien element in her system but which

the shaman, calling upon myth, will re-integrate within a whole where everything is meaningful (Lévi-Strauss 1963: 197).

Quesalid's explanations, and the insights acquired by his patients, need not have been true to occasion therapeutic improvement: they needed only to satisfy certain minimal non-cognitive requirements of plausibility, coherence, and explanatory economy, as well as certain minimal requirements of inter-subjective agreement. To the extent that his patient's disorders are problems of causal opacity—of suffering from the unintelligible and alien nature of illness—it could be expected that a number of similarly qualified explanatory fictions and clinical interventions would have similar degrees of therapeutic efficacy. Lévi-Strauss claims that cure by magic is a consensual phenomenon (1963: 169). This does not mean that *any* consensually endorsed belief is curative. A myth will not regenerate amputated limbs. Nor will group consensus alone cure an illness. Short-lived changes in public opinion about what counts as symptomatic and nonsymptomatic, and pathological and normal, will not alter the underlying physiological status of an illness. Lévi-Strauss' point is that group consensus is one of the primary factors determining the status and power of the healer, and contributing to the patient's belief in the healer's authority and knowledge. This is one of the essential components of thera-peutic improvement. 'Quesalid did not become a great shaman because he cured his patients; he cured his patients because he had become a great shaman' (1963: 180).

Janet's Theriac

Placebos are rarely used deliberately in contemporary clinical psychology and psychotherapy. Unlike Quesalid, clinical psychologists and psychotherapists do not train with a view to debunking their craft and unveiling the placebic nature of their treatment methods. Most do not deliberately supply their clients with explanations they know to be fictions. And most do not resort to deception or other practices of intentional ignorance to help clients get better. The vast majority of clinical psychologists support the principles of informed consent and respect for client autonomy, and they find broad (and often poorly explained) institutional support for their beliefs in the ethics guidelines of major national and international associations (for example, the American Psychological Association's *Ethical principles of psychologists and code of conduct* (American Psychological Association 2002), and the World Medical Association's *Declaration of Helsinki* (World Medical Association 2001).

It was not always so. In the late nineteenth and early twentieth century, some clinical psychologists were as skeptical about their treatment methods and explanations as Quesalid was about his own. Some resorted to deceptive practices that were as benevolently paternalistic as Quesalid's practices. The French psychiatrist Pierre Janet was one of these. Janet used persuasion, suggestion, deception, and the psychological equivalent of sugar pills to great effect. He treated his patients by fabricating stories about their condition and persuading them that the stories were *bona fide* psychological explanations. But Janet's motivation was not, like Quesalid's, to debunk psychological healing; it was to help patients in need, using whatever techniques seemed to work. His stance to psychotherapy was mainly pragmatic. Psychotherapy for Janet was a grab bag of tools, some workable and some not: 'it is a sort of psychological theriac... [O]ne should not be surprised if they do not always succeed or that such treatments are considered as lotteries by official science' (Janet 1925). The tools in Janet's grab bag included hypnosis, suggestion, 'monoideism', moral education, guided imagery, and the deliberate manipulation and reconstruction of patient's memories. All of these avowedly directive techniques stood in sharp contrast with Freud's ostensibly non-directive exploratory techniques. Where Freud was convinced that it was the patient's talking that cured, Janet was convinced that it was the patient being *talked to* that cured (Borch-Jacobsen 1996: 3–5); and where Freud was convinced that he had found a method that cured by enabling patients to discover the truth about their pasts and their unconscious motivations, Janet knew that he was deliberately misleading his patients in order to cure them (Hacking 1995: 195–196). Janet was unabashed about the paternalistic authority implied by the use of therapy-induced deceptions:

> [My] belief is that the patient wants a doctor who will cure; that the doctor's professional duty is to give any remedy that will be useful, and to prescribe it in the way in which it will do most good. Now, I think bread pills are medically indicated in certain cases, and that they will act far more powerfully if I deck them out with impressive names. When I prescribe such a formidable placebo, I believe that I am fulfilling my professional duty, and that I am keeping with my real though tacit undertaking with my patient; and I am quite sure that if he gets well he will bear me no grudge. But you believe, says the objector, that the action of the remedy is psychological, and yet you allow the patient to believe that its action is chemical; you are infringing the general obligation to be absolutely sincere! Perhaps I am. We are faced here with one of those conflicts between duties which are continually arising in practical life; and, for my part, I believe that the duty of curing my patient preponderates enormously over the trivial duty of giving him a scientific lecture which he would not understand and would have no use for... Can we be sure that this [rule—hiding nothing from the patient, and saying nothing that is not true] is a good rule? I knew a woman who went mad because the doctor told her bluntly that her husband's case was hopeless, and that he would be buried before the fortnight was out. The statement was perfectly true, but would not the doctor have done better to veil the truth a little? If truth be a virtue, must we not also recognize that discretion and tact are virtues? Did not our

forefathers speak of 'medical tact'? That is what we are concerned with here. There are some patients to whom we must tell the whole truth; there are some to whom we must tell part of the truth; and there are some to whom, as a matter of strict moral obligation, we must lie. (1925, 1: 338)

Janet's use of placebos, suggestion, and deception is evident in his account of the effects of traumatic events on psychological functioning—one of the first systematic accounts ever developed. The directive treatment strategies he devised for trauma clearly illustrate the important role he assigned to fabrication, deception, and explanatory fictions in psychological healing, as well as the important role he assigned to having patients believe that the diagnoses and interpretations with which he supplied them were true. Janet was the first psychologist to hold that dissociation is the main psychological mechanism in the production of a wide variety of what are currently designated as post-traumatic symptoms (van der Kolk *et al.* 1989a: 366; see also van der Kolk *et al.* 1989b, 1989c).

The central argument of Janet's *L'Automatisme Psychologique* (1889) is that the experience of overwhelming emotions results in memories that cannot be adequately accommodated into the patient's psychological economy. When this occurs, the offending memories become split off (or dissociated) from conscious awareness, only to recur later as a partial re-experiencing of the traumatic event in the form of somatic states, emotions, images, and behaviors. The re-experience of the traumatic event produces adaptive or quasi-adaptive symptoms, such as the narrowing of conscious awareness, avoidance behaviors, withdrawal, and rigid or primitive reactions to further traumatizing situations. Corresponding to these symptoms is arrested personality development and reduced vitality. 'Unable to integrate the traumatic memories, they seem to have lost their capacity to assimilate new experiences as well. It is as if their personality which definitely stopped at a certain point cannot enlarge any more by the addition or assimilation of new elements: all patients seem to have had the evolution of their lives checked: they are attached to an unsur-mountable obstacle' (Janet 1925: 660).

Traumatization occurs when people fail to take effective action against a perceived external threat. The event precipitating what Janet called a 'vehement' emotional reaction could, in itself, be quite minor; what matters, however, is the subjective reaction to the event. In one famous case involving a nineteen-year-old woman suffering from impetigo and hysterical blindness, and regarded by most doctors as insane, the precipitating event had occurred years earlier in childhood, when the patient was forced to sleep beside a girl with impetigo on the entire left side of her face (Janet 1889: 436–40). Prefiguring later developments in psychodynamic psychotherapy, Janet main-tained that one of the most critical components of effective action against potentially traumatizing events is the formulation of a verbal representation of the experience. When this fails to occur, as it did in the case of his patient when she was a young child, trauma often follows. Patients, he observed, quite often told themselves that the situation was not as threatening as they had initially experienced it to be, and thus not worthy of further articulation (Janet 1904); but later they were caught unawares with post-traumatic amnesias and hyperamnesias, having failed to transform traumatic experiences into less frightening narratives. 'The individual, when overcome by vehement emotions, is not himself. [The] characteristics which have been acquired by education and moral development may suffer a complete change under the influence of emotion. Forgetting the event which precipitated the emotion has frequently been found to accompany intense emotional experiences in the form of continuous and retrograde amnesia' (Janet 1909: 1607). Fugues, amnesias, reduced interest and vitality, constricted affect, and abulias, were the symptoms of the involuntary intrusive reliving of the trauma.

Janet's treatment of post-traumatic stress disorder involved recovering, neutralizing, and integrating the offending memories into the patient's entire psychological economy, using a variety of psychological tools, including benevolent deception: essentially, reconstructing their past with the help of credible fictions. Before this could occur, however, it was essential for the psychotherapist to establish a therapeutic rapport with the patient. Janet observed that at a certain stage in the therapy, patients performed an 'act of adoption', thereby signaling their willingness to settle down and talk seriously about their troubles (Janet 1925: 1154). This involved patients accepting the psychotherapist's authority, expertise, and moral guidance. At the same time, however, he stressed that the psychotherapist must try to minimize control over the patient, to avoid becoming a parent surrogate or omnipotent protector. Therapeutic rapport, like the later Freudian concept of transference, could be either a vehicle for cure or a symptom of illness. Janet found that trauma victims such as his nineteen-year-old patient were especially liable to develop transient pathological fixations on their psychotherapists, and a pathological need for guidance. The 'somnambulistic influence' of the psychotherapist would disappear when patients became aware of and ashamed about the degree of their dependence.

Psychotherapy with patients suffering from post-traumatic stress involved three stages of intervention: stabilization and symptom reduction, the identification and modification of traumatic memories, and relapse prevention. In the second stage, Janet resorted to a variety of directive techniques to help patients gain access to their memories, including hypnosis, visual imaging techniques, and automatic writing. Once accessed, he used manipulative techniques such as mnemonic neutralization, substitution, and reframing, with a view to getting patients to relive and verbalize the traumatic event.

One of Janet's most well-known case histories using these techniques was the case of Justine, a forty-year-old woman who suffered from a debilitating fear of cholera (Janet 1894; see also Ellenberger 1970). Janet's study of Justine is a study in the dynamics of 'psychological automatism', the phenomenon in which complex, situation-sensitive, and goal-directed actions are performed without full conscious awareness. Janet treated Justine for three years, during which time she demonstrated—according to Janet—significant therapeutic improvement. One of her characteristic pathological behaviors would begin with her crying out 'Cholera, it's taking me!' after which she would experience an hysterical crisis. Janet learned that when Justine was a child she had developed a morbid fear of death, because she had been forced to accompany her mother—a nurse—as she treated dying patients. During this time Justine first saw the bodies of cholera victims.

Janet found it impossible to engage Justine during her hysterical crises. As she was unresponsive to his presence as a psychotherapist, Janet adopted a role in the crisis as one of the actors, complete with a voice of his own. When Justine cried out 'Cholera! He will take me!' Janet replied 'Yes, he holds you by the right leg'—thereby prompting Justine to withdraw her leg. Janet then asked, 'Where is your cholera?' to which she replied 'Here! See him, he's bluish, and he stinks!' The strategy opened up a dialogue through which Janet gleaned first-hand reports about the hallucinatory picture that occupied her mind, and this in turn allowed him to gradually transform the crisis into an ordinary hypnotic state. In the crisis state Justine reported seeing two corpses propped up nearby her, the closest of which was an ugly, naked, putrefying, green-tinged man. She also reported hearing bells toll, and shouts of 'Cholera! Cholera!' After the crisis had faded, she forgot every detail of the scene except the idea of cholera, which became a fixed idea.

Janet discovered that direct commands given to the hypnotized patient were of limited use. The dissolution of the hallucinatory picture required the use of substitutive suggestive methods: that is, gradually making her believe things that were not the case. Using suggestion, Janet convinced Justine that the naked corpse had clothes, and that it resembled a Chinese general whom she had seen recently in the Paris Universal Exposition. He also convinced her that the general was not terrifying but comical. With this revisualization the hysterical attack was transformed into cries followed by fits of laughter. Eventually the cries disappeared, and the pictures of cholera occurred only during dreams. These too dissolved when Janet used suggestion to produce innocuous dreams. After one year of treatment using suggestive methods, Janet observed the patient still absent-mindedly whispering the word 'Cholera!' to herself while engaged in other activities. Again using hypnotic suggestion, Janet suggested that 'Cho-le-ra' was the name of the Chinese general. Overall, Justine's treatment lasted another three years.

Quesalid and Janet were successful healers. And yet their treatment methods traded in explanatory fictions. What then could explain their success? How can a psychological treatment be effective if it does not somehow help people gain access to what is real in themselves? Both Quesalid and Janet supplied their patients with believable explanations for unintelligible and frightening symptoms; they instilled hope; they gave disorders a name; and they provided their patients with coping procedures or rituals that called for their active involvement, and which they (and others in their community) believed were the primary means of the restoration of health. From a clinical point of view, it was irrelevant that the explanations with which Quesalid and Janet supplied their patients were false, or served as elaborate explanatory fictions that mapped out imaginary causal pathways. The explanations were therapeutically effective as long as their patients *believed* that they were true. In this sense they were powerful placebos.

Contemporary Research on Placebos

The hypothesis that exploratory psychotherapy has the potential to generate interpretations and insights that are the psychological equivalent of sugar pills and placebo surgeries in physical medicine raises broader conceptual questions: What precisely *is* a placebo? How are placebos distinguished from nonplacebos?

To begin answering these questions, it is worth listing the myths and misconceptions surrounding placebos and the placebo effect (Brown 1994).

- ◆ Because placebos are physiologically inert, they can have no effect on physiological function.
- ◆ Placebos only have an effect on psychological symptoms (or, conversely, if a placebo relieves symptoms, then it shows that the symptoms were unreal, imaginary, or 'psychosomatic').
- ◆ Some people more than others are placebo responders, because of certain personality characteristics.
- ◆ Placebo use is unethical because it always involves tricking or deceiving patients.
- ◆ Almost any medical condition can respond to placebo.
- ◆ Placebo use is ineffective if patients are told they are receiving placebos.

With the exception of the last point (see Chapter 7), these misconceptions have slowly collapsed under the weight of scientific investigation. Beginning with

Beecher's (1955) famous article 'The powerful placebo', placebo research today includes a wide variety of approaches and methods, a wide variety of explanatory models, and a wide variety of research agendas (Gliedman *et al.* 1957; White *et al.* 1985; Harrington 1997; Guess *et al.* 2002; Moerman 2002a; Gorsky and Spier 2004). The research fronts include: the neurobiology of the placebo response, the ethics of giving placebos, conflicting models of placebos, the relevance of placebos for understanding the mind-body relation, placebo responsiveness and personality factors, placebo effects versus statistical regression to the mean, placebos and pain analgesia, and methodological issues about the use of placebos in clinical trials.

Beecher's Powerful Placebo and Placebo Confounds

The scientific study of placebos has its origins in battlefront medicine. During World War II, Henry Beecher served as a field hospital anesthetist in Europe, working with injured soldiers arriving from the front lines (Evans 2003). With uncertain supply lines near the battle front, operations had to be performed sometimes without morphine. This was a dangerous procedure, not only because of the extreme pain, but because of the risk of fatal cardiovascular shock. On one occasion when supplies of morphine ran out, a nurse working with Beecher injected a severely wounded soldier (who was about to undergo emergency surgery) with a saline solution, without telling him what it was. Beecher was astounded with the result: the patient calmed down, appeared to experience little pain during the operation, and did not go into shock. Beecher repeated the procedure with considerable success when supplies of morphine ran low, and returned to the USA convinced about the efficacy of placebos. He later observed that on the battlefront, injected saline solution was 90% as effective as morphine in the alleviation of pain from acute injuries, whereas in civilian hospitals it was 70% as effective as morphine in reducing postoperative pain (Beecher 1959). This was one of the first indications that the effectiveness of placebo is dependent on context and other variables.

Beecher's 1955 paper 'The powerful placebo' is perhaps the most influential paper in the history of placebo research, marking a widespread change in attitude to placebos in medical research (Kaptchuk 1998a, 1998b; Harrington 2002). Using a new approach that had been developing in a handful of biomedical research centers since 1946 (Gold *et al.* 1937; Gold 1946, 1954; Shapiro and Shapiro 1997a; Kaptchuk 1998a, 1998b), it was the first study to rigorously quantify the effects of placebos across a variety of diseases and disorders. Applying recently developed meta-analytic methods to the data sets of fifteen clinical trials involving 1082 patients, with a view to quantifying precisely the patient responses to placebos, Beecher concluded that the placebo effect is powerful, pervasive, and more than merely a psychological phenomenon. Placebos, he argued, cause measurable physiological changes in patients, and some of these were greater than those caused by pharmacological agents or medical interventions. Beecher estimated that approximately 35% of patients in all medical treatments responded to placebo treatments.

Because of its power and pervasiveness, Beecher warned that clinicians and experimenters needed to be careful about the potentially confounding effects of placebos when attempting to determine the effectiveness of a drug or medical treatment. The most effective method to sift out placebo responders from nonplacebo responders is through randomized placebo controlled clinical trials—the so-called gold standard of clinical research, and a newly emerging methodology in the 1950s. 'Any hidden placebo effects operating in an active treatment arm could then be unmasked by measuring the magnitude of the effect in the placebo control arm—and could then be subtracted from your active treatment data' (Harrington 2002: 42).

In the relatively short span of ten years, from World War II to 1955, the placebo underwent a profound transformation from a harmless tool aimed at placating anxious patients—a 'humble humbug', in the words of the editor of a leading medical journal—to a powerful therapeutic intervention and a centerpiece of the randomized controlled trial (Kaptchuck 1998a). This brought in its wake other profound transformations. Corresponding to the new way of thinking about placebos was a new way of conceiving therapeutic efficacy. Prior to the randomized placebo-controlled trial, therapeutic efficacy was tied to beneficial outcomes, using the patient's original condition as a baseline from which to measure improvement. With the advent of the randomized placebo-controlled trial, therapeutic efficacy was relativized to placebo outperformance. 'No longer was it sufficient for a therapy to work: it had to be better than placebo. For the first time in history... method became more important than outcome' (Kaptchuck 1998a: 1724; Kaptchuck 2002). This was not the only major transformation. Corresponding to this new way of conceiving therapeutic efficacy was a new approach to medical ethics, with the emphasis placed squarely on the informed consent of patients rather than on the principle of beneficence.

Beecher's paper, however, was as influential as it was flawed. One of the problems was statistical in nature. In some instances, what appears to be therapeutic change due to placebo is really no more than an artifact of the *measurement* of therapeutic change: that is, regression to the mean. Diseases and disorders are rarely static: they tend to wax and wane over time. This complicates their measurement, and hence the statistical inferences made on the basis of those measurements. People suffering from a disease or disorder tend to seek medical help when the symptoms are at their worst; they tend not to seek help when their symptoms are waning. In randomized placebo-controlled clinical trials involving large patient populations, it is not uncommon for patients to be screened and selected for the trial precisely when their presenting symptoms are waxing. It is also not uncommon for patients whose symptoms are waning to fail to meet the inclusion criteria for the trial. Thus when the first objective measurements of the patients' conditions are taken, in order to establish baseline states, it is often the extreme symptoms that are recorded. Statistically, however, it is quite common for later measurements to be less extreme than the earlier measurements. It may seem then that the therapeutic improvement of those patients assigned to the placebo group is a clear case of the placebo effect. Without further evidence, however, this would be an unfounded inference. The appearance of placebo-driven therapeutic improvement might in fact be a case of regression to the mean: 'the phenomenon that a variable extreme on its first measurement will tend to be closer to the center of the distribution for a later measurement' (Davis 2002; see also Davis 1976; Senn 1988). Galton (1886; cited in Davis 2002) first described regression to the mean, or what he called 'regression toward mediocrity', in his study of hereditary stature: 'It is some years since I made an extensive series of experiments on the produce of different seeds of different size but of the same species... It appeared from these experiments that the offspring did not tend to resemble their parent seeds in size, but to be always more mediocre than they were—to be smaller than the parents, if the parents were larger; to be larger than the parents, if the parents were small.' Galton concluded that 'the filial regression towards mediocrity was directly proportional to the parent deviation from it'.

Regression to the mean is a purely mathematical property of correlated data. It is a statistical artifact of measurement that has nothing to do with the quirks of human psychology or physiology. Nonetheless, it can be confounded with placebo effects in clinical trials, especially in those trials (and meta-analyses) that do not include no-treatment arms. The confound occurs when a statistical phenomenon that affects all measurements of large patient populations is interpreted as a placebo effect. Some statisticians have argued that *most* clinical trials have skewed results, because they attribute to placebo effect what is really regression to the mean (McDonald *et al.* 1983). This may be overstating it. But it points to an important conceptual distinction that needs to be integrated into the design of clinical trials, and into any discussion of placebo effects. 'Any research designed to measure a placebo effect must carefully consider how regression to the mean might influence the results... Future studies to quantify the magnitude of the placebo effect in various settings can benefit from study designs and data-analytic methods commonly used to estimate treatment effects in randomized, double-blind, controlled clinical trials in the presence of regression' (Davis 2002: 165).

Confusing regression to the mean with the placebo effect was just one of the flaws in Beecher's meta-analysis. Perhaps the most significant problem with his meta-analysis of the fifteen clinical trials is that all but one of the trials failed to include a no-treatment control group. Without this, it is not possible to conclude definitively that there was *any* clear placebo effect, since the improvement of patients in the placebo control groups might have been caused by the random fluctuation of symptoms or the natural history of the (untreated) disease or disorder, rather than by the placebo (Kiene 1993a, 1993b; Ernst and Resch 1995; Kienle and Kiene 1997; Kaptchuk 1998a, 1998b). One of the clinical trials reviewed by Beecher, for example, showed that after taking a placebo medication, 35% of patients with colds (that had started six days earlier) felt better within two days. But people with colds often get better within six to eight days without any treatment at all, so some of those patients who got better after taking the placebo medication may have improved anyways, without the placebo. Any conclusions about the 'powerful placebo', in other words, must first show that placebos outperform the no-treatment condition. Beecher's error is not uncommon. Just as credit is sometimes falsely assigned to medical interventions for changes that would have occurred anyways, or that have been caused by factors that have been overlooked and not controlled for, so credit is sometimes falsely assigned to placebo interventions for changes that would have occured anyways, or to other disguised factors. The response that is seen in the placebo arm of a clinical trial is commonly taken to be the true placebo effect: but without controlling for the effects of a number of disguised or neglected therapeutic agents, including the natural history of the disease or disorder, this is an unwarranted inference.

Not surprisingly, a number of trenchant criticisms of Beecher's original placebo study have focused precisely on confounds such as these (Kaptchuk 1998a, 1998b). Kienle and Kiene (1997), for example, identify ten factors, all overlooked by Beecher, that could create the false impression of a powerful placebo effect. These factors include: the natural course of the disease (including spontaneous improvement, fluctuation of symptoms, regression to the mean, habituation), additional treatment, observer bias (including conditional switching of treatment, scaling bias, poor definition of drug efficacy), irrelevant response variables, subsiding toxic effects of previous medication, patient bias (including answers of politeness and experimental subordination, conditioned answers, neurotic or psychotic misjudgment), no placebo given at all (including psychotherapy, psychosomatic phenomena, voodoo medicine), uncritical reporting of anecdotes, misquotation, and false assumption of toxic placebo effects created by everyday symptoms, misquotation, and persistence of symptoms (see also Kiene 1993a, 1993b).

Similarly, Ernst and Resch (1995) distinguish between the true placebo effect and the perceived or apparent placebo effect. Like Kienle and Kiene, they identify a number of potentially confounding variables that could easily lead participants and clinicians to make false inferences about the power of the placebo. These include: the natural course of the disease, regression towards the mean, time effects (such as improved investigator skills from one intervention or measurement to the next, seasonal changes, and decreases in 'white coat hypertension' in patients), and unidentified parallel interventions.

Confounding variables such as these do not present insuperable methodological obstacles; nor do they justify the eliminativist conclusion that once these variables are fully taken into account, the placebo effect vanishes into thin air, as little more than a medical fiction (Kienle and Kiene 1997). To reduce the chances of these confounds occurring, Ernst and Resch advocate the use of *three-arm* designs in placebo-controlled trials, with one arm devoted to the no-treatment condition ('provided that there are no ethical objections'). Three-arm controlled clinical trials would allow a comparison of the progress of the experimental (or 'verum') group (which receives the experimental treatment) against the progress of a placebo control group and the progress of a no-treatment control group. The therapeutic effect of the experimental treatment would then be estimated by subtracting the therapeutic effect of the placebo treatment; and the therapeutic effect of the placebo would be estimated by subtracting the rate of autonomous response that is displayed by the no-treatment control arm from the placebo effect. The no-treatment arm would thus help to reveal the effects of the confounding variables. Kirsch and Sapirstein (1998) go one step further: they recommend that clinical trials should adopt a balanced *four-arm* strategy to account for the so-called 'active placebo effect': the experimental group, the placebo control group, the no-treatment group, and the active placebo group. This latter group would receive a placebo that lacks the key ingredients of the experimental treatment, but contains other active substances that produce identical side effects.

These solutions to the problem of confounding variables are promising, and clearly show that more research is needed in the design and implementation of multiple arm clinical trials. Three-arm and four-arm clinical trials that include no-treatment control arms are relatively uncommon. In one literature search conducted by Ernst and Resch (1995), for example, it was found that *fewer than 4 %* of the 318 clinical trials and meta-analyses between 1986 and 1994 included both placebo controls *and* no-treatment controls. The search parameters they used on MEDLINE were sufficiently broad: namely, all clinical trials and meta-analyses published during 1986–1994 that included the words 'placebo' and 'untreated' in their summary. In another literature search, part of a meta-analytic study about the efficacy of antidepressant medications versus placebo in the treatment of depression (Kirsch and Sapirstein 1998), no studies were found that used no-treatment controls. Despite wide-ranging inclusion criteria, and a computer search of PsychLit and MEDLINE databases from 1974 to 1995 using the search terms *drug-therapy* or *pharmacotherapy* or *psychotherapy* or *placebo* and *depression* or *affective disorder*, Kirsch and Sapirstein reported that they were 'not… able to locate any studies [of the efficacy of antidepressant medication] in which pre- and post-treatment assessments of depression were reported for both a placebo group and a no-treatment or wait-list control group. For that reason, we turned to psychotherapy outcome studies, in which the inclusion of untreated control groups is much more common'. But even the literature review of psychotherapy studies of depression that used no-treatment and wait-list controls bore little fruit. The same search of PsychLit and MEDLINE databases from 1974 to 1995 produced only 19 psychotherapy studies that met the inclusion criteria, which included the following: a) the sample was restricted to patients with a primary diagnosis of depression; b) sufficient data were reported or obtainable to calculate within-condition effect sizes; c) data were reported for a wait-list or no-treatment control group; d) participants were assigned to experimental conditions randomly; and e) participants were between the ages of 18 and 75.

Randomized placebo-controlled trials are no longer in their infancy. Given that the first randomized controlled trials were conducted in the 1930s, when placebos and double-blind conditions were joined together in the Gold *et al.* study (1937) of xanthines versus placebo (Gold 1946, 1954; Shapiro and Shapiro 1997a), they can now be considered well into adulthood. Why then are there so few three or four-arm clinical trials that include no-treatment control groups in addition to placebo control groups? Why has such a promising trial design been overlooked in favor of the more conventional two-arm controlled clinical trials? The main causes of the absence are twofold, one methodological and one ethical.

The methodological challenges in the design and measurement of no-treatment control groups appear to be as daunting as those facing placebo control groups. The purpose of no-treatment control groups is the observation of people who receive no treatment of any sort: no experimental treatments, no placebo treatments, and no parallel hidden treatments. The disease or disorder is allowed to follow its natural course, thus providing a baseline against which the interventions used in the experimental group and the placebo group can be measured. But what is it to receive no treatment? Is there such a thing? And is there such a thing as a natural history of disease? The act of recruiting and assigning participants to no-treatment control groups may itself have positive or negative effects, thereby altering the otherwise natural course of the observed disorders or diseases. This is true of diagnosis as well. If diagnosis is itself a kind of treatment (Brody and Waters 1980), then the act of screening and diagnosing participants for studies in which they might be assigned to a no-treatment control would itself constitute a kind of treatment, albeit a degraded or incipient one. This too would violate the condition that participants receive no treatment. Conversely, assignment to a no-treatment control group might exacerbate feelings of hopelessness in some people, especially those suffering from depressive disorders (Kirsch and Sapirstein 1988). This too could alter the course of the depression in ways that would not have occurred had participants not been exposed to any treatment. Again, if assignment to a no-treatment control involves placement on a wait-list, then the expectation of future treatment could trigger a placebo response (Frank and Frank 1991). Participants assigned to no-treatment control groups are not blind to the experimental conditions, and so like the participants in the experimental and placebo control groups, they may come to form expectations about their condition and their treatment which bias the results in ways that would not have occurred had they not been assigned to any group at all. No-treatment controls, in other words, are vulnerable to some of the same confounding variables and sampling biases to which placebo controls are vulnerable.

Given these difficulties, it would be easy to conclude with Moerman that 'except under the most extraordinary circumstances, it is logically and conceptually impossible to have a no-treatment group' in randomized controlled trials (2002a: 26). 'While these people [assigned to no-treatment control groups] have not had pills, they have had a good deal more than 'nothing'(2002a:26; see also Kleinman et al. 2002: 15). The only true no-treatment control group, Moerman argues, would be one in which participants did not know that they had been assigned to a no-treatment control group: the recruitment, diagnosis, and assessment of participants would proceed without their awareness, and therefore without their consent. This is not a practical impossibility, but the ethical consequences, Moerman suggests, could be as disastrous as those seen in the infamous Tuskegee Syphilis Study (Jones and Tuskegee Institute 1981).

This brings up the second reason why there are relatively few no-treatment controls in the history of clinical trials: in cases where there are available proven treatments for the disease or disorder under investigation, experimenters and physicians must withhold available proven treatments from participants if they are to observe the disease or disorder in its natural state. But this violates the principle of beneficence, namely, that one 'helps others further important and legitimate interests and abstains from injuring them' (Beauchamp and McCullough 1984: 27). With serious or life-threatening conditions, withholding or delaying treatment could be harmful, or even fatal. With less serious conditions, it could result in needless suffering and hardship—even if participants have given fully informed voluntary consent. Withholding or delaying treatment also restricts physicians' efforts to help patients pursue their own best interests.

Two points are in order. First, Moerman's conclusion that it is logically and conceptually impossible ('except under the most extraordinary circumstances') to have a no-treatment group in randomized controlled trials is overstated. The conclusion rests on two premises: first, that no-treatment is identical to the *absolute absence* of *all* forms of treatment intervention; and second, that only participants who are unaware of having been assigned to no-treatment control groups count as true recipients of no treatment. Both premises are false.

According to the first premise, anything less than the absolute absence of treatment counts as a form of treatment, thus resulting in a distortion of the natural history of a disease or disorder. But there is no need to make the criterion of no-treatment so stringent in order to have a clinically informative comparison group. The idea that there is a state of absolute no-treatment against which no-treatment control groups could be measured for purity is a theoretical fiction, on the same order as the idea (in physics) of a center of gravity or an absolutely flat surface. Nothing could possibly count as a state of absolute no-treatment; even the slightest self-maintaining activity in (say) the experience of a cold would count as treatment (e.g. using a handkerchief for a sneeze or a thermometer to take one's temperature). A more relaxed and clinically realistic criterion of no-treatment would allow that there are grades of treatment and no-treatment, with absolute treatment and absolute no-treatment serving as fictional–theoretic end-points of a continuum. Once treatment is regarded as a matter of more or less rather than all-or-nothing, it is clear that there are significant differences between the treatments participants receive in the experimental group and the 'treatments' they receive in the no-treatment control group. In the latter case, participants 'have had a good deal more than 'nothing' (Moerman 2002a: 26): preliminary contact with experimenters, followed by screening and diagnosis. But they have also had a good deal less than the treatment that is administered to their counterparts in the experimental groups and the placebo groups: no pills or interventions, and weeks with little or no contact with experimenters.

According to the second premise of Moerman's argument, participants assigned to no-treatment control groups must be unaware of their assignment and observation, in order that the condition of no-treatment be satisfied. Anything less than this violates the condition of no-treatment. This is an unnecessarily strict requirement. With many diseases and disorders, onset, course, and duration occur independently of whether participants are aware of being recruited, assigned, and diagnosed for a control group.

The second point concerns the claim that withholding or delaying treatment violates the principle of beneficence, and thus is ethically impermissible. (Such a view would be consistent, for example, with the World Medical Association's *Declaration of Helsinki* (2001). While the *Declaration* does not address the specific issue of no-treatment controls, it equates the use of placebo controls with the withholding of treatment). Is it ethically impermissible to withhold or delay treatment? There are, clearly, cases where it is: life-threatening conditions, irreversible fatal diseases, conditions where there would be irreversible harm without treatment, vulnerable patient populations, and patients who are too incapacitated to give fully informed consent. But is it ethically impermissible to withhold or delay treatment in all cases and for all health conditions? Withholding or delaying treatment occurs every day. Patients routinely make well-informed decisions to not receive medical treatment for non-life-threatening conditions such as irritable bowel syndrome, allergies, headache, colds, phobias, anxiety, and depressive moods (Temple 2002). A much smaller subset of patients even make well-informed decisions to forego medical treatment for life-threatening conditions. The reasons justifying these decisions are various: skepticism about the efficacy of available treatments, the preference to let self-limiting symptoms run their course, the desire to avoid the side effects of treatments, and so on. When these decisions are not the result of coercion, irrational beliefs or fears, or economic hardship, and when they are based on a reasonable understanding of the health consequences and the level of suffering that might be entailed, they can be considered to be expressions of patients' autonomy. If patients are capable of making these autonomous decisions about their own health care, once certain minimal conditions have been fulfilled, there is no reason why they cannot make similarly autonomous decisions about participation in no-treatment control groups in clinical trials. Temple makes a similar point with respect to patients enlisting in trials using placebo controls: 'if patients are not able, and cannot be trusted, to make the decision to defer symptomatic treatment of a condition they are usually very familiar with, they are no better prepared, ethically, to participate in an active control trial (giving up assured standard therapy in favor of a less tested agent)' (Temple 2002: 212).

What are the minimal conditions that must be fulfilled? a) Patients must be fully informed of the health consequences of participation in a no-treatment control group; b) patients must not be deceived or coerced; c) there must be no potential for irreversible harm to patients; d) patients must not be suffering from life-threatening conditions, irreversible fatal diseases, or conditions of serious morbidity; e) there must be early escape mechanisms for opting out of the trial once a pre-established level of discomfort has been reached.

Explanatory Approaches

As is typical with core explanatory concepts in the medical sciences, there has emerged since Beecher's famous paper a rich proliferation of explanatory theories of the placebo effect, coming from disciplines as diverse as biomedicine, neurobiology, cognitive neuropsychology, psychoneuroimmunology, medical anthropology, social psychology, evolutionary psychology, psychiatry, and the history and philosophy of medicine. Harrington identifies a number of explanatory approaches that have appeared since the 1950s (Harrington 1997, 2002):

- The individual differences approach. Some early placebo researchers argued that placebo responsiveness could be correlated with certain types of personality. So-called 'placebo reactors' were characterized by different researchers in this tradition as highly suggestible, neurotic, highly hypnotizable, weak in reality testing skills, repressive, hysterical, and submissive. Few clear results have emerged from this research tradition.

- The interpersonal dynamics approach. Some placebo researchers argued that rather than focusing only on the patient as the site of the placebo effect, the placebo effect must be understood in terms of the complex interpersonal dynamics of the physician–patient relationship. Shapiro (1969) and Brody (1997), for example, argued that physicians were themselves powerful placebos, independently of the specific treatments they provided patients. Frank and Frank (1991), Strupp (1972a, 1972b, 1979) and others argued that interpersonal emotions such as hope, trust, caring, and compassion, which play a central role in all healer–patient relationships, are central components of the placebo response.

- The perceptual filtering approach. Some placebo researchers who were skeptical of reports about the physiological changes putatively induced by placebos argued that the placebo effect could be explained in terms of patients' perceptual filtering and misattribution. According to this approach, patients who respond to placebos are typically motivated to get better and to please their physicians, and in doing so they tend to foreground beneficial changes, which they attribute to the placebo, while filtering out negative changes (Gibbons and Hormuth 1981; Ross and Olson 1981). Placebos affect subjective states of awareness, but not physiological states.

◆ The neurobiological approach. Some placebo researchers argued that the placebo effect, particularly analgesic placebo response, can be understood in neurobiological terms as the activation of endorphins, the brain's own natural painkillers (Levine *et al.* 1978). With the development of functional imaging techniques, positron emission tomography, functional magnetic resonance imaging, and other methods for mapping brain states, more and more of the placebo effect is yielding to neurobiological explanation, and is appearing to be a function of endogenous pharmaceutics (Fields and Price 1997; Benedetti *et al.* 2005).

◆ The conditioning approach. Some placebo researchers have argued that the placebo response resembles the response to a conditioned stimulus. The various psychoneuroimmunological processes involved in the 'training' or 'learning' of the immune system as it is affected by both active and inert substances can be explained in terms of classical conditioning theory or nonconscious associative learning processes (Ader 1997; Ader and Cohen 1975).

◆ The meaning making approach. Some medical anthropologists and philosophers have argued that placebo effects can be understood in terms of cultural practices of meaning making (Brody 1997; Hahn and Kleinman 1983; Moerman 2002a, 2002b, 2002c). The placebo effect is a meaning response, which can activate biological processes and enhance the effectiveness of *bona fide* medications. 'The meaning response is the psychological and physiological effects of meaning in the treatment of illness' (Moerman 2002a: 14).

◆ The logic of expectation approach. Some placebo researchers have argued that placebo effects can be explained in terms of a logic of expectation in which cultural conceptions of the effectiveness of medications, or imagined expectations, can override their pharmacological action (Montaigne 2003; Kirsch 1985, 1997, 1999, 2005; Humphrey 2002; Kihlstrom 2003; see also Benedetti *et al.* 2003). Patients' knowledge about and expectations of a therapy affect the therapy outcome.

One *apparently* useful way to frame these multiperspectival approaches to the study of the placebo effect is to see them as straddling the divide between two radically different approaches to the human and behavioral sciences: the interpretive approach, which focuses on the meanings and intentions of agents, and the natural scientific approach, which focuses on the causal mechanisms of natural processes. Using this conceptual frame, the interpersonal dynamics approach and the meaning making approach would fall into the former category (with certain exceptions: see Brody 1997), and the neurobiological approach and conditioning approach would fall into the latter category. Harrington (1997: 8) for instance hints at this: 'because placebos as a phenomenon seem to hover ambiguously at the crossroads between these two perspectives, they are at once a frustration and a wonderful challenge'.

This way of carving up intellectual geography into meaning versus mechanism, and understanding versus explanation, is an old one, with roots in nineteenth-century thought, especially Dilthey's distinction between the *Geisteswissenschaften* and the *Natuurwissenschaften*. Iterations of the distinction are found in the writings of Wittgenstein, Winch, Geertz, Taylor, Sartre, Ricoeur, Gadamer, Luria and others.

A simplified and highly generic version of the interpretive approach holds that human beings are fundamentally different from the law-governed processes of nature; and that natural scientific methods, and natural scientific standards of observation, measurement, and explanation do not apply to the study of human beings. The understanding of human beings must be couched in terms of the language of intentions and meanings, which are not the same as, or reducible to, causes. Entirely different explanatory standards must therefore apply. By contrast, a simplified and generic version of the natural scientific approach holds that the scientific methods used in the study of natural processes can be applied successfully to the study of human beings; and that the explanatory and observational standards of natural science are applicable to the human and behavioral sciences.

But the distinction between the interpretive and the natural scientific approaches is a useful conceptual frame in appearance only, not only because the distinction proves difficult to draw when examined up close (Held 2007), but because the frame itself can give the misleading impression that *only* these two approaches exist, and that there must be a forced choice between them. Uncritical adoption of the frame can interfere with seeing other perhaps less dichotomous ways of making sense of the placebo phenomenon (Kleinman *et al.* 2002). In a later publication Harrington (2002: 50–51) suggests going beyond this distinction altogether: 'something that started out as a humble humbug in medicine [the placebo] just could end up being an impetus both for a foundational rethinking of legacies that no longer work, and for the imaginative development of new research programs that have more room for all of what we are as human beings, inside and outside, mind and body, meaning and mechanism'.

Not surprisingly with such a wide proliferation of explanatory theories, definitions of the placebo and the placebo effect also proliferate. There is no universally agreed-upon definition (or concept) of the placebo and the placebo effect. Narrow definitions of the placebo effect, for example, run the risk of being overly restrictive: they omit a large realm of placebo phenomena. Wide definitions, on the other hand, run the risk of smuggling in theories of causation and mechanism (Brody 1997), thereby falling prey to question-begging assumptions. To complicate matters, there is no universal agreement about which clinical phenomena even ought to be designated as placebo effects. Even the attempt to characterize the placebo effect by enumeration of prototypical examples is fraught with difficulties. Take for example some of the following brief definitions, arranged chronologically.

- Shapiro (1964) defines a placebo as a procedure that is without specific activity for the condition being evaluated.
- O'Leary and Borkovec (1978) define the placebo as a condition for which there is 'no currently supported theoretical reason why...[it] would influence the behavior under question'.
- Critelli and Newman (1985) define placebo factors (in psychotherapy) as factors that are common to most types of therapy, such as expectancy of improvement, credibility of rationale, and perceived belief by therapists in their treatment procedures.
- Grünbaum (1994) defines a placebo as a therapy for which none of the characteristic factors are remedial for the specified target disorders, but the target disorders are nonetheless improved because of the effect of the therapy's incidental factors.
- Moerman (2002a, 2002b, 2002c) defines the placebo effect as a meaning response, which is the psychological and physiological effect of meaning in the origin and treatment of illness.
- Bootzin and Caspi (2002) define the placebo effect as a dynamic, constantly changing variable co-varying with other variables, both psychological and physical, that operate in the therapeutic process. The interaction of variables is not predictable, but they operate synergistically in active treatments.

Not only is there no universally-agreed-upon definition of the placebo and the placebo effect: there is also widespread disagreement about the precise psycho–physical status of placebos and placebo effects, and their bearing on the mind–body relation. Some placebo researchers deny that placebos can bring about 'real' changes to physical conditions: the placebo effect, it is claimed, is an entirely psychological phenomenon. Others have taken the placebo effect as evidence that psychological states such as expectation, hope, and faith can somehow interact with neurochemical pathways. More radically, some have even denied that placebo effects exist. Hróbjartsson and Gøtzsche (2001), for instance, claim that the placebo effect is little more than a medical legend.

To add to the difficulty, placebo effects have proven elusive to study under controlled experimental conditions, despite the widespread use of placebos in randomized controlled clinical trials to test the effectiveness of medications. One reason for this elusiveness is that controls would be needed to rule out alternative explanations of the effects of placebos. That is, just as placebo controls are routinely called upon to identify a drug's effects, so another control group would be needed to show that changes in the placebo control are due to the placebo, and not to non-placebic factors such as spontaneous remission or regression to the mean (Cardena and Kirsch 2000). But this other control group would have to receive neither the drug being tested nor the placebo.

Grünbaum argues that the standard technical vocabularies used to define placebo therapies and experimental placebos are confusing and obscure, and sorely in need of conceptual rigor: 'the medical and psychiatric literature on placebos and their effects is conceptually bewildering, to the point of being a veritable Tower of Babel' (1986: 19). There is no doubt that a greater degree of conceptual rigor needs to be brought to placebo research. But the price should not be a conceptual or definitional straitjacket. The proliferation of definitions (and imbedding explanatory theories) may be confusing, but it is also a valuable source of conceptual growth and disciplinary cross-fertilization. This is a virtue rather than a lamentable flaw, given the dynamic nature of the field of placebo research. Conceptual proliferation is especially important as more comes to be learned about the psychoneuroimmunological conditions of placebo effects, and their interaction with social, cultural, and symbolic conditions. As with all core concepts and categories, the concepts of placebo and placebo effect have what might be called graded structure. At the center of the field are concepts based upon prototypical cases; at the margins are less well-defined or controversial cases (Neisser 1987). Among the proto-typical cases are sugar pills and saline solution injections. These clearly demonstrate the power of inactive substances or procedures to stimulate the native healing processes of patients. But the graded structure of concepts is characterized by a continuum of category representativeness, rather than by black-and-white class membership. This means that there is room for disagreement about the more atypical instances of placebos and placebo effects. The graded structure of these concepts is fluid, so much so that changes at the margins of the field can put pressure on what are considered to be core or prototypical cases.

In addition to displaying graded structure, the concepts of placebo and placebo effect display a dynamic structure. They are, as Critelli and Newman (1984) have argued, 'constructs in transition', with ancient beginnings

(Shapiro and Shapiro 1997a), a turbulent adolescence (once they entered medicine), and an uncertain future. Like other core concepts in medicine, they have evolved and devolved over time, with emerging conceptualizations going hand in hand with emerging medical technologies, emerging methods of medical measurement, and emerging conceptions of therapeutic efficacy, all of which in turn go hand in hand with emerging cultural understandings of illness and health. To complicate the search for adequate definitions even more, it is conceivable that culturally dominant definitions of placebo themselves influence placebo effects at the clinical level. That is, with changes in the conceptualization of placebo from one generation to the next go changes in the nature and scope of the placebo effect from one generation of patient to the next. The idea of a single finalized definition of placebo and placebo effect is an abstract philosophical ideal.

With these qualifications in mind, consider now the definitions of placebo developed by Shapiro, Grünbaum, and Brody. Each one offers a robust and clear account of the placebo, each one builds upon the other, and each one addresses the concern that placebo research is a bewildering Tower of Babel.

Shapiro's Definition of Placebo

Shapiro's (1964) and Shapiro and Morris' (1978) definition of placebo is one of the most well-known definitions in circulation—so much so that it has also become well-established in medical literature. Versions of it appear, for instance, in Goodman and Gilman's (Nies 1990) text on pharmacological therapeutics, and in Dorland's *Illustrated Medical Dictionary*. The definition seems to capture a number of the more prototypical features of the phenomena. Moreover, the central distinction contained in the definition—between specific and nonspecific effects—is *prima facie* plausible.

In one of his earliest papers on the subject, Shapiro (1964) writes: 'A placebo is defined as any therapeutic procedure (or a component of any therapeutic procedure) which is given i) deliberately to have an effect, or ii) unknowingly and has an effect on a symptom, syndrome, disease, or patient but which is objectively without specific activity for the condition being treated. The placebo is also used as an adequate control in research. The placebo effect is defined as the changes produced by placebos'.

Shapiro and Morris (1978) revise this early definition of placebo slightly. A placebo is defined as 'any therapy or component of therapy that is deliberately used for its nonspecific, psychological, or psychophysiological effects, or that is used for its presumed specific effect, but is without specific activity for the condition being treated' (Shapiro and Morris 1978: 371–372). A placebo *control* is defined as 'a substance or procedure that is without specific activity for the condition being evaluated'. A placebo *effect* is defined as 'the psychological or psychophysiological effect produced by placebos'. This definition too has undergone slight modifications in response to critics (Shapiro and Shapiro 1997a, 1997b).

Shapiro and Morris add qualifications to their definition. They note that some therapeutically effective specific treatments contain placebo components, and some therapeutic results are a function of the combination of both placebo and nonplacebo effects. Thus they distinguish between pure placebos, which are treatments that have no active and specific components, and that may be considered to serve as prototypical exemplars, and impure placebos, which are therapies that contain some nonplacebo components, and are located at the margins of placebo phenomena. Between these two end-points lies a continuum that measures grades of placebo representativeness. Those treatments that have specific components but exert their effects primarily through non-specific mechanisms are placebo therapies.

Shapiro and Morris claim that until relatively recently, the history of medical treatment has really been a history of placebo effects. As with all medical treatments, the pharmacological substances and surgical interventions of ancient, medieval, and early modern medicine were used for their presumed specific effects on target disorders. These disorders were identified under the relevant therapeutic theories and nosological categories of the time. Most of the treatments exerted no discernible specific activity for the conditions they treated. And most of the explanatory theories were false. Whatever effectiveness displayed by the treatments was thus a function of nonspecific, psychological, or psychophysiological effects.

The concept carrying most of the burden in Shapiro and Morris' definition of placebo is that of 'specific activity'. This is also the weakest part of the definition. Specific activity is characterized vaguely as 'the therapeutic influence attributable solely to the contents or processes of the therapies rendered. The criterion for specific activity (and therefore the placebo effect) should be based on scientifically controlled studies' (1978: 372). The specific activity of a drug such as aspirin, for example, produces specific, nonplacebo effects on a specified target disorder (e.g. a headache). Psychological factors, such as the arousal of hope, the expectation of cure, or physician charisma, produce nonspecific, placebo effects on a specified target disorder.

Shapiro and Morris' characterization of the placebo effect is a useful first approximation, and it has some bearing on the current hypothesis about psychodynamic placebos. But it leaves a number of questions unanswered. What *precisely* is 'specific activity?' What is a 'specific effect?' On what grounds is specific activity distinguished from non-specific activity? What is the role of the therapist's intentions in the administering of a placebo? Are placebos always deliberate, or are some inadvertent? One obvious problem with the definition is that placebos do have specific effects, and do appear to exert a specific activity for certain conditions. They are far from inert.

Grünbaum's Definition of Placebo

Grünbaum's (1994) analysis of the concept of placebo addresses some of these questions. It adds a further degree of conceptual clarity to Shapiro and Morris' characterization, and captures several other prototypical features of the concept.

Grünbaum uses the term 'incidental' to characterize the relevant placebo components of a therapy, rather than the more ambiguous term 'nonspecific', which connotes indistinctness. There is good reason for this: the effects of placebos can be just as sharply defined and delimited as the effects of nonplacebos; and they can be just as precisely described as the effects of nonplacebos. For example, the therapeutic effect of a sugar pill placebo on a headache can be just as specific as the effect that would have been produced by an active drug such as aspirin (1994: 308). To describe it as nonspecific is misleading. According to Grünbaum, the distinction between placebos and nonplacebos is not based on the distinction between nonspecificity and specificity, but on the question of whether the therapy's putatively characteristic factors play a therapeutic role for the target disorders.

Grünbaum also notes that it is not only patients who are unaware that the treatments they are receiving are placebos. The physicians who administer placebos may mistakenly believe that they are administering therapeutically effective treatments, when in fact they are administering placebos. There is therefore a distinction between intentional placebos and inadvertent placebos— a distinction not captured by Shapiro and Morris' definition. Something counts as an *intentional* placebo if: i) none of the characteristic constituents of the therapy (as specified by the therapeutic theory) are remedial for the disorder; ii) if the physician or therapist believes that none of the specific constituents are remedial; and iii) if the physician or therapist believes that the treatment method is remedial by virtue of other incidental aspects of the treatment. By contrast, something counts as an *inadvertent* placebo if: i) none of the characteristic constituents of the therapy are remedial for the disorder; ii) if the therapist believes that the treatment method is remedial for the disorder by virtue of its characteristic constituents (as specified by the therapeutic theory); and iii) if the patient believes that the treatment method is remedial for the disorder by virtue of its characteristic constituents. The distinction between inadvertent and deliberate placebo is not fixed: a placebo treatment that is considered inadvertent by one therapeutic theory may be considered an intentional placebo by another.

Grünbaum's analysis of the concept of placebo is summarized in the following diagram, which depicts both placebo and nonplacebo therapies. The diagram shows two poles connected by lines representing causal relations. Located at one pole of the dyadic relation is the therapeutic theory ψ, the therapy t, the characteristic factors F of t, and the incidental factors C of t. At the other pole is the patient, his or her target disorders D, and other facets of the patient's health.

The therapeutic theory ψ is the overarching theory under which the patient's disease or disorder is diagnosed, explained, and treated: for example, the theory of classical Freudian psychoanalysis. The therapeutic theory ψ recommends a particular treatment t for a particular target disorder D, which is identified in terms of theory ψ's nosology, and explained in terms of ψ's etiology. The therapeutic treatment t is not homogeneous in structure and function: it contains a spectrum of different ingredients or treatment factors, which can be divided roughly into two classes. Some ingredients are 'characteristic factors': that is, what the therapeutic theory ψ identifies as the defining characteristics of a given type of therapy t, without which the therapy would not be distinguishable from other therapies. The therapeutic theory ψ also allows that the treatment t contains ingredients that are not defining characteristics: that is, incidental factors. This includes factors that have not yet been identified *as* incidental.

Located at the other pole of the dyad are the patient's life processes, the target disorders D, and other facets of the patient's health. While the target disorders are conceptually distinguished from the rest of the patient's life processes, there may be an unavoidable degree of vagueness in establishing clear boundaries between the two.

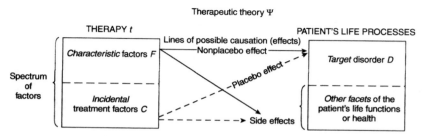

Fig. 4.1 Illustration of therapeutic theory ψ, used in clarifying the definition of 'placebo'. Reproduced with permission from A. Grünbaum (1986). The placebo effect in medicine and psychiatry. *Psychological Medicine (England)*, **16**, 19–38.

Between the two poles (the therapy t, and the patient's life processes) is a web of causal relations, with arrows representing the possible causal influences that may result from the two sets of treatment factors. The characteristic factors F of therapy t follow three possible causal pathways: they may be remedial for D, they may have no effect on D, or they may have deleterious effects on other facets of the patient's functions. Similarly, the characteristic factors F may have these same influences on other facets of the patient's health. These count as side effects.

A therapy counts as a nonplacebo if one or more of the characteristic factors F have a positive therapeutic or remedial effect on the target disorder D. A therapy counts as a placebo if none of the characteristic factors F are remedial for target disorders D, but the target disorders D are nonetheless improved because of the effect of incidental factors C. (The incidental factors C may or may not have positive or negative effects on D; they may also have desirable or undesirable effects outside of D, which are side effects). Thus the question of whether or not a positive therapeutic effect on the target disorder D is a placebo effect 'depends on whether it is produced by the incidental treatment factors or the characteristic ones' (Grünbaum 1994: 293).

On Grünbaum's analysis, then, a necessary and sufficient condition for something being a placebo is that *none* of the characteristic treatment factors F of the treatment t are remedial for target disorders D. What is significant here is that the concept of placebo effect is relativized to a particular therapeutic theory and to a particular disorder. Placebo effects only make sense in terms of a particular therapeutic theory which hypothesizes that factors xyz are characteristic factors, and which hypothesizes that such-and-such is a disorder. Independently of such theories, there are no such things as placebo effects. If, *per impossibile*, human history had evolved in such a way that there were no therapeutic theories (and by implication no theorists), then there would be no placebo effects. A treatment gain counts as a placebo effect with respect to a particular therapeutic theory ψ only when the remedial effect is caused by treatment factors other than those which ψ hypothesizes to be characteristically efficacious for the disorder.

Grünbaum's definition of placebo has been criticized for: i) failing to give an adequate place to patient and therapist expectancies, considered by some theorists to be the defining feature of the placebo effect; and ii) failing to acknowledge that placebo control treatments must be theoretically conceived and constructed in terms of factors considered to be characteristic from the point of view of an alternative therapeutic theory (Greenwood 1996, 1997; see Grünbaum 1996 and Erwin 1996b for replies to Greenwood). Moreover, Grünbaum's definition may have the unwanted effect of ruling out certain marginal placebo phenomena as nonplacebos, or admitting certain core nonplacebo phenomena as marginal placebos. Take, for example, a medication M with fifteen characteristic factors F, and fifteen incidental factors C. Only one characteristic factor F is remedial for D; the rest are inert. But suppose that the one active factor F is weak. It exerts only a very slight remedial effect on D. All fifteen incidental factors C, however, are active. According to Grünbaum's analysis, the medication M would be considered a nonplacebo, because at least one characteristic factor F is remedial. But this is a case where it would be ill-advised to consider the medication a nonplacebo. M is *mainly* a placebo. Grünbaum's definition may be better served by distinguishing between grades of remedial activity; and by locating grades of remedial activity on a continuum. Some characteristic factors F display low degrees of remedial activity; some display none at all; others display very high degrees.

Despite these problems, Grünbaum's analysis of the concept of placebo is helpful for understanding how some psychodynamic insights and interpretations might function as placebos. A psychodynamic psychotherapy is characterized by an overarching therapeutic theory ψ (e.g. the theory of classical Freudian psychoanalysis, the theory of Horneyian psychoanalysis) that recommends a specific treatment method t (e.g. analysis) for a particular target disorder D (e.g. neurotic anxiety)—insofar as disorder D is identified under the nosological component of the therapeutic theory. The treatment t identifies both characteristic factors F (e.g. analysis, free association, dream analysis, analytic interpretations, analysand insight and so on) and incidental factors C (e.g., a charismatic analyst, the payment of a high fee for the analysis, and any number of common therapeutic factors that may serve as catalysts for the patient's receptivity to the treatment).

According to the Standard View's principle of exploratory validity, and the principle of therapeutically effective insight, one of the characteristic factors of the treatment method of psychodynamic psychotherapy is the client's acquisition of veridical insights into the etiology of the target disorders D. A psychodynamic psychotherapy would count as a nonplacebo if one or more of its characteristic factors F have a remedial effect on the target disorders D. Thus, if the acquisition of veridical insights had a remedial effect on D, the therapy would count as a nonplacebo. Grünbaum's example of classical Freudian psychoanalysis illustrates this: 'the patient's correct, affect-discharging insight into the aetiology of his or her affliction is the one quintessential ingredient that distinguishes the remedial dynamics of his treatment modality from any kind of treatment by suggestion. Treatments by suggestion, [Freud] charged, leave the pathogenic repressions intact, and yield only an ephemeral cosmetic prohibition of the symptoms' (Grünbaum 1994: 295).

According to Grünbaum's definition of placebo, a psychodynamic psychotherapy would count as a placebo if none of the characteristic factors F of the treatment method had a positive therapeutic or remedial effect on the target disorders D, but the disorders nonetheless improved because of the effect of incidental factors C. If the acquisition of veridical insights into the etiology of the disorders—one of the characteristic factors of t, according to the principle of therapeutically effective insight—does not have a remedial effect on the target disorders, and yet the treatment has a remedial effect on them, then the therapy counts as a placebo. More specifically, if the acquisition of veridical insights into the etiology of the target disorders D has remedial effects on D for reasons other than the truth-value of the insights (e.g. aesthetic considerations, doctrinal compliance), then the insights count as placebos. Similarly, if the acquisition of false or fictitious insights into the etiology of target disorders D has remedial effects on D, then the insights count as placebos.

Brody's Definition of Placebo

Brody (1980, 1985) offers another important definition of the concept of placebo, one which captures certain dimensions of the phenomenon not captured by Shapiro and Grünbaum's definitions, and one that diverges in important ways from both in its relativization of the concept of placebo to belief states. Brody notes the shortcomings of Grünbaum's definition: it does not define the term 'remedial', and it does not define the term 'placebo effect', other than claiming that it is the effect produced by placebos. Brody keeps the definition of the two terms separate, and makes the definition of the placebo effect the central definition (rather than vice versa).

Brody's (1985) definitions of placebo and placebo effect are as follows:

1. t is a therapy for target disorder D if and only if it is believed that the administration of t to a person with D increases the empirical probability that D will be cured, relieved, or ameliorated, as compared to the probability that this will occur without t.

2. t is a specific therapy for D if and only if:
   a) t is a therapy for D;
   b) there is a class A of conditions such that D is a subclass of A and that for all members of A, t is a therapy;
   c) there is a class B of conditions such that for all members of B, t is not a therapy; and class B is much larger than class A.

3. A 'placebo effect' occurs for person V if and only if:

   a) V has condition D;

   b) V believes that he or she is within a healing context (i.e. the sociocul-turally approved setting, with its associated rituals and practitioners, that is identified by V as a healing context);

   c) V is administered a particular treatment t as part of that context, where t is either the total active intervention or some component of that intervention;

   d) target disorder D is changed;

   e) the change in D is attributable to the symbolic import of t and not to any specific therapeutic effect of t or to any known pharmacological or physiological property of t.

4. A 'placebo' is:

   a) a form of medical therapy, or an intervention designed to simulate medical therapy, that at the time of use is believed not to be a specific therapy for the condition for which it is offered and that is used either for its psychological effect or to eliminate observer bias in an experi-mental setting;

   b) (by extension from a) a form of medical therapy now believed to be inefficacious, though believed efficacious at the time of use.

One of the primary differences between Grünbaum's definition and Brody's definition focuses on the role of belief. Grünbaum's definition labels as the generic objective *property* of being a placebo the failure of a treatment to be remedial for a particular target disorder by means of any of the characteristic factors of the treatment. The term 'remedial' is undefined. The failure of a treatment to be remedial is an objective property: a treatment is remedial regardless of what patients or practitioners believe about a treatment. Brody's definition on the other hand takes patient and practitioner belief as central: whether a treatment t is a placebo depends on whether it is *believed* by patient and practitioner at the time to be efficacious or not. This has the virtue of incorporating references to the symbolic effects of treatment, and the treat-ment's influence on the patient's imagination, beliefs, or emotions. It also recognizes the relativity of the placebo effect to the dominant biomedical theory, to physician beliefs, and to patient beliefs.

With its emphasis on the belief states of patients and physicians, Brody's definition falls within the broad meaning model of placebos (Brody 1980; Brody 1997; Moerman 2002a). According to this model, the placebo response occurs when: a) the *meaning* of the illness experience for the patient is altered in a positive manner, given the patient's belief system and world view;

b) the patient is supported by a caring group; and c) the patient's sense of mastery and control over the illness is restored or enhanced.

Like Shapiro and Grünbaum's definitions, Brody's definition of placebo helps to cast light on how psychodynamic insights and interpretations might function as placebos. A psychodynamic psychotherapy consists of a particular treatment modality t for a particular target disorder D. It would count as a nonplacebo if the change in the client's disorders is attributable to some specific therapeutic effect of the treatment. The placebo effect would occur, however, when the client is administered a particular treatment t (e.g. analysis), and experiences a change in D—and yet the change is attributable to the symbolic import of the treatment and not to its specific therapeutic effects. Therapeutic change could come, for example, from the symbolic import of psychodynamic insights and interpretations, rather than from their truth value and psychological accuracy. A psychodynamic psychotherapy would count as a placebo if it were designed to simulate therapy that, at the time of use, is believed not to be a specific therapy for the condition for which it is offered and that is used for its psychological effect; or if it were a therapy now believed to be inefficacious, though believed efficacious at the time of use.

A Cognitive Definition of Placebo

The following definition of the placebo follows Brody's and Moerman's definition insofar as it focuses attention on the *beliefs, feelings*, and *cognitions* of the patients who experience the placebo effect; in addition, it focuses on the beliefs and cognitions of the dispensers of placebos (i.e. doctors, nurses, experimenters), and the cultures in which they exist. Unlike Brody's definition, however, the focus here is primarily on thinking, feeling, and experiencing *subjects* as belief holders, and the resultant interactions between subjects, rather than belief states *per se*. Thinking, feeling, and experiencing subjects, and not belief states, are taken to be the most basic units of analysis in making sense of the placebo effect; and the relation between two or more subjects—namely, doctor and patient—is taken to be one of the most basic units of analysis in making sense of all forms of healing, including placebo treatments. For the sake of economy in the following definition, the term 'subject' will be used instead of the more cumbersome term 'thinking, feeling, and experiencing subject'.

The logical order of dependence in the following definition of the placebo effect is roughly as follows: the placebo effect depends upon cognition (conceived broadly as beliefs, attitudes, thoughts, expectations, memories) and affect, cognition and affect depend upon subjects and subjectivity, and subjects and subjectivity depend upon communities of subjects. This definition adds a further layer to Brody's belief-oriented definition of the placebo effect: namely, the acts of cognition, recognition, and identification that make placebo effects, and medical treatments in general, an interaction *between subjects*. This is not a complete or final definition of the placebo effect; nor is it intended to supplant or exclude other definitions. Rather, it supplies one further dimension to the understanding of the concept of placebo effect, like an additional layer superimposed upon a layering of photographic negatives. The schematic steps in the definition are as follows.

A placebo effect occurs if and only if:

1. The patient is a thinking, feeling, and experiencing subject.
2. The patient is a member of a culture.
3. The patient presents symptoms.
4. The patient stands in a special relation with others who are recognized by the surrounding culture, and by the medical culture, as expert healers or medical authorities.
5. The patient is administered a treatment for his or her disease or disorder by a medical authority or expert healer.
6. The patient's disorder or disease is changed.
7. The change in the disorder or disease is not caused by the hypothesized or theorized characteristic factors of the treatment.
8. The change in the disorder or disease is caused by the incidental factors of the treatment (which could include the patient's belief that he or she will improve with the treatment, or his or her expectation of improvement, or his or her interaction with a medical authority or expert healer).

The expanded definition of placebo effect is as follows.

A placebo effect occurs if and only if:

1.0 The patient is a thinking, feeling, and experiencing subject (i.e. inanimate objects, insects, plants, and some animals do not respond to the administration of placebo).

1.1 The patient is a thinking, feeling, experiencing, and conscious subject (i.e. someone who is asleep, unconscious, or in a comatose state does not respond to the administration of placebo).

1.2 The patient is a holder of robust or nontrivial beliefs (i.e. someone who does not or can not hold beliefs, such as a neonate or someone in a comatose state, does not respond to the administration of placebo).

1.21 The patient is a holder of robust or nontrivial beliefs about themselves, including beliefs about their current and future state of well-being (i.e. a neonate, or someone with severe cognitive impairment does not respond to the administration of placebo).

1.22 The patient has a functioning memory (i.e. someone suffering from dense anterograde and retrograde amnesia, or extensive short-term memory impairment, does not respond to the administration of placebo).

1.23 The patient is capable of experiencing affects such as desires, moods, and emotions (i.e. someone who is incapable of experiencing desires, or emotions such as fear or hope, is not capable of responding to the administration of placebo).

2.0 The patient is a member of a culture (i.e. a hermit or a wild child does not respond to the administration of placebo).

2.1 The patient is recognized as a thinking, feeling, and experiencing subject by others (i.e. someone who loses his or her status as a thinking, feeling, and experiencing subject, or who is excluded from all communities of subjects, or who is regarded only as a thing, is not a possible subject of interpersonal relations).

2.11 The patient recognizes others as thinking, feeling, and experiencing subjects.

2.2 The culture in which the patient belongs has a robust cultural and symbolic history (i.e. someone in a pre-symbolic or nonsymbolic culture would not respond to the administration of placebo).

2.21 The culture's history includes a history of medical treatments (i.e. there are no placebos in cultures devoid of medicine or medical treatments, such as cultures prior to the Neolithic Age (prior to about 8000 BC, when the first surgical procedure (trepanning) was performed and the first evidence of medical theorizing occurred).

3.0 The patient presents symptoms.

3.1 The patient is suffering from symptoms (i.e. someone who is symptomatic but not suffering from symptoms does not respond to the administration of placebo).

3.11 The patient is conscious of suffering from symptoms (i.e. someone who is conscious but not experiencing any significant degree of suffering from symptoms does not respond to the administration of placebo; and someone who is unconscious and suffering from symptoms does not respond to the administration of placebo).

3.2 The patient is suffering from a condition that is recognized and defined as a disease or disorder of such and such a type by the surrounding culture, and by the surrounding medical culture (i.e. a patient does not respond to the administration of placebo for a disorder or disease that is not considered to exist).

4.0 The patient stands in a special relation with others who are recognized by the surrounding culture, and by the medical culture, as expert healers or medical authorities (i.e. someone who has no relation to healers or medical authorities is not in a position to be administered a placebo).

4.01 The patient's relation with the expert healer or medical authority is an emotionally charged relationship, and involves trust and confiding (Frank and Frank 1991).

4.1 The patient believes that he or she is within a healing context (what Brody [1985]) calls the socioculturally approved setting, with its associated rituals and practitioners, that is identified with healing by the patient).

4.2 The patient is recognized by the medical culture and by the attending medical authority or expert healer as a patient.

4.21 The patient recognizes and identifies with the role of patient (i.e. someone who does not recognize, identify with, or find credible the role of patient, does not respond to the administration of placebo).

4.3 The patient is diagnosed as suffering from a specific condition (or conditions) by the medical authority or expert healer (i.e. someone who is not diagnosed as suffering from any specific condition is not in a position to be administered a placebo for that condition).

4.31 The patient believes that he or she is suffering from a specific disease or disorder insofar as it is recognized and defined as such by the medical authority or expert healer, and by the medical culture (i.e. someone who does not believe that he or she is ill, or who regards the diagnosis of his or her condition as incredible, or who lacks the concept of disease, is not in a position to respond to the administration of placebo).

4.32 The patient is given a prognosis of his or her condition (i.e. someone who is given no prognosis is not in a position to form beliefs or hold expectations about a potential treatment's effect on the future course of his or her disease or disorder).

4.4 The patient's condition is such that it is recognized as falling below a baseline state that is considered by the medical culture and by the medical authority or expert healer to be a state of health (i.e. someone who is considered to be well is less likely to respond to the administration of placebo than someone who is considered to be unwell).

4.41 The patient believes that his or her condition falls below a baseline state that is defined as a state of health (i.e. someone who does not consider himself or herself to be unwell (even when 4.4 holds) is less likely to respond to the administration of placebo than someone who considers himself or herself to be unwell).

5.0 The patient is administered a treatment for his or her disease or disorder by a medical authority or expert healer (i.e. someone who is not given a treatment for a diagnosed condition is not in a position to respond to the administration of placebo).

5.01 The treatment involves ingesting certain substances, and/or the performance of a defined sequence of actions, that are recognized by the medical culture and the medical authority or expert healer to be efficacious treatments for the cure or amelioration of the diagnosed condition.

5.02 The treatment consists of a set of factors that the medical authority or expert healer, and the immediately surrounding medical culture, believe, hypothesize, or theorize to be the characteristic factors of the treatment, without which the treatment would not be distinguishable from other treatments (Grünbaum 1986).

5.03 The treatment also consists of a set of factors that the medical authority or expert healer, and the medical culture, believe, hypothesize, or theorize to be the incidental factors of the treatment (Grünbaum 1986).

5.1 The patient recognizes something as a treatment for the cure, relief, or amelioration of his or her condition (i.e. someone who does not identify, recognize, or understand that something is a treatment or potential treatment is not in a position to respond to the administration of placebo).

5.11 The patient believes that he or she has received a treatment for his or her condition (i.e. someone who does not believe that he or she has received any treatment, or who has forgotten that he or she has received a treatment, or who holds significant doubts about whether a treatment has been administered, is not in a position to respond to the administration of placebo).

5.12 The patient believes that the treatment is efficacious for the specific disorder or disease from which he or she suffers (i.e. someone who recognizes a treatment as a treatment, but who holds significant doubts about the treatment's efficacy for his or her specific disorder, is not in a position to respond to the administration of placebo).

5.13 The patient expects that the treatment will be effective in his or her particular case (i.e. someone who believes that he or she has received a treatment that is effective for his or her disorder, but who on other grounds holds no expectations of improving from the treatment, is not in a position to respond to the administration of placebo).

6.0 The patient's disorder or disease is changed (i.e. someone who continues to have symptoms, and continues to suffer from symptoms, has not responded to placebo, if the treatment was a placebo).

6.1 The patient's primary presenting symptoms remit for a period of time that is considered by the culture and the medical culture, and by the attending medical authority or expert healer, to be indicative of the cure, relief, or amelioration of the presenting symptoms.

6.2 The patient is conscious of relief from symptoms.

6.21 The patient believes that the treatment has been efficacious.

6.3 The patient's condition is such that it is recognized as approximating a baseline state that is considered by the medical culture and by the attending medical authority or expert healer to approximate a state of health (i.e. someone who is considered to continue to suffer from the diagnosed disease or disorder has not responded to placebo, if the treatment given was a placebo).

6.31 The patient believes that his or her condition approximates the baseline state that is defined as a state of health (i.e. someone who considers himself or herself to continue to be unwell following a treatment has not responded to placebo).

7.0 The change in the patient's disorder or disease is not caused by the hypothesized or theorized characteristic factors of the treatment (i.e. with pharmaceutical or surgical interventions, the change is not caused by the class of pharmacological or physiological properties believed to be the characteristic factors of the treatment; with psychological interventions, the change is not caused by the class of psychological properties believed to be the characteristic factors of the treatment).

7.1 The change in the patient's disorder or disease is not caused by factors such as the natural course of the disease or disorder, or the random fluctuation of symptoms.

7.2 The change in the patient's disorder or disease is not caused by unidentified parallel interventions.

7.3 The change in the patient's disorder or disease is not confounded with factors such as regression to the mean, observer bias, irrelevant response variables, subsiding toxic effects of previous medications, patient bias (such as answers of politeness and experimental subordination, conditioned answers, neurotic or psychotic misjudgment), and time effects (such as improved investigator skills from one intervention or measurement to the next, seasonal changes, and decreases in 'white coat hypertension' in patients) (Ernst and Resch 1995; Kienle and Kiene 1997; Kaptchuk 1998a, 1998b).

8.0 The change in the disorder or disease is caused by the incidental factors of the treatment (which could include the patient's belief that he or she will improve with the treatment, or his or her expectation of improvement, or his or her interaction with a medical authority or expert healer).

8.1 The patient holds the (mistaken) belief that the change is caused by the characteristic factors of the treatment (i.e. the patient does not believe that the change was caused by his or her believing or expecting that the treatment would be effective, or that it was caused by interacting with a medical authority or expert healer).

8.2 The medical authority or expert healer who administers the treatment either believes that the change in the patient's disorder or disease is caused by the pharmacological or physiological properties of the treatment (an inadvertent placebo), or believes that it is not caused by the pharmacological or physiological properties of the treatment (an intentional placebo).

To summarize, the placebo effect occurs if and only if: 1) the patient is a thinking, experiencing, conscious, belief-holding subject; 2) the patient is a member of a culture; 3) the patient has symptoms; 4) the patient stands in a special relation with others who are recognized by the surrounding culture, and by the medical culture, as expert healers or medical authorities; 5) the patient is administered a treatment for his or her disease or disorder by a medical authority or expert healer; 6) the patient's disorder or disease is changed; 7) the change in the patient's disorder or disease is not caused by the hypothesized characteristic factors of the treatment; 8) the change in the disorder or disease is caused by the incidental factors of the treatment.

There are several advantages of this definition over Shapiro's, Grünbaum's, and Brody's. First, it recognizes (with Bootzin and Caspi [2002]) the synergistic, multidimensional, and interpersonal nature of the placebo effect. A placebo is not a static and discrete thing like a sugar pill; it is more like an event than a thing. Moreover, the placebo effect is not, strictly, 'inside the head' of the patient. It is a culturally situated and interpersonally constituted event; no one responds to placebos in a social and cultural vacuum. Second, the definition preserves the centrality accorded to patients' beliefs in the placebo effect, while also emphasizing (unlike the other definitions) the role of patient affect and conscious awareness; the placebo effect is made possible by the complex interplay of belief, hope, expectation, and emotions, among other variables. Third, the definition is more explicit than the other definitions in what it rules out as possible placebo responders. Anything that is not a conscious, experiencing, belief-holding and culturally situated subject is not a placebo responder. Fourth, the definition offers a more robust and detailed account of what Grünbaum sparingly calls patients' 'life processes' and what Brody sparingly calls 'healing context'.

Chapter 5

Insight Placebos

Pseudo-Insights

Psychodynamic psychotherapy is sometimes bad medicine. The very treatment methods that are designed to help clients end up harming them (Strupp *et al.* 1977; Mays and Franks 1985). Psychological exploration can leave clients feeling more sad, confused, depressed, or anxious than before they began the treatment. The damage wrought by the treatment may go beyond emotional damage. Clients can also be left with false beliefs, illusions, or cognitive distortions, which they nonetheless regard as true. This can wreak havoc with their interpersonal lives, their plans for the future, and their judgments about practical and moral matters.

Take, for example, some of the more well-documented emotional risks of engaging in dynamic analytic therapy. During the course of analytic therapy it is not uncommon for clients to experience increasing levels of distress and anxiety. As the analysis advances, the accreted layers of defense mechanisms habitually deployed by clients to deal with unwanted feelings and thoughts are gradually exposed and deciphered. Anxiety continues to increase as the treatment encourages exploratory 'regressions' to putatively earlier ways of experiencing. During this period psychotherapists must monitor their clients closely. As they are exposed to the 'reawakening' of unwanted or unexpected archaic emotions, clients are liable to become increasingly prone to impulsive actions that might jeopardize their well-being. Here, the goals of exploratory psychotherapy must always be balanced against the need to preserve a degree of emotional stability and adaptiveness. Prudence is sometimes the better part of therapeutic exploration.

Another obvious and well-documented risk in exploratory psychotherapy is the risk of inducing false memories (Loftus *et al.* 1989a; Loftus *et al.* 1989b; Crews 1990; Loftus 1993; Loftus and Ketchum 1994; Hacking 1995; Conway 1997). Clients may find themselves having vivid memories of traumatic childhood events that never occurred. The results, as is well known, can be extremely destructive.

There are also less obvious and less debated—but equally harmful—cognitive distortions, with complex epistemic characteristics. Pseudo-insights fall into this class of distortions: that is, insights that in fact are false or fictitious but nevertheless appear to refer to real psychological or behavioral forces, entities, and states. Pseudo-insight occurs when clients believe they are insightful as a result of exploratory psychotherapy, and *appear* to command a psychologically sophisticated vocabulary that seems to be well fitted to the contours of their psychology, emotions, personality, and behavior; and yet clients are in fact mistaken, ignorant, or deceived about themselves. Pseudo-insights thus resemble false memories in a number of respects: they are plausible, persuasive, and capable of exerting powerful influences over behavior, emotion, and judgment; and they can be harmful to a client's well-being, and to his or her interpersonal relationships. Pseudo-insights also tend to be more comprehensive than false memories, targeting wider dimensions of a client's psychology, personality, and behavior. Moreover, their epistemic status as false or spurious is less easily established than the epistemic status of false memory claims. Some partial degree of corroboration of memory claims can always be achieved by appealing to second and third person accounts of the past, by cross-checking memory claims with independent reports of historical fact, and by matching them against objective historical evidence. Such measures are not as readily available with insight claims.

Unlike the problem of false memory, the risks of pseudo-insights and pseudo-self-knowledge have received little recognition by theoreticians in the psychodynamic psychotherapies. Perhaps this is because of the uniquely epistemic dimension of the risk—a dimension, as it was argued in Chapter 2, that is often overlooked in theoretical discussions of psychodynamic psychotherapy. Perhaps the uncritical assumption at work here is that such risks do not exist in a properly conducted psychotherapy. When clients at a sufficiently advanced stage of a properly conducted exploratory psychotherapy report feeling insightful, and their behaviors and symptoms have improved in ways consistent with the contents of their insights, then—so the assumption goes—their insights must be valid. At a certain point in the progress of the treatment, any residual skepticism that psychotherapists might hold about the veridicality of the claims their clients make is simply unreasonable. Meehl illustrates this position in his brief account of a psychoanalytic case history (see Chapter 2, section i): 'I think most fairminded persons would agree that it takes an unusual skeptical resistance for us to say that this step-function in clinical status was 'purely a suggestive effect', or a 'reassurance effect', or due to some other transference leverage or whatever (75th hour!) rather than that the remote memory was truly repressed and the lifting of repression efficacious' (Meehl 1983: 358).

Behind these assumptions are weighty clinical considerations. To view clients as equally fallible at all stages of the psychotherapy could be counter-therapeutic, because it could infantilize them and hold them in a state of long-term dependence. Exploratory successes need to be acknowledged and endorsed, as they build upon each other and provide encouragement to clients contemplating the termination of treatment. But weighty clinical considerations do not eliminate epistemic doubts: they simply postpone them.

A number of philosophers have pointed out the epistemic risks of cognitive distortions. Both Grünbaum (1984) and Farrell (1981), for example, argued that because of the pressures of suggestion and expectation, pseudo-insights that masquerade as *bona fide* insights are not as uncommon in psychoanalysis as is commonly thought; and that these insights can contaminate the clinical data used by psychoanalysts to confirm their hypotheses, thus resulting in self-confirming clinical hypotheses. In a different psychotherapeutic context, Hacking (1995) borrowed the term 'false consciousness' from Marxist social theory to describe the unwanted cognitive effects exerted by powerful treatment methods on the malleable memories and self-understandings of sufferers of multiple personality disorder. Hacking (1995: 266) writes of certain cautious skeptics (such as himself) who 'fear that multiple therapy leads to a false consciousness... There is a sense that the end product is a thoroughly crafted person, but not a person who serves the ends for which we are persons. Not a person with self-knowledge, but a person who is the worse for having a glib patter that simulates an understanding of herself... False consciousness is contrary to the growth and maturing of a person who knows herself. It is contrary to what the philosophers call freedom. It is contrary to our best vision of what it is to be a human being'.

While Grünbaum, Farrell, and Hacking defend quite divergent critiques of the logic and epistemology of psychotherapy, one of the points they have in common is their insistence on the distinction between appearance and reality in matters involving insight claims. What appears to be insight may in reality be something else: false insight, or false consciousness that mimics self-understanding. The distinction between appearance and reality in reflexive matters cannot be collapsed or dropped if any sense is to be made of the relations between self-knowledge, self-misunderstanding, self-deception, and self-ignorance (Jopling 2000).

How do pseudo-insights arise? Part of the explanation can be found in the nature of the psychotherapeutic encounter itself, which is a highly volatized interpersonal encounter unlike many other interpersonal relations. The powerful emotional and cognitive forces that are at play between psychotherapist and client (Strupp 1972a, 1972b; Frank and Frank 1991) tend to increase clients' suggestibility, and their levels of expectation and credulity. From a sufficiently robust platform of suggestibility and heightened credulity, clients are in a position to be convinced that their insights are true, when in fact they are mistaken, false, or incomplete.

Psychological suggestibility is a well-explored phenomenon. A number of experimental, clinical, and theoretical research traditions are devoted to the study of suggestion and its close relatives—hypnosis, persuasion, coercion, and brainwashing (Gheorghiu 1989). Within the psychotherapeutic context, psychological suggestibility manifests itself as the disposition of clients to form strong emotional ties to their psychotherapists, and to be more receptive to their psychological influence than they would otherwise be. Clients who are psychologically suggestible tend to confer on their psychotherapists greater authority than they would normally be inclined to do, and tend to be less critical or questioning (Gheorghiu 1989). Freud was particularly cognizant of this: the analysand's affectionate help-seeking compliance 'clothes the doctor with authority and is transformed into belief in his communications and explanations' (Freud SE 1917, 16: 445).

Epistemic suggestibility is a much less explored phenomenon than psychological suggestibility. Victims of epistemic suggestion are rendered suggestible about knowing practices, objects of knowledge, standards of knowledge, distinctions between knowledge, belief, and opinion, and evidentiary criteria. Epistemic suggestibility often goes unrecognized in psychodynamic psychotherapy. Consider two of the ways in which it might operate. At one level, clients might be rendered suggestible about the immediate targets of psychological exploration. That is, their attention might be focused on targets they would not otherwise have taken as epistemically significant: namely, those psychological objects, events, or forces that are regarded by their psychotherapists as psychologically and behaviorally salient. Many of these targets diverge sharply from common sense or folk psychology. Thus, from a wide range of possible psychological issues, only certain types of memories, desires, feelings, or personality traits, and certain types of causal patterns, are regarded as worthy of exploration; others are backgrounded, or downgraded in explanatory power.

There is also a higher order level of epistemic suggestibility. Clients might be rendered suggestible not only about the immediate targets of psychological exploration, but about the epistemic standards that are applied to these targets. Everyone uses epistemic standards of one sort or another, even if few people are explicitly aware of them. To grow up in a community of language users and knowers is to acquire rough working models or prototypes of what counts as good and bad reasoning, good and bad evidence, good and bad judgment, and good and bad interpretations. Everyone can provide simple relevant examples of how these models are applied in everyday contexts. It is doubtful if thinking and discourse could proceed without epistemic standards of any sort.

Psychodynamic psychotherapy has its own norms of reasoning, norms of evidence, and norms of epistemic responsibility. These emerge from common-sense epistemic norms, but they do not mirror them; the divergences are sometimes quite sharp. Clients might be so influenced by exploratory psychotherapy that the epistemic norms they bring to it from outside are challenged or eroded. They might find themselves revising their ideas about what counts as a plausible belief about the nature of psychological makeup, psychopathology, behavior, and personality; what counts as epistemically responsible; and what counts as explanatorily salient.

One example of epistemic suggestibility is what Ehrenwald (1996) calls doctrinal compliance. This occurs when clients alter their beliefs about their psychology, behavior, emotions, and personality in ways that conform to the theoretical orientations of their psychotherapists. Clients may come to think of themselves, for example, as suffering from an Oedipal complex; or they come to regard their current problems as having originated with some childhood trauma. What clients accept as true about themselves may in fact be true, but its truth is not the reason why it is accepted as true; it is accepted as true because it happens to be the theoretical orientation of the psychotherapist. But what clients accept as true about themselves may in fact be false, inexact, or trivial. This counts as a case of cognitive distortion that is caused by the treatment itself.

Doctrinal compliance is found in classical Freudian psychoanalysis. Freud worked strenuously to convince analysands about the theoretical extrapolations and retrodictions of the traumatic events they allegedly suffered in their early childhood, even when they professed to have no recollection of the events in question (Freud SE 1920, 18: 18). He tried not only to change analysands' beliefs about the course of past events (through, for example, powerful leading questions [Fish 1986]), but also to change their standards for evidentiary fitness and plausibility, and their ideas about the range of what is knowable and psychologically plausible.

One of the unfortunate consequences of epistemic suggestibility is the phenomenon of pseudo-insight. Pseudo-insights are false psychological observations and discoveries, and false causal self-attributions, that conform to the theoretical orientations and clinical expectations of psychotherapists. For example, clients who claim to acquire insights into childhood events that did not in fact occur, and who claim to detect in themselves vestiges of childhood thoughts and feelings that are really artifacts of the treatment method, rather than accurate descriptions of historical and psychological fact, are suffering from pseudo-insights. Pseudo-insights are epistemically insidious. Clients regard them as authentic, and take their acquisition as signs of therapeutic progress. Their failure to see them for what they are might suggest that some form of brainwashing is occurring (Grünbaum 1984). But this explanation, as will be discussed later, is too narrow. One reason for clients' failure to distinguish truth from falsity is that the evidentiary and interpretive criteria that they bring to psychotherapy from their pre-clinical and extra-clinical epistemic practices have been progressively weakened by continued exposure to the pressures of the therapeutic situation, and their psychotherapists' theoretical orientations and epistemic practices.

The risk of pseudo-insight poses a serious threat to the empirical base of the theories of the psychodynamic psychotherapies. Clients' insights—including their self-reports, introspective deliverances, causal self-attributions, and claims of interpretive assent—are often called upon as evidence to validate some of the developmental and etiological theories of the psychodynamic psychotherapies. But if these insights are really pseudo-insights, then their evidentiary status is dubious. Contaminated evidence is not completely useless: it can still reveal important information, if it is sufficiently decontaminated and interpreted properly; but it is of much less decisive value than uncontaminated evidence. Before claiming confirmatory support, then, the onus is squarely on psychodynamic psychotherapists to find ways to neutralize the effects of contamination.

This is the central thrust of Fliess's critique of Freudian psychoanalysis. Fliess argued that psychoanalysis is based upon spurious clinical confirmation, because psychoanalysts induce their suggestible clients to supply the very clinical material that is used to confirm psychoanalytic theories of personality and etiology. Fliess argued that Freud projected his own schematic ideas onto his clients, and manipulated their clinical productions—including their insights and recollections—by suggestion and leading questions. Whatever clinical material was produced during the course of the analysis was not allowed to flow unimpeded, as the method of free association ostensibly encouraged. Rather, clients were rendered cognitively and emotionally compliant in the face of the analyst's interpretations and leading questions, and this generated the conditions under which they produced memories and other relevant clinical material that conformed to the analyst's expectations, and to the broad outlines of the analyst's interpretations (Freud 1954: 334–337; Marmor 1970; Meehl 1983; Grünbaum 1984). From this potent mix of epistemic contamination and therapeutic artifact arose analysand insight, or something *appearing* to be insight.

Fliess' point is that classical Freudian psychoanalysis—and by implication, non-psychoanalytic psychodynamic psychotherapies—is not as different from the suggestion therapy of Bernheim and Delboeuf of the Nancy School as Freud claimed. Rather, it is a disguised and complex version of suggestion therapy, complicated by the fact that it claims to be non-directive and truth-tracking. Freud was acutely aware of the dangers pointed out by Fliess (Meehl 1983; Grünbaum 1984), acknowledging that 'there is a risk that the influencing of our patient may make the objective certainty of our findings doubtful. What is advantageous to our therapy is damaging to our researches' (Freud SE 1917, 16: 452). However, Freud consistently denied that suggestion could contaminate the progress of analysis—as long as the analysis was carried out properly. 'The danger of our leading the patient astray by suggestion, by persuading him to accept things which we ourselves believe but which he ought not to, has certainly been enormously exaggerated. An analyst would have had to behave very incorrectly before such a misfortune could overtake him; above all, he would have to blame himself for not allowing his patients to have their say. I can assert without boasting that such an abuse of 'suggestion' has never occurred in my practice' (Freud SE 1937, 5: 363–4; see also Meehl 1983; Bowers and Farvolden 1996).

Fliess is not the only one to have pointed out the epistemic damage caused by suggestion. The suggestion hypothesis is also a central component of Grünbaum's (1984) well-known critique of psychoanalysis. Grünbaum argues that unless the analysand's compliance with the analyst's expectations, and his or her doctrinal acquiescence to the analyst's theoretical orientation, can be adequately neutralized, the analyst risks inducing in analysands 'fanciful *pseudo*-insights persuasively endowed with the ring of verisimilitude' (Grünbaum 1984: 130). This is a weighty criticism. If the probative value of analysands' putatively truth-tracking insights is undermined by suggestion and doctrinal compliance, then Freudian analysis 'might reasonably be held to function as an emotional corrective *not* because it enables the analysand to acquire *bona fide* self-knowledge, but instead because he or she succumbs to proselytizing *suggestion*, which operates the more insidiously under the pretense that analysis is *non*directive' (Grünbaum 1984: 130).

The concept of pseudo-insight in Fliess and Grünbaum's critiques is important for understanding the problematic epistemic status of the claims to empirical confirmation that are made by classical Freudian psychoanalysis. But it has much wider implications: it is important for understanding how pseudo-insight and pseudo-self-knowledge are a threat to the *entire range* of psychodynamic psychotherapies. It is also important for understanding how other forms of exploratory psychotherapy are at risk of self-fulfilling clinical validation of their central theoretical constructs by the epistemic contamination of clinical data through suggestion and client compliance. Psychoanalysis is not alone in generating a spurious empirical base of clinical material: those psychotherapies that are committed to the Standard View also have the potential to induce in suggestible clients pseudo-insights that masquerade as *bona fide* insights.

The concepts of pseudo-insight and pseudo-self-knowledge, however, remain largely unanalyzed. Grünbaum for instance characterizes pseudo-insight simply as consisting of pseudo-memories (1984: 132, 277), as resembling brainwashing (1984: 135), and as requiring the indoctrination of the analysand to become an ideological disciple of the therapeutic theory (1984: 137). But this leaves unanalyzed many of the important epistemic and hermeneutic characteristics of pseudo-insight. Similarly, it leaves unanalyzed the concepts of veridical insight and veridical self-knowledge. Grünbaum characterizes self-knowledge as the veridical disclosure of the patient's hidden conflicts (1984: 136). But this is unavailing: it says little about what counts as true and false insight, what criteria are used to establish truth and falsity, what counts as the proper object of insight, and what kinds of evidence count as supportive of true and false insights. These are not fatal omissions, but the concepts involved are so robust and complex that filling them out adequately will almost certainly alter the thrust of the epistemic criticisms they serve to underwrite.

What then is pseudo-insight? What distinguishes pseudo-insight from *bona fide* insight? How does pseudo-insight function, and what role does it play in clients' psychology and behavior? What are the varieties of pseudo-insight?

First, pseudo-insight is not psychobabble insight. Psychobabble is an outgrowth of some of the alternative psychotherapies, such as *est*, rebirthing, and primal therapy (Rosen 1977; Beyerstein 2001; Lilienfeld *et al.* 2003a, 2003b; Singer and Nievod 2003), as well as the new-age therapies that blend together versions of mysticism, spiritualism, and occultism. The term 'psychobabble' is misleading. Psychobabble is not *mere* babble. Clients who use psychobabble idioms to articulate feelings, make sense of behaviors, and explain psychological states, are not using words randomly or capriciously; nor are they using words entirely devoid of meaning. They are following certain rules of linguistic practice that have been established by relatively small communities of therapeutic practitioners: rules for which there are roughly correct and incorrect ways of going on, and rules which ostensibly link words to certain putative referents (the psychological events, states, or objects picked out by the relevant explanatory theory).

To an uncritical eye, it might seem that psychobabble idioms provide legitimate tools for deep psychological analysis, and a ready medium for deep insight. But the appearance of explanatory power and descriptive validity is an appearance only. Psychobabble idioms are meaningful in a loose sense; but they are explanatorily empty, in the same way that 'folk physics' explanations are meaningful but empty, or that cartoon depictions of the chemistry of household cleansers (a staple of television advertisements for soaps and shampoos) are meaningful but empty. This is because they are compatible with any state of psychological affairs whatever. They have the 'power' to explain every phenomenon in the fields to which they refer. Typically, those using psychobabble explanations see confirming evidence everywhere. But the price for this expanded explanatory power is unfalsifiability. Few behaviors or events could contradict psychobabble explanations. Any evidence that might count as disconfirmation can be explained away with the help of rescuing ad hoc strategies (Popper 1963). Psychobabble explanations fall squarely within the category of what Popper (1963) called pseudo-science.

Psychobabble insights and interpretations are empirically impoverished and imprecise. Typically, they are pitched in terms of an obfuscating technical jargon that glosses over psychologically and experientially complex phenomena with terms that are inappropriately vague and referentially malleable.

Compared to psychobabble insights, pseudo-insights in the psychodynamic psychotherapies hold out more explanatory promise. They are, among other things, relatively robust and precise. Pseudo-insights are characterized by: i) misidentified and/or misdescribed observations about the target disorders (and their relation to the broader range of the client's behaviors and psychological states); ii) false, fictitious, or spurious explanations about the causes of the disorders (and their relation to the broader range of the client's behaviors and psychological states); and iii) widespread explanatory and predictive failures. Pseudo-insights are analogous to pseudo-explanations in the natural and medical sciences in two respects: first, insofar as the postulated explanatory entities (e.g. ether, demons, humors) identified under an explanatory theory are eventually rejected as non-existent, even if for a time they are considered to be similar enough to valid explanatory entities to be taken as serious candidates for explanation; and second, insofar as the putative causal relations specified by the theory (e.g., causal relations between pathogens, symptoms, and treatment agents) are eventually rejected as non-existent, even if they are for a time considered to be similar enough to actual causal relations to be taken as serious candidates.

On the face of it, pseudo-insights look like true insights. Both share certain formal similarities. Pseudo-insights involve:

i) an understanding of target disorders D as specified by therapeutic theory T—but without the client's awareness of T's actual status as false, misclassified, or fictitious;

ii) an understanding of symptoms S of the target disorders D, as specified by the therapeutic theory T—but without the client's awareness that T's symptomatology is false or fictitious;

iii) an understanding of the causes C of target disorder D, as specified under T, but without the client's awareness of T's etiology as false or fictitious;

iv) an understanding of treatment method M, and its specific mechanisms of alleviation A, as specified under the treatment method T, but without the client's awareness of the status of M (and A) as misconceived or fictitious;

v) an understanding of the relation R of symptoms S, causes C, and treatment method M to the client's life processes, but without the client's awareness of R's actual status as misdescribed or fictitious;

vi) the integration of M into a definite and realizable course of action, directed towards the attainment of therapeutic goals G, but without the client's awareness of the misconceived or fictitious status of this integration.

To put flesh on the bare-bones of this formal model of pseudo-insight, consider how new advances in the scientific understanding of psychological disorders bring with them new revelations about the explanatory poverty of what were once considered valid insights, as well as new revelations about the therapeutic poverty of what were once considered valid clinical interventions. More than once across the history of psychology, disorders thought to have been psychological in origin and nature have been discovered to be organic. When this occurs, the insights people thought they had gained into their disorders through psychological treatments are rendered invalid. Take, for example, Tourette syndrome, an organic disorder of the central nervous system characterized by physical tics, and in some cases echolalia and coprolalia. The failure to understand the neurophysiological basis of Tourette syndrome has caused a great deal of suffering across the history of psychology. People with the syndrome have been misdiagnosed, misprognosed, and mistreated. They have been 'diagnosed' as possessed by demons, and subjected to 'treatments' such as exorcism (Hines 1988). More humane treatments followed from the psychoanalytic explanations of the syndrome that dominated psychiatry from the 1920s to the 1950s. But these explanations were pitched at the level of psychology rather than neurophysiology, and thus tracked nonexistent or irrelevant causal pathways, and identified nonexistent or irrelevant causes. In so doing, psychoanalytic explanations obscured the real nature of the syndrome, and interfered with the clients' progress toward accurate insights. The psychoanalytic interpretations clients were given, and the insights they gained into the unconscious origins of their disorders, were false or fictitious: in effect, they were pseudo-insights.

In one psychoanalytic case history of Tourette syndrome, for example, it was claimed that the analysand was 'reluctant to give up the tic because it became a source of erotic pleasure to her and an expression of her unconscious sexual strivings' (Shapiro *et al.* 1978). In another, the analysand's tics were regarded as 'stereotyped equivalents of onanism... The libido connected with the genital sensation was displaced into other parts of the body'. In another, tics were regarded as 'a conversion symptom at the anal–sadistic level'. In another, the analysand displayed a 'compulsive character, as well as a narcissistic orientation': tics represented 'an affective syndrome, a defense against the intended affect'. Interpretations such as these may seem to be psychologically plausible. They may even capture some of the subjective meanings built up around the symptoms. But they are etiologically and nosologically false. Thus whatever insights the analysands developed on the basis of these interpretations were far removed from the truth: they were, in effect, pseudo-insights. Shapiro *et al.* write: 'Psychoanalytic theorizing of this kind in effect leaves no base untouched. Tics are a conversion symptom but not hysterical, anal but also erotic, volitional but also compulsive, organic but also dynamic in origin... These psychological labels, diagnoses, and treatments were unfortunately imposed on patients and their families, usually with little humility, considerable dogmatism, and with much harm... These papers, because of their subsequent widespread influence, had a calamitous effect on the understanding and treatment of this syndrome' (Shapiro *et al.* 1978: 39–42, 50, 63).

The fact that the explanatory entities, causal relations, and taxonomic divisions picked out by pseudo-insights are irrelevant or non-existent does not mean that pseudo-insights are entirely bereft of *instrumental* value. Pseudo-insights may serve as useful cognitive tools and heuristic devices, helping to shape the way in which the clinical material is investigated, generating useful predictions and retrodictions, and serving as robust working hypotheses from which *bona fide* insights may eventually develop. By stimulating further inquiry, in other words, they may point the way to the truth (Wisdom 1967). Not only is it more cognitively instrumental for clients to think about their disorders, symptoms, and etiology with *some* minimally coherent form of explanation—even if it is false or fictional—than it is to think about them without *any* form of explanation at all; it is also emotionally instrumental. Pseudo-insights offer to clients *hope* that their otherwise unintelligible disorders are identifiable and understandable.

The instrumental value of pseudo-insights is also reflected in the instrumental value of pseudo-interpretations and pseudo-explanations. Mahrer claims that detailed 'operating instructions' are an essential component of any theory of psychotherapy: 'The theory provided a working manual of conditions—operations—consequences. If a theory did not include this component, the therapist would not know what to do, or when to do what, or what to try to do it for' (Mahrer 1989: 50). A working manual based on false explanations is better than having no working manual at all, just as having an inadvertently false or fictitious 'higher order framework' (Mahrer 1989: 50) is better than having no framework at all.

Instrumental value, however, is no reason to throw epistemic caution to the wind. The fact that pseudo-insights *may* serve these ends is not enough to put to rest all further doubts about their usefulness. Just as pseudo-insights may serve as useful cognitive tools, so they may serve as unhelpful, harmful, or ethically inappropriate tools; just as they may point the way to the truth, so, as the case of psychoanalytic explanations of Tourette syndrome illustrates, they may point away from the truth. An instrumentalist justification of demonological explanations of psychosis, for instance, carries little or no weight. Instrumental value alone is no guarantee that truth is being tracked, or even pointed to.

Philosophical Pseudo-Insights

Many psychodynamic psychotherapies defend conceptually rich theories of mind and general models of human nature; and many uphold conceptually rich norms of well-being, normalcy, and health. While not explicitly philosophical, these theories can naturally trigger philosophical inquiry in clients, especially those who are psychologically minded and aware of the range of possible theoretical orientations. Sometimes, clients engaged in psychological exploration end up acquiring insights that have a degree of philosophical content. The insights revolve around such weighty topics as the soul, fate, determinism, moral responsibility, death, human nature, wisdom, or the meaning of life. Such insights are not abstract and technical; they are pitched at a practical level that helps clients to see their lives in new light. These insights might be considered a beneficial side effect of psychodynamic treatment, an unwanted form of intellectualization, or a simple annoyance.

Just as the logic and epistemology of psychodynamic psychotherapy is often downplayed by psychodynamic researchers and clinicians as relatively unimportant, so the role of philosophy in psychodynamic treatment is often downplayed as unimportant, incidental to the real engine of therapeutic change, or just plain exotic. This is the case even if clients' philosophical insights follow directly from exploratory psychotherapy. Why this happens is open to speculation. It may be an indication of disciplinary hubris on the part of psychology; or a symptom of the historical short-sightedness that afflicts contemporary psychology and psychotherapy (Chandler and Holliday 1990): that is, an ignorance of the roots of contemporary psychotherapy in the tradition of practical philosophy that started in the ancient world, thrived in the Renaissance, and that carried on at the edges of academic philosophy throughout the early modern and modern periods (Gill 1985; Chandler and Holliday 1990; Nussbaum 1994; Hadot 1995).

Take the concept of fate. While it is not one of the central building blocks of classical psychoanalytic theory and clinical practice, Freud's discussion of *Ananke*—the view of death as destiny, and the inexorable and tragic sense of life this view suggests—clearly reaches beyond the domain of empirical psychology into speculative and practical philosophy. Versions of this view, and its relevance to the philosophical ideal of wisdom, are defended in ancient Stoic philosophy (Hadot 1995); and the view is discussed by philosophers such as Montaigne, Spinoza, Schopenhauer, Wittgenstein, and some twentieth-century existentialist philosophers. Ricoeur (1970) characterizes the Freudian conception of *Ananke* (fate) as a symbol of 'a wisdom that dares to face the harshness of life'. It is an acceptance of the necessity of one's death, 'resignation to the inexorable order of nature', and the art of bearing the burden of existence (1970: 328). It is likely that the concept of *Ananke* infiltrated some of Freud's clinical practice, through for instance the interpretations he offered to analysands, his remarks about the long-term goals of psychoanalysis, and his own clinical behaviors. It is also likely that with some analysands, the concept of *Ananke* exerted a degree of influence on the contents of interpretations and insights.

Some philosophical insights may prove therapeutically beneficial. They may, for example, help to break exploratory impasses, stimulate new avenues of exploration, and frame psychological problems in a new light. Even a low-level degree of acquaintance with rudimentary philosophical ideas and methods (such as the analysis of concepts, critical thinking, and philosophical argument) may help to give clients a slightly greater degree of intellectual autonomy than they had before. But the potential therapeutic benefits need to be balanced against the risks, the most obvious one of which is intellectualization. Philosophy is an ideal candidate to be pressed into service as part of a larger strategy of denial or resistance, or as an intellectualized form of self-deception. Pursuing philosophical insights for their own sake could easily degenerate into a flight from or a defensive reaction to highly emotional material that needs to be confronted head-on, without the distorting lens of philosophy. Moreover, the symptoms of organically-based depression, for example, may lend themselves to philosophical reinterpretation as signs of an ontological mood such as existential anxiety, resulting in misdiagnosis and mistreatment (Kramer 1993; Jopling 1998).

There are other risks too. What passes for philosophical insight may really be a complex form of pseudo-insight: that is, an insight that is deceptively similar to authentic philosophical understanding, and that to clients *seems* authentic, but is really sophisticated patter with little intrinsic philosophical content. The symptoms of philosophical pseudo-insight are not unlike those of psychobabble insight. In addition to vapid quasi-philosophical slogans, they include sloppy reasoning, misrepresentation of philosophical issues, obscurantism, oversimplification of philosophical issues with vague terms stretched to the point of vacuity, and confused *ad hoc* amalgams of technical terminology (i.e. jargon). Philosophical pseudo-insights may be a sign that clients are over-philosophizing their psychological problems, or creating new artifactual problems where none before existed: that is, creating philosophical problems that were not part of the original complex of psychological problems that first prompted entry into therapy. Bishop Berkeley's (1710/1982) warning that philosophers have the bad habit of kicking up a dust and then complaining that they cannot see applies equally well to those clients in exploratory psychotherapy who regard therapeutically salient events as displaying latent philosophical significance. With philosophical over-interpretation, the non-philosophical dimensions of life are dismissed as instances of ignorance, or as incipient philosophical problems waiting to be uncovered. Philosophy is sometimes bad medicine.

Insight Placebos

Insight placebos are a subset of the larger class of pseudo-insights. Like pseudo-insights, they consist of false or fictitious explanations of psychology, behavior, emotions, and personality—explanations that nonetheless appear to client and psychotherapist as authentic and truth-tracking. Like pseudo-insights, they do not trace any known causal pathways, and they refer to imaginary or nonexistent psychological entities, forces, events, or relations. But insight placebos do something more than pseudo-insights: they trigger the placebo effect. By contrast, pseudo-insights lack therapeutic efficacy.

In the class of non-placebic pseudo-insights are:

a) pseudo-insights that make no noticeable difference to the client's target disorders (i.e. they are epiphenomenal with respect to the underlying target disorder);

b) pseudo-insights that make only marginal or transient differences that are causally dependent upon the operation of other more powerful therapeutic factors;

c) pseudo-insights that are temporally coincident with the remission of symptoms, which clients and psychotherapists mistakenly identify as causally active;

d) pseudo-insights that are *ex post facto* rationalizations of therapeutic changes;

e) pseudo-insights that are counter-therapeutic, or nocebo insights (where the content of the client's insight consists of anticipated negative outcomes, which themselves are a cause of illness (Hahn 1997)).

Insight placebos are not merely vehicles for other placebological factors; that is, they are not epiphenomenal with respect to underlying placebo mechanisms that are not related to insight. They are in themselves placebos: that is, their contents and meaning function as placebos. They stand to psychological disorders as sugar pills and sham treatments stand to somatic disorders. Just as somatic placebos 'uncork the internal pharmacopeia which all humans possess as a biologically programmed tool for self-healing' (Brody 1997), so insight placebos unleash the mind's natural powers to heal itself.

As with sugar pills and sham treatments, insight placebos go undetected *as* placebos. Clients do not experience them as unreal, fake, or as confabulations: they experience them as real insights, and as having a therapeutic efficacy that comes from their appearing to correspond faithfully to the contours of the psychological and behavioral reality they putatively explain. To clients, they seem to exert specific therapeutic effects on target disorders, like a key opening a lock.

Viewed in this epistemically uncritical light, insight placebos appear to satisfy the Standard View, particularly the principle of therapeutically effective insight. In actuality, however, insight placebos have no significant explanatory power and descriptive validity. But like their cousins in physical medicine, they are far from inert or powerless (Harrington 1997; Guess *et al.* 2002; Moerman 2002a). Whatever degree of therapeutic efficacy they possess is placebological in nature. Their therapeutic agency can be explained by factors that have less to do with the trajectory of truth-tracking therapeutic exploration than with the psychological mechanisms governing suggestibility, deception, self-deception, heightened expectation, and heightened credulity.

Insight placebos are not readily identifiable as consisting of false or psychologically fictional explanations. They are well disguised. Just as therapeutic suggestion is considerably more subtle and undetectable than crude persuasion that targets symptoms (e.g. 'your anxiety will abate if you count to fifty'), so insight placebos are considerably more sophisticated and less detectable than simple-minded fictions, such as those found in psychobabble idioms. Insight placebos are characterized by psychological robustness and complexity; and they are informed by the psychotherapist's sophisticated technical terminology. The identifiability of insight placebos is made more difficult by the fact that prolonged exposure to a treatment method and theoretical orientation tends to sensitize clients to the importance of a narrow range of psychological and behavioral issues that exclude other potential issues. This in turn predisposes clients to expect that those issues will be addressed *only* by those treatment methods and exploratory styles to which they are currently exposed. Once an advanced stage of exploratory psychotherapy has been reached, clients and psychotherapists alike are highly motivated to endorse insights as authentic.

The following case history illustrates how a placebo interpretation can lead to insight placebos. The case involves a psychoanalyst who deliberately misled one of his analysands with a false interpretation in order to effect a temporary therapeutic change and a temporary but therapeutically expedient self-understanding (Mendel 1964). As a result of the analyst's interpretation, the analysand acquired a number of false or fictitious insights which contributed to his therapeutic progress. R was a thirty-seven-year-old pharmacist who initially entered analysis reporting difficulties in his relationship with his twelve-year-old stepson. He had been married ten years and had two children. His wife also had a child from a previous marriage. R had grown unhappy in his marriage, and had not had sexual relations with his wife for two years. He had stayed in the marriage for the sake of his children and because of his strict Catholic background. After one hundred hours of analysis, R had a brief extra-marital affair, which he reported having enjoyed. Soon after the affair, however, he had a terrifying dream accompanied by anxiety attacks and heart palpitations. In his dream R was riding in a train full of soldiers who, for no apparent reason, killed his two children but spared him and his stepson. In an emergency therapy session the next day R produced a number of associations about the dream: i) he enjoyed the affair, felt no guilt, and wished he could continue it; ii) he felt sexually renewed by the affair; iii) he felt trapped in his marriage; iv) he felt he owed it to his children to stay in the marriage, and that they were the only reason for remaining in it; v) one of his friends had stayed unhappily married for the same reasons for twenty-three years before finally getting divorced, and then reported that his decision to remain married was the biggest mistake in his life; and vi) he claimed to love his children, and the horrible dream had made no sense to him.

Given R's high level of agitation, and given the fact that he was leaving the following day for an extended business trip that would interrupt the momentum of the analysis, the psychoanalyst decided that it would be therapeutically expedient to concoct a false interpretation of the dream. The psychoanalyst felt that his client would be unable at that stage in the analysis to handle an accurate interpretation, which would have required the client to finally confront a truth he had systematically denied—namely, his growing hostility toward his children, who were keeping him in a loveless marriage. This would have been a highly sensitive part of the analysis, and a cursory and premature treatment of it would have easily interfered with the client's otherwise good progress. Moreover, premature exposure to the psychoanalyst's interpretation of the dream would not have helped R's anxiety or his day-to-day functioning. The psychoanalyst thus opted for benevolent paternalistic deception— a plausible fiction—rather than a confrontation with the truth.

The false interpretation the psychoanalyst gave to R was relatively simple: 'In the dream, the children are in fact part of you; the children are the impulses which have caused you to do things of which you do not entirely approve; you have punished them by having them killed by the soldiers' (Mendel 1964: 187). This is neither psychologically implausible nor obviously false. It offers a simple explanation of an otherwise puzzling dream; it deploys rudimentary psychoanalytic theory; and it refers to certain psychological forces or entities that appear to have causal power. But like Frank's interpretation (Frank and Frank 1991: 205–10; see Chapter 2), the interpretation is noticeably lacking in detail and interpretive robustness. While not quite a one-size-fits-all interpretation, its basic explanatory structure could fit a number of roughly similar cases. The interpretation, in other words, does not 'follow from' the total mass of clinical material presented during the course of the analysis with the requisite degree of clarity and precision that would presumably characterize a truth-tracking interpretation. It stretches and force-fits some of the clinical material, it edits out certain salient parts, and it fills in noticeable gaps with conveniently configured narrative overlays.

But R did not notice these shortcomings; or if he did, he pretended not to notice them; or he noticed them but failed to attend to them and spell them out; or he fooled himself about their validity, and fell prey to a kind of self-deception (see Chapter 6). Why did he not notice them? He had already formed a close bond with the analyst. Intensive exploratory analysis was already past the one-hundred-hour mark, enough time for a platform of suggestibility and doctrinal compliance to have been established. R's response was clear and pronounced: he immediately recognized the interpretation as true, immediately identified with it, and was inwardly affected by it. He acquired a number of insights into his dream, and then experienced a marked reduction in anxiety. The interpretation and the insights helped to dispel the fears occasioned by the dream, and they helped to alter his behavior, since he then decided not to make a habit of having extra-marital affairs. R's insights are insight placebos: they are therapeutically beneficial explanatory fictions.

Why would a false or fictitious interpretation be therapeutically beneficial? First, it was well timed. It presented R with an immediate opportunity for problem solving (and, to a certain extent, reality testing). It gave R the experience of a small measure of therapeutic success, upon which foundation future therapeutic successes could also be built. This in turn gave him hope of relief and increased his expectations for improvement; and this in turn made him more amenable to further treatment of the same kind. The acceptance of the interpretation, moreover, was preceded by intense emotional arousal, which rendered R more suggestible and less critical than he would otherwise have been. The interpretation also helped him overcome a sense of self-alienation and confusion, and gave him the feeling that he was understood, and that his problems were not entirely mysterious. Finally, it triggered in R a number of new insights into his motives and desires, and moved along his explorations in new directions. All this therapeutic progress occurred despite the fact that the interpretation and the insights following upon it were false.

Mendel provided further support for his hypothesis that inexact or false interpretations have therapeutic efficacy with the following clinical study, one that paralleled early versions of the social psychology experiments on the Barnum effect (Ulrich *et al.* 1963). Four clients involved in psychodynamic psychotherapy were given the same one-size-fits-all interpretation on six occasions, at one-month intervals. The gist of the interpretations was as follows: 1. You seem to live your life as though you are apologizing all the time. 2. Much of what you say now seems to be related to the difficulties you have with men. 3. You seem hesitant in the exploration of your strong points. 4. Apparently, you have always felt that you had to take on the burdens of all the family. 5. You seem frightened of the effect your expression of feelings has on me and others. 6. Much of what you say seems to be related to the difficulties you have with women (Mendel 1964). When fleshed out with detail and imbedded within the clinical context, each of these interpretations could function as placebos. That is, false or fictitious explanations of psychology, emotions, behavior, and personality could be powerful enough to rally the client's native healing powers.

Despite different psychological histories and personalities, the clients in the study tended to agree with the interpretations and to respond to them with a significant reduction in anxiety in twenty of the twenty-four instances. In only two instances did clients decisively reject the interpretation, and in only two other instances did they express doubts. While there are problems in the design and implementation of the study, Mendel concluded that psychodynamic interpretations do not need to be accurate in order to promote therapeutic changes: they need only be able to confer meaning on otherwise puzzling behaviors, feelings, and thoughts.

Mendel's examples illustrate a phenomenon that is also observable in clinical medicine: namely, diagnosis as treatment. For many non-life-threatening diseases and disorders, a clear diagnosis, physician–patient agreement about the nature of the problem, and an assurance of improvement are enough to facilitate recovery—even without any specific treatment intervention. Brody and Waters (1980), for example, describe a case history analogous to Mendel's to illustrate the therapeutic effects of diagnosis. A 44-year-old lawyer presented with sharp chest pains, fully expecting that he would suffer a massive fatal heart attack. His symptoms followed no discernible pattern, there was no family history of heart disease, and further testing revealed no underlying organic pathology. Upon further consultation, however, it was discovered that the patient lost his only brother to cancer ten months before the chest pains began. It was apparent to the physician that the patient had not yet mourned his loss, because until two weeks before the chest pains he had been kept fully occupied with probate as the executor of his brother's will. The first chest pains occurred the night the probate process came to an end. During the consultation the patient wept profusely, and recognized the delayed mourning. The physician encouraged him to mourn actively, after which time the chest pains subsided. 'In [this] case the diagnosis *in itself* exercised a therapeutic effect for the patient inasmuch as it provided an understandable, acceptable explanation for his behavior. A formerly mysterious symptom was given meaning... If a symptom can be discussed in objective terms, and even drawn in a diagram, it may be seen as a manageable entity for which alternative solutions exist, instead of the shadowy specter it seemed before' (Brody and Waters 1980: 446). Frank also notes that 'an effectively reassuring explanation simultaneously promotes patients' feelings of mastery and offers hopes of recovery' (Frank and Frank 1991:128).

Diagnosis is treatment even if the diagnosis is incorrect, scientifically unfounded, empirically impoverished, or speculative. Diagnoses in alternative medicine, for example, provide patients with theoretical explanations that make sense of their experiences. 'Inevitably, since the alternative [medicine] world is not as constrained by the dichotomy of objectivity and subjectivity, the chiropractor will find the subluxation, the acupuncturist will detect the yin–yang disharmony, and the health food advocate will identify the transgression that makes sense of the patient's life world... When it is considered that 40% to 60% of patients may never receive a firm diagnosis in conventional medicine, an alternative diagnosis may be a potent form of nonspecific healing that changes the circumstances under which the patient exists, including reducing the dysphoria of uncertainty' (Kaptchuk 2002).

Insight Artifacts

The social and behavioral sciences are in the business of discovering the regularities of human behavior and psychology. Under ideal investigative circumstances, the evidence for these regularities is uncontaminated by theory, observer bias, context effects, and transient social influences. Under less than ideal circumstances, however, the evidence may fall short of this high grade, with the result that the replication of scientific experiments and the confirmation and disconfirmation of scientific hypotheses is placed in jeopardy. One of these less than ideal circumstances occurs when the methods and tools of inquiry generate data infected with methodological artifacts: that is, patterns, structures, or properties of behavior that are not naturally present in the behaviors or psychological states under investigation, but are produced *during* the course of inquiry by extrinsic agents such as observational interference, measurement instruments, or quirks of the methodological design (e.g. a study's limited population, unrepresentative sampling, skewed or leading questionnaires). Methodological artifacts are not *unreal*; they are determinate events or states, with properties that are just as real as the pre-measurement properties. Nor are they generated *de novo*, without any grounding in pre-existing psychological or behavioral conditions. But they are a source of experimental contamination.

Some of the more well-known factors that generate methodological artifacts in the social and behavioral sciences are the Hawthorne effect, the experimenter effect, the novelty effect, the disruption effect, pre-test and post-test sensitization, regression to the mean, and experimenter bias.[1] Often these are factored out or reduced with careful experimental design, thereby minimizing the chances for unwanted confounds, contaminated data, and self-fulfilling predictions (Jones 1977). But the failure to take the requisite precautionary measures can result in data that bear the imprint of the measurement instruments or the observational contexts. Take self-reports, one of the more commonly used measurement instruments in the social, behavioral, and clinical sciences. Sometimes, people's reports about their behaviors or mental states are influenced by the idiosyncratic properties of the questionnaires that elicit the information (Schwartz and Sudman 1992, 1994, 1996; Schwartz 1999). That is, the questions determine the answers that are received, and this results in data that are more reflective of the categories of the experimental tasks than the experimental participants' relevant behaviors or mental states. Interference such as this jeopardizes efforts to generalize the results of the experiment beyond the narrow confines of the relevant sample population and the idiosyncratic experimental conditions; moreover, it jeopardizes efforts to confirm or disconfirm scientific hypotheses.

If methodological artifacts are found in the social and behavioral sciences, then it is likely that they have analogs in the clinical sciences. The analogy between the two disciplinary fields is close, because the conditions under which patients are investigated and treated bear a number of deep similarities to the conditions under which participants are investigated in the social and behavioral sciences. Both groups, for instance, display some property, condition, or symptom set that merits investigation, and both groups, as a consequence, are placed under observation by so-called experts in human behavior or health. Both groups, moreover, are aware that they are under observation. Again, both groups submit to various forms of testing and measurement, and thus are vulnerable to pre-test and post-test sensitization effects, disruption effects, and experimenter or clinician bias. Finally, both groups are subjected to causal explanations of behavior, mental states, or symptoms that are framed in experience-distant terms.

If the analogy is a valid one, then similar evidentiary and confirmatory problems can be expected to arise because of the potential for contamination of data. (For the sake of terminological parsimony, the general term 'clinical artifact' will be used to denote all forms of clinical analog, and the specific term 'psychotherapeutic artifacts' will be used to denote those analogs found only in psychotherapy and clinical psychology.) Just as methodological artifacts have the potential to interfere with the confirmation and disconfirmation of hypotheses in the social and behavioral sciences, and to threaten the ideal of theory-independent, public, and uncontaminated evidence, so psychotherapeutic artifacts have the potential to interfere with the confirmation and disconfirmation of hypotheses in clinical psychology and psychotherapy. Similarly, both fields present methodologists with multiple challenges in creating effective preventative measures and decontamination strategies.

But the problems with psychotherapeutic artifacts go deeper still, reaching right down to the level of individuals trying to deal with their own psychological problems, and entangling them in unwanted epistemic confusion. Psychotherapeutic artifacts do not merely make an appearance after the fact, in psychological research and theorizing; they become part of clients' experience. Artifact and fact are liable to be confounded, for example, in psychodynamic insights and interpretations. In some cases, what clients take to be discoveries of fact are actually encounters with artifact. While insights and interpretations appear to refer to psychological, behavioral, or historical facts about the client, they refer in some cases to artifacts that have been generated by the very conditions of treatment and exploration that make such insights and interpretations possible in the first place.

But how is this possible? The psychodynamic psychotherapies are characterized as exploratory therapies. Clients make important discoveries about themselves during the course of treatment (i.e. the Standard View's principle of exploratory validity). What is discovered—feelings, desires, personality traits, and memories, as well as unconscious forces, resistances, repressions, denials, displacements, sublimations, and their behavioral analogs—is *already there*, awaiting discovery; it is not made up during the activity of exploration, by the exploratory tools themselves. Exploratory psychotherapy, in other words, does not fabricate its own objects of exploration: it deals with psychological, historical, and behavioral facts, not methodological or treatment artifacts.

This is an important conceptual claim, and it guides a great deal of theorizing and clinical practice in psychodynamic psychotherapy. But it is far from self-evident. The distinction between making and finding the real is a central one in metaphysics and epistemology, and tends (along with a number of other deep conceptual distinctions) to separate realists from anti-realists and constructivists. But the distinction is freighted with weighty assumptions, and it should be properly considered more like a tentative hypothesis than a settled fundamental principle. For the sake of convenience, this particular version of the principle of exploratory validity will be called Hypothesis A. Streamlined, it runs as follows: the objects of psychodynamic exploration, interpretation, insight, and theoretical explanation (i.e. feelings, desires, memories, behaviors, personality traits, as well as depressions, anxieties, and phobias) have determinate properties, yield determinate forms of evidence, and exist antecedently to the psychodynamic theories that explain them and the treatments that work upon them. They are not clinical artifacts that are manufactured by psychotherapeutic treatment methods themselves; nor are they merely theoretical constructs.

The lock and key metaphor adds further color to Hypothesis A. The treatment methods of the psychodynamic psychotherapies operate directly upon target disorders like a key opening a lock. Just as the ridges and grooves of a key fit precisely onto the tumblers of a lock, so the uniquely molded contours (or characteristic factors) of psychodynamic treatment methods fit precisely onto the contours of the target disorders, and exert upon them precise counterforces. And just as there are certain properties about a key that are incidental with respect to its specific unlocking agency—the weight and material of the key—so there are certain factors in each psychodynamic treatment that are incidental with respect to the presumed therapeutically efficacious factors. However divergent their accounts of the characteristic factors that are presumed to drive treatment, most of the psychodynamic psychotherapies are committed to some version of Hypothesis A, and some version of the characteristic versus incidental factor distinction.

Consider now Hypothesis A1 which, with the help of some counterintuitive physics, stands the lock and key metaphor on its head: just as the tumblers of some locks are made to conform to the grooves and ridges of some keys, so some of the objects of psychodynamic treatment are made to fit the unique contours of the treatment methods that are brought to bear upon them. If this hypothesis is valid, then some of the objects targeted by psychodynamic insight and interpretation are artifacts. This would not be a long step from what has already been shown to be at least conceptually possible: namely, that insights and interpretations do not always refer to the things that clients and psychotherapists think they do, or what the Standard View claims they do. Consider now some simple examples that offer empirical support for this hypothesis: artifactual dreams, artifactual beliefs, and artifactual symptoms.

Artifactual Dreams

It is not uncommon for clients in psychodynamic psychotherapy to report dreams to their psychotherapists. It is also not uncommon for psychotherapists to construe dreams as part of the ever-growing bundle of relevant clinical material, and to offer clients interpretations of their dreams. In turn, these interpretations can trigger and influence more dreams, thereby supplying yet more clinical material for further interpretation; and so on. If Hypothesis A is correct, then dreams and dreamwork count as real psychological events or forces, which display determinate properties and yield determinate forms of evidence. Dreams and dreamwork exist independently of psychodynamic treatment methods, and the real meaning of dreams awaits discovery and deciphering at the hands of skilled interpreters. Nothing about dreams and dreamwork is contrived or unnatural. (According to classical Freudian psychoanalysis, moreover, the very idea of a *completed* dream interpretation makes sense.)

This picture is naïve in a number of ways (see Wittgenstein 1982). For one, it does not take the phenomenon of artifactual dreams seriously enough. It is not uncommon for dreams to be influenced on a number of levels by psychodynamic treatment methods. Not only do clients have dreams about their psychotherapists, or about the events of previous or anticipated therapy sessions; they can even 'come to dream in imagery that accords with their therapists' theories' (Frank and Frank 1991: 178). After many hours of analysis devoted to deciphering their dreams, for instance, some clients begin to have dreams, and to have *memories* of dreams, and to provide *reports* of their dreams, that fit the theoretical expectations of the very dream analysis they are undergoing, and that 'take a form that will best please the analyst' (Frank and Frank 1991: 194). Their dream images, for example, come to be populated with symbols that are freighted with psychodynamic meanings, and which clients would not otherwise have encountered oneirically. Similar things can happen to oneiric thematization. Some of the emotionally charged issues that make an appearance during the waking hours of treatment, and that are construed by the psychotherapist as being highly relevant for further work (e.g. memories of distant childhood events such as traumas and sexual feelings), come to acquire a certain oneiric prominence, while those that are not similarly targeted during the treatment recede in oneiric significance. In the dream state, in other words, certain themes are developed and transformed in ways that make them much more receptive to dream analysis than they would otherwise have been (Wittgenstein 1982); other themes are backgrounded. Some clients in dream analysis, in other words, begin to have psychodynamic dreams. Much of this influence, however, and the artifactuality to which it leads, goes unnoticed. Clients typically experience their dreams as spontaneous and unbidden; they are not aware of the tell-tale markings of artifice, context effects, or clinician bias. To psychotherapists, moreover, dreams typically appear to provide more or less uncontaminated (or easily decontaminated) evidence of the psychopathogenic force of repressed wishes and unconscious urges, triggered during sleep by prior conscious experiences and now seeking vicarious fulfillment in the dimension of sleep.

If, as Frank and Frank (1991) suggest, analysands in psychoanalytic dream analysis sometimes have psychoanalytic dreams, the same is true for other kinds of psychodynamic dream analysis. Clients in Jungian analysis sometimes have Jungian dreams, and have Jungian *memories* of dreams, and provide Jungian *reports* of dreams; clients in Kleinian analysis sometimes have Kleinian dreams, and have Kleinian *memories* of dreams, and provide Kleinian *reports* of dreams; and clients in Adlerian psychotherapy sometimes have Adlerian dreams, and have Adlerian *memories* of dreams, and provide Adlerian *reports* of dreams; and so on. There may even be substantive similarities between the dreams of clients being treated by the same psychotherapist; and substantive differences between the types of dreams dreamed by clients who move from one modality of psychodynamic treatment to another. Dreams, in other words, are not independent of the treatment methods brought to bear upon them, such that they would have occurred in more or less unaltered form if clients were not exposed to any psychodynamic treatment methods at all. While dreams are not so psychically plastic that they can be influenced in any which way, changes in treatment method and theoretical framework can still bring about systematic changes in oneiric content, imagery, symbolism, and structure, which in turn can bring about systematic changes in the kinds of *insights* that clients acquire about the meaning of their dreams.

The production of artifactual dreams thus leads to a problematic evidentiary feedback loop that undermines the claims to objectivity of dream analysis. Take the case of psychoanalytic dream analysis. When analysands report (during free association) having had dreams that display the very sorts of themes, images, and symbols that are predicted by psychoanalytic dream analysis, then psychoanalysts will tend to see confirmation of their theoretical approach, and evidence that their particular treatment strategy is successful (Farrell 1981). Naturally, psychoanalysts are encouraged to continue with the same treatment methods which yielded such opportune results, rather than to try out different methods, test alternative or differential explanations, or seek falsifying evidence. Encouraged by the apparent success of their dream analysis, analysands will continue to supply their psychoanalysts with oneiric material that bears the imprint of the methods of the dream analysis. And so on. Thus the treatment method helps to produce some of the very clinical material that confirms—or at least *seems* to confirm—the validity of the method; and the insights clients acquire into the meaning of their dreams, with the help of their analyst's dream interpretations, are insights into treatment artifacts rather than naturally occurring dreams. This wreaks havoc with the objectivity of dream insights and dream interpretations.

Freud's account of dreams supports a version of Hypothesis A: the idea that the objects of psychological exploration, interpretation, insight, and theoretical explanation are psychically real in their own right, with determinate properties and determinate forms of evidence. If dreams, as Freud wrote, are 'the royal road to a knowledge of the unconscious activities of the mind' (SE 1900 5: 608), then there is little about them that can be artificial or contrived. Naturally, Freud had to account for the phenomena of corroborative or compliance dreams (what he called 'obliging dreams') and, by implication, oneiric artifacts. He did this by distinguishing between manifest and latent dream content. The manifest content of dreams, Freud conceded, often bears the marks of analyst persuasion; but the latent content of dreams, and the dreamwork that operates over the latent material, is not vulnerable to the psychoanalysts' expectations and suggestions (Freud SE 1923, 19: 114-15): 'In fact, in many dreams which recall what has been forgotten and repressed, it is impossible to discover any other unconscious wish to which the motive force for the formation of the dream can be attributed. So that if anyone wishes to maintain that most of the dreams that can be made use of in analysis are obliging dreams and owe their origin to suggestion, nothing can be said against that opinion from the point of view of analytic therapy' (SE 1923, 19: 117; see also Grünbaum 1984: 237–8). Comments or cues from the psychoanalyst, in other words, could serve as triggers to dreams, just as could comments from other persons not directly involved in the dream analysis. The dreamwork itself, however, is a purely internal activity that is not open to external influence: it is protected by a kind of psychic *cordon sanitaire*. But the idea that there is a sharp division and one-way interaction between latent and manifest content is not unproblematic. It is not clear from Freud's account, for example, how something that is so immune to external influence could continue to remain immunized during its nightly engagement with manifest material that is subject to external influence. There is no doubt that part of Freud's reluctance to admit to anything but the most superficial role for therapeutic influence (such as suggestion) in dream analysis and in the use of free association can be explained by the unflattering model he held of the suggestion therapy of his predecessors: viz. therapeutic suggestion amounted to charismatic and domineering hypnotists overwhelming docile clients with crude commands. This model greatly oversimplifies the actual dynamics of suggestion therapy as practiced by Janet and others.

Artifactual Beliefs

At the simplest level, psychotherapeutic artifacts arise through the transmission of *cognitive* influence: that is, clients' *beliefs* about their personality, psychological make-up, and behaviors, and more specifically about their target disorders and their causes, can be influenced by the theoretical orientations of the psychotherapies under which they are treated (Ehrenwald 1966; Frank and Frank 1991). Clients in the psychodynamic psychotherapies are not indifferent to or ignorant of the theories governing their treatments: what they know about these theoretical orientations, or believe about them, makes a difference to their clinical productions and to the treatment outcomes. Clients are selected for psychodynamic psychotherapy in part because they tend to be psychologically-minded. They tend to approach psychotherapy with background assumptions about what works, what differentiates one psychotherapy from another, and what therapeutic treatment method best fits their own outlooks, values, and norms of well-being. Moreover, long-term exposure to their psychotherapist's theoretical orientation tends to modify these background assumptions, and in turn to modify the beliefs clients hold about the nature of their disorders, and the therapeutic progress they are making. Thus analysands in Freudian psychoanalysis hold beliefs about their psychological make-up, behaviors, emotions and personality that are framed in Freudian terms, just as clients in Kleinian psychotherapy hold beliefs about themselves that are framed in Kleinian terms, and clients in Kohutian psychotherapy hold beliefs about themselves that are framed in Kohutian terms; and so on. These are examples of doctrinal compliance at the level of belief production, and they result in belief artifacts.

Frank notes another vehicle for belief artifacts: client self-reports, which are solicited by measurement instruments, tests, outcome studies, or even in informal contexts. 'The kind of improvement patients report tends to confirm their therapist's theories. Patients in psychoanalysis, which relates mental health to the extent of the patient's self-knowledge, express increasing awareness of unconscious material as therapy progresses. Those who report improvement in client-centered therapy report that the discrepancy between their perceived and ideal selves has been reduced... Therapists who consider that the ability to sense and directly express feelings as a sign of progress find that their patients are better able to do this as therapy progresses... Evocative therapies influence patients' productions' (Frank and Frank 1991: 193).

Yet another vehicle for belief artifacts is first-person psychological self-explanation. In one study of clients in psychoanalytic, non-directive, and Adlerian therapy (Heine 1953), for example, it was found that clients tended to explain their symptoms and therapeutic progress in terms that were consistent with the theoretical orientation of the psychotherapy under which they were treated, often using sophisticated technical concepts drawn from the therapeutic theory's nosology and etiology (e.g. 'repression', 'superego'). Heine speculates that the degree of theoretical influence is such that knowing in advance the psychotherapist's theoretical orientation would support fairly accurate predictions of the content and nature of the clients' insights.

The transmission of cognitive influence that leads to belief artifacts is noticeable in the use of free association in psychoanalysis. It might seem that the method of free association yields more or less spontaneous and uncontaminated clinical material, rather like a spigot from which flows unimpeded a tangled mass of psychoanalytically meaningful material. Even the conscious distortions, editing, and framing that analysands introduce into their associations count as fully interpretable and decontaminable clinical material. In his later writings, however, Freud openly acknowledged the use of directive techniques of suggestion to mold the beliefs and memories produced by analysands in the course of freely associating about their pasts. At the same time, however, he denied that the use of such techniques resulted in irrevocably contaminated clinical data. The use of suggestion, he claimed, is at best a secondary and derivative technique that rides on the shoulders of the analysis. The analyst, he asserted, does not *manipulate* the transference relation that is so crucial in bringing about the analysand's new self-understanding, but instead *analyzes* it.

In his discussion of the sexual character of early childhood trauma, for instance, Freud appealed to the use of suggestive techniques in free association to generate clinical material about historical events for which there is little contemporary evidence: 'If the first-discovered scene is unsatisfactory, we *tell* our patient that this experience explains nothing, but that behind it there *must* be hidden a more significant, earlier experience; and we *direct* his attention by the same technique to the associative thread which connects the two memories—the one that has been discovered and the one that has still to be discovered'. (SE 1896, 3: 195–196 (italics added)). Because of the fragmentary and incomplete mnemonic evidence of early childhood traumas, the analyst must resort to suggestive techniques to help fill in the blanks. The goal here is not to deceive analysands about their pasts, but to manoeuvre them into a position from which they can begin to understand the etiology of their problems; and, ultimately, to put them into a position from which they can begin to understand that their resistances and defense mechanisms are maladaptive because they are based on infantile fantasies that have long since outlived their usefulness.

But Freud went one step further. In addition to allowing that analyst suggestion plays a robust compensatory role where the available clinical material from free association was wanting, he allowed that the etiological understanding developed by analysands as a result of suggestive compensation could aid in therapeutic improvement *even if it were inexact or false*. This is an open admission that the agent of therapeutic change is not always the *truth* of the analyst's interpretations of the clinical material yielded by the method of free association, nor the truth of the analysand's understanding and insights, but the analysand's *belief* in the veridicality of the relevant interpretations and insights. 'Quite often we do not succeed in bringing the patient to recollect what has been repressed. Instead of that, if the analysis is carried out correctly, we produce in him an assured conviction of the truth of the construction which achieves the same therapeutic result as a recaptured memory' (Freud SE 23: 265–6). This admission creates a number of problems. If analysands are free to develop 'assured convictions' about what is in fact a false (yet *prima facie* plausible) insight, and if psychological fictions can be as therapeutically effective as veridical insights, then the line of demarcation between psychoanalytic therapy and suggestion therapy, which Freud tried so assiduously to defend, is blurred. Grünbaum notes:

> Notoriously, neurotics are quite suggestible. By the same token their beliefs are quite malleable. Thus, often enough, patients do claim to confirm the etiologic interpretations and sundry causal attributions made by their analysts. But… such purported confirmations can be warrantedly explained by the well-attested doctrinal compliance of patients with the subtly communicated theoretical expectations of the healing authority figure to whom they have turned for help. As Freud himself appreciated all too keenly (SE 1917, 16: Lectures 27 and 28), there are myriad ways in which he can unconsciously but persuasively mold the analysand's convictions and engender a compliant pseudocorroboration (1984: 31).

Freud tried to rule out the possibility of belief malleability as a serious threat to the evidential base called upon in the clinical validation of psychoanalysis.

When applied scrupulously, and with an eye to its potential suggestive interference, the method of free association would (Freud claimed) yield a vast amount of *bona fide* clinical material, through which the analyst could then sift for clues of hidden causal connections. Free association 'guarantees to a great extent that… nothing will be introduced into it by the expectations of the analyst' (SE 1925, 20: 41). So effective is free association considered to be in allowing uncontaminated repressed material to come to light spontaneously that some psychoanalysts have even likened it to an investigative instrument of the same order of power as the microscope and the telescope (SE 1955, 2: xvi; Eissler 1969: 461). While the analogy clearly illustrates the degree of confidence some psychoanalysts have in the method of free association, it is a misleading analogy because of the vast differences in the nature of the objects targeted by the two kinds of instruments. Unlike human beings, objects such as microscopic organisms do not engage investigators in conversation. Nor are such objects consciously aware that they are under investigation with a particular method, and thereby capable of making (conscious or unconscious) adjustments to their behaviors to conceal or reveal what they consider to be salient in the investigation.

The method of free association brings with it unavoidable interference effects and observer effects that influence the content of clinical material yielded by analysis. These effects include such things as the analyst's expectations, verbal and nonverbal cues, strategies of interpretive 'filling in' and 'smoothing over' in the construction of interpretations, and the subtle rewards and punishments given to compliant or noncompliant behaviors (Farrell 1981).[2] Exaggerated methodological rigor does not eliminate these interference effects. Analysts who try to suppress every element of interpersonal influence in their application of the method—by eliminating gestures and spontaneous reactions, speaking in emotionally flat tones, withholding comments on the analysand's behaviors, refusing to offer opinions or advice—have simply substituted one kind of interpersonal influence with another more artificial one. In the face-to-face transactions of the psychotherapeutic encounter, 'the expressions on the therapist's face, a questioning glance, a lift of the eyebrows, a barely perceptible shake of the head or shrug of the shoulder all act as significant cues to the patient. But even *behind* the couch, the 'uh-ohs' as well as our silences, the interest or the disinterest reflected in our tone of voice or our shifting postures all act like subtle radio signals influencing the patients' responses, reinforcing some responses and discouraging others' (Marmor 1962: 291–292).

Artifactual Symptoms

Cognitive influence leads to one kind of psychotherapeutic artifact. But there is more to it than the molding of beliefs, opinions, and other cognitive states in response to the psychotherapist's theoretical orientations and expectations: some *symptoms* are receptive to theoretical influence, such that clients produce complex behavioral, psychological, and phenomenological material that appears to indicate the presence of the theoretically postulated symptoms (e.g. symptoms of an Oedipal complex, or castration anxiety, or a collective unconscious, or feelings of inferiority). In his essay on the imagination, the sixteenth-century French writer Michel de Montaigne (2003: 109–120) anticipated the contemporary logic of expectation model of placebo action (Kirsch 1985, 1997, 1999; Benedetti *et al.* 2003; Kihlstrom 2003) with a description of how some symptoms of illness are produced by the imagining and expectation of them. Where Kirsch, Benedetti and others who defend the logic of expectation model focus mainly on how the patient's *knowledge* about a treatment affects the treatment outcome, Montaigne focused on how the patient's imagination and affective states—which in some cases are more powerful than knowledge—affect treatment outcome. '*Fortis imaginatio generat casum.* [A powerful imagination generates the event] as the scholars say. I am one of those by whom the powerful blows of the imagination are most strongly felt. Everyone is hit by it, but some are bowled over' (2003: 109). Montaigne's point is that the way that some illnesses are imagined and anticipated influences the nature of symptoms themselves, and can result in symptoms that are neither entirely artificial nor entirely natural, but artifactual. Montaigne also observed that symptom remission is just as much influenced by imagination and expectation as symptom onset and duration: that is, how the treatment is *imagined* affects the therapy outcome. 'Why do doctors first work on the confidence of their patient with so many fake promises of a cure if not to allow the action of the imagination to make up for the trickery of their potions? They know… that there are men for whom it is enough merely to look at a medicine for it to prove effective.' (Montaigne 2003: 116-117; see also Melmed *et al.* 1986; Humphrey 2002).

Montaigne's insight that symptoms are malleable and receptive to influence receives support from a number of quarters. In a series of experiments about the placebo–opiate link, for example, Benedetti and others (Amanzio *et al.* 2001; Benedetti *et al.* 2003; Benedetti *et al.* 2005) showed that the patient's knowledge about a therapy (namely, the treatment of pain) affects the therapy outcome. Patients suffering from pain who know that they are receiving treatment (even if it is a placebo such as saline solution) tend to do better than those who do not know they are receiving treatment.

The phenomenon of symptom suggestibility also illustrates Montaigne's insight. In some cases, physicians' adherence to the principle of informed consent has the unwanted effect of bringing on adverse reactions in patients who have been given negative prognoses or negative information. Having been informed about the negative side effects of a treatment, some patients develop those side effects because they have been told about them, and not because of the treatment itself. Loftus and Fries (1979) write: 'An examination of the medical evidence demonstrates that... not only can positive therapeutic benefits be achieved by suggestion, but negative side effects and complications can similarly result. For example, among subjects who participated in a drug study after the usual informed consent procedure, many of those given an injection of a placebo reported physiologically unlikely symptoms such as dizziness, nausea, vomiting, and even mental depressions. One subject given the placebo reported that...these effects were so strong that they caused an automobile accident. Many other studies provide similar data indicating that to a variable but often frightening degree, explicit suggestion of possible adverse effects causes subjects to experience these effects. Recent hypotheses that heart attack may follow coronary spasm indicate physiological mechanisms by which explicit suggestions, and the stress that may be produced by them, might prove fatal. Thus the possible consequences of suggested symptoms range from minor annoyance to, in extreme cases, death'. Loftus and Fries conclude that informed consent may be dangerous to the health of patients.

Another type of symptom artifact that serves to illustrate Montaigne's insight is nosological self-scrutiny (Hahn 1997). In some cases, the mere awareness of nosological categories causes intensified self-scrutiny and self-diagnosing behaviors, which in turn cause the development of symptoms consistent with the expected or imagined disease, or high levels of hypochondriacal anxiety about it, despite the absence of underlying organic pathology. One well-known form of nosological self-scrutiny is cardiophobia, or cardiac neurosis. This occurs when the persistent fear of heart attacks and other cardiac problems leads to symptoms that closely mimic the symptoms of heart disease, which are forceful and involuntary. Patients with cardiophobia may seem to be suffering from heart disease, but no organically based disease processes are detectable. It might seem that nosological self-scrutiny is a rare occurrence affecting only a small population; but this remains to be determined, as there are few empirical studies of it. In at least one study (Woods *et al.* 1966) it was found that 79% of medical students reported having suffered from 'medstudentitis' at some time during their medical education. Symptoms abated within two to four weeks for most of the medical students in the study, but 15% of the students continued to have a 'phobic avoidance of both study and clinical contacts related to the disease in question' (Woods *et al.* 1966: 787).

Hahn (1997) classifies nosological self-scrutiny as a kind of nocebo effect: that is, the expectations of sickness and the affective and imaginary states associated with such expectations actually cause sickness. 'Not only are professional, folk, and lay nosologies, symptomatologies, and explanatory models *descriptions* of sickness events—as they are most often viewed—but a nosology is also a *sickness repertoire*, available for performance by those persons who have gained awareness through cultural participation. Knowledge that symptoms such as fainting exist provides a role or script available to be performed. In addition, nosologies may be *licenses* (insofar as they certify the cultural legitimacy of the condition) or *prescriptions* (insofar as they define expected sequences of occurrence)' (Hahn 1997: 69). This might seem implausible: how could the mere anticipation and imagination of disease produce real physiological effects or real symptoms? But 'nocebos increase the likelihood that the sickness they refer to will occur. However, nocebo acts need not be—and most appear not to be—deliberate, voluntary, or fully conscious' (Hahn 1997: 59). They are causal in the same way that other pathogens such as cigarette smoke and tubercular mycobacterium are causal.

The nineteenth-century British author Jerome K. Jerome (1899/1964) gives a comical sketch of nosological self-scrutiny and its associated symptom artifacts in the comic novel *Three Men In A Boat*:

> I knew it was my liver that was out of order, because I had just been reading a patent liver-pill circular, in which were detailed the various symptoms by which a man could tell when his liver was out of order. I had them all.
>
> It is a most extraordinary thing, but I never read a patent medicine advertisement without being impelled to the conclusion that I am suffering from the particular disease therein dealt with in its most virulent form. The diagnosis seems in every case to correspond exactly with all the sensations that I have ever felt. I remember going to the British Museum one day to read up the treatment for some slight ailment of which I had a touch—hay fever, I fancy it was. I got down the book, and read all I came to read; and then, in an unthinking moment, I idly turned the leaves, and began to indolently study diseases generally. I forget which was the first distemper I plunged into—some fearful, devastating scourge, I know—and, before I had glanced half down the list of 'premonitory symptoms', it was borne in upon me that I had fairly got it.
>
> I sat for a while frozen with horror; and then in the listlessness of despair, I again turned over the pages. I came to typhoid fever—read the symptoms—discovered that I had typhoid fever, must have had it for months without knowing it—wonder what else I had too; turned up St Vitus's Dance—found, as I had expected, that I had that too—began to get interested in my case, and determined to sift it to the bottom, and so started alphabetically—read up ague, and learnt that I was sickening for it, and that the acute stage would commence in about another fortnight... I plodded conscientiously through the twenty-six letters, and the only malady I could conclude I had not got was housemaid's knee. I felt rather hurt about this at first; it seemed somehow to be a sort of slight... I reflected that I had every known malady in pharmacology, and I grew less selfish, and determined to do without housemaid's knee. Gout, in its most malignant stage, it would appear, had seized me without my being aware of it; and zymosis I had evidently been suffering from boyhood. There were no more diseases after zymosis, so I concluded there was nothing else the matter with me...

Then I wondered how long I had to live. I tried to examine myself. I felt my pulse. I could not at first feel any pulse at all. Then, all of a sudden, it seemed to start off. I pulled out my watch and timed it. I made it a hundred and forty-seven to the minute. I tried to feel my heart. It had stopped beating... I patted myself all over my front, from what I call my waist up to my head, and I went a bit round each side, and a little way up the back. But I could not feel or hear anything...

I had walked into that reading-room a happy healthy man. I crawled out a decrepit wreck.

I went to my medical man... He opened me up and looked down me, and clutched hold of my wrist, and then he hit me over the chest when I wasn't expecting it—a cowardly thing to do, I call it—and immediately afterwards butted me with the side of his head. After that, he sat down and wrote out a prescription, and folded it up, and gave it to me, and I put it into my pocket and went out.

I did not open it. I took it to the nearest chemist's, and handed it in. The man read it, and then handed it back.

He said he didn't keep it.

I said: 'You are a chemist?'

He said: 'I am a chemist. If I was a co-operative stores and family hotel combined, I might be able to oblige you. Being only a chemist hampers me'.

I read the prescription. It ran:

'1 lb. beefsteak, with

1 pt. bitter beer

every 6 hours.

1 ten-mile walk every morning.

1 bed at 11 sharp every night

And don't stuff up your head with

Things you don't understand'.

I followed the directions, with the happy result—speaking for myself—that my life was preserved, and is still going on. (Jerome 1899/1964: 2–5)

If symptom artifacts occur in physical medicine, then it is likely that their psychological analogs are to be found in psychological interventions.[3] If they do, then just as somatic symptom artifacts appear to be natural and unbidden, so psychological symptom artifacts would appear to be natural and unbidden, despite the fact that they are not based on any underlying disorders, and do not follow known causal pathways. Consider for example the symptom artifacts that may be caused by psychologically-oriented nosological self-scrutiny. Sensitized to the nosological categories in terms of which they have been diagnosed, or to the symptom profiles of psychological disorders targeted by their treatments, some clients in psychotherapy may fall into patterns of psychological self-monitoring and self-scrutinizing. As with 'medstudentitis' and cardiophobia, this can lead to the development of symptoms that are consistent with the psychological theories and treatment methods to which they are exposed—what has been called symptomatological self-identification (Borch-Jacobsen 1996).[4] For example, after an initial socialization process that includes learning about the onset, course, duration, symptom profiles, and remission patterns of the primary disorders treated by the psychodynamic psychotherapies, clients may become increasingly psychodynamically self-scrutinizing, and may develop symptoms that mimic the symptoms predicted by the relevant psychodynamic theory and targeted by its associated treatment method. These would not count as cases of malingering, because they are not deliberate or well-planned. Clients may experience their symptoms as real and intrusive, and may appear to be sincerely unaware of (or selectively inattentive to) the artifactual character of their symptoms. It does not occur to them that the diagnostic and treatment methods to which they are subjected have influenced some of the very symptoms they are experiencing.[5]

What are the effects of artifactual symptoms on the client's acquisition of insight? With the psychodynamic emphasis on exploration and discovery, the artifactual symptoms may seem so real to clients that they feel that they have made important 'discoveries' about themselves, the objects of which discoveries they mistakenly interpret as having existed prior to psychotherapeutic intervention. They thus construe their exploratory psychotherapy as a process of *bona fide* psychological discovery. What is actually happening, however, is that the treatment method has generated an overlay of artifactual symptoms that looks surprisingly like the symptoms predicted by the therapeutic theory's etiology and symptomatology. As with artifactual dreams, this too results in a feedback loop, and a psychotherapy whose central theoretical claims are to a certain extent self-confirming.

*

Beliefs, dreams, and symptoms are some examples of psychological states that can become psychotherapeutic artifacts. They are the clinical analog to the methodological artifacts that appear in the social and behavioral sciences. There may be other psychotherapeutic artifacts, ranging more extensively over target disorders, behaviors, psychological states, and personality attributes. Frank, for example, cites a number of studies that suggest that clients' *values* tend be influenced by, and correspond increasingly to, those of their psychotherapists, particularly as the duration of treatment increases. The studies show, moreover, that psychotherapists tend to evaluate their clients as displaying improvement the more clients' values come to resemble their own (Frank and Frank 1991: 174–5). As psychotherapeutic artifacts multiply, the clinical material that is considered relevant for interpretations and insights becomes increasingly geared to the theoretical framework that first influenced it. In turn, as Marmor observes, the clinical material tends to confirm more and more of the theory: 'Depending upon the point of view of the analyst, the patients of each [rival psychoanalytic] school seem to bring up precisely the kind of phenomenological data which confirm the theories and interpretations of their analysts! Thus each theory tends to be self-validating. Freudians elicit material about the Oedipal complex and castration anxiety, Jungians about archetypes, Rankians about separation anxiety, Adlerians about masculine strivings and feelings of inferiority, Horneyites about idealized images, Sullivanians about disturbed interpersonal relationships, etc'. (Marmor 1962: 289).

The behavioral and cognitive mechanisms that give rise to psychotherapeutic artifacts are also at work in other dimensions of human conduct: for example, in some educational settings, and in religious, military, and ideological training. And they have not gone unnoticed. The complex links between self-attribution, suggestion-driven psychological artifact, and the crystallization of incipient or ambiguous mental states have long been a subject of psychological speculation and literary description;[6] and they have long been the target of experimentation and hypothesis testing in social and cognitive psychology.[7] The psychotherapies, in other words, represent only one particularly focused forum in which these mechanisms are activated (Strupp 1972a, 1972b), with different psychotherapies accessing and realizing them in different ways. In the psychodynamic psychotherapies, for instance, mechanisms of suggestion and disambiguation are pressed into service to create information-rich interpersonal environments that help clients to understand complex, confused, or ambiguous internal states – but only by shaping or crystallizing those very states in ways that conform to the psychotherapy's theoretical orientation. Those states are crystallized into new forms that would not otherwise have occurred, and that nonetheless have the appearance of having existed prior to therapeutic intervention.

Psychodynamic exploration does not always conform carefully and sensitively to the unique contours of the client's psychology—although this is what the Standard View suggests. Rather, it has the power to sometimes transform clients so that they come to fit the treatment methods, by manufacturing some of the very facts about the clients that they putatively uncover (Farrell 1981). Because therapeutic exploration is an activity that itself generates some of the evidence that supports the therapeutic theory, clients' acquisition of insight becomes part of a self-confirming feedback loop. Much more is occurring than straightforward exploration and discovery. There is rather a dynamic interchange between the treatment methods and the psychological and behavioral material upon which they operate—a dialectic of forming and conforming. It is not as if the facts of a client's psychology, behavior, and personality are simply awaiting discovery, which will be occasioned only by means of a precisely applied treatment method that fits those facts snugly like a key opening a lock; rather, psychotherapists use the therapeutic situation to change clients to fit their theoretical orientation and treatment methods (Farrell 1981: 126–127).

Thus the familiar analogy between psychodynamic psychotherapy and archaeological excavation is misleading. Rather than careful layer-by-layer archaeological excavation of well-preserved hidden treasures, the psychodynamic psychotherapies are more like methods of digging that in their very operation sometimes confuse and fuse the layers of disturbed earth with the original remains. Or, switching metaphors, clients in their therapeutic explorations are more like explorers whose very steps forward alter the landscape they are exploring.

This contrasts sharply with the view that differences between psychodynamic psychotherapies are largely differences of detail and emphasis—as if they are like different windows opening out over the same field of facts. According to this view, one psychodynamic approach might emphasize certain aspects of a client's personality structure as explanatorily salient with respect to certain disorders, while another might emphasize certain aspects of a client's developmental history. But both are referring to and working upon the same personality, and tracking and converging upon the same underlying psychological and behavioral facts.

This view—call it the convergence view—greatly oversimplifies matters. If there are such things as psychotherapeutic artifacts, then different exploratory psychotherapies generate different psychological and behavioral artifacts. Rather than convergence upon the same underlying facts, there is pronounced divergence in the generation of artifacts.

The psychoanalyst Erik Erikson defends a version of the convergence view. Erikson argues that the differences between widely divergent therapeutic systems are less substantial than the similarities; and that despite vastly different treatment methods and explanatory theories, alternative forms of psychotherapy ultimately refer to and work upon the 'same forces'.

> In northern California I knew an old shaman woman who laughed merrily at my conception of mental disease, and then sincerely—to the point of ceremonial tears— told me of her way of sucking the 'pains' out of her patients. She was as convinced of her ability to cure and to understand as I was of mine. While occupying extreme opposites in the history of American psychiatry we felt like colleagues. This was based on some joint sense of the historical relativity of all psychotherapy: the relativity of the patient's outlook on his symptoms, of the role he assumes by dint of being a patient, of the kind of help which he seeks, and of the kinds of help which are eagerly offered or are available. The old shaman woman and I disagreed about the locus of emotional sickness, what it 'was', and what specific methods would cure it. Yet, when she related the origin of a child's illness to the familial tensions existing within her tribe, when she attributed the 'pain' (which had got 'under a child's skin') to his grandmother's sorcery (ambivalence), I knew she dealt with the same forces, and with the same kinds of conviction, as I did in my professional nook. This experience has been repeated in discussion with colleagues who, although not necessarily more 'primitive', are oriented toward different psychiatric persuasions. (Erikson 1958: 55)

Erikson holds that psychoanalysis and shamanism—and, by implication, many other forms of psychological healing—use different concepts to refer to the same primary psychological disorders and the same primary psychological treatment mechanisms. This is an important claim. But it is unclear from Erikson's account what precisely remains the 'same' for psychoanalysis and shamanism once the linguistic and conceptual differences have been factored out: causal pathways, symptom profiles, disease entities, or treatment methods— or something even more basic?

One thing that Erikson does not mean is that the technical terminologies of shamanism and psychoanalysis have the same basic *meanings*. The shamanistic concept of sorcery, for instance, does not carry the same meanings, nor does it fit in the same network of conceptual and logical relations, as the psychoanalytic concept of ambivalence. Superficially, it might seem that Erikson's claim that both systems refer to the 'same forces' is a claim that could be settled by empirical investigation. Showing that the referent of the term 'pain' is the same as the referent of the term 'ambivalence' would not be unlike showing that the term 'evening star' refers to the same thing as the term 'morning star'. But there are three reasons why this is doubtful.

First, the history of psychotherapy is a fractionated history. Few empirical discoveries have played a significant role in settling disagreements between the rival psychotherapeutic schools about the basic concepts and principles underlying etiology, symptomatology, nosology, and treatment. Similarly, few empirical discoveries across the history of psychotherapy have resulted in substantive convergences or cross-theoretic reductions of conceptual terminology between competing psychotherapies. The failure of theoretical convergence also shows up on the clinical level. Not only is there healthy disagreement between psychotherapists of competing schools on what counts as an accurate description of a client's symptoms, and what counts as an accurate account of etiology (see Corsini *et al.* 1991); more significantly, there is often robust disagreement about what *sorts* of empirical considerations would come to count as potentially decisive and criterial.

Second, it is unclear from Erikson's account precisely what remains the 'same' for the psychotherapist and the shaman once surface terminological differences are suspended, because attributions of sameness and difference are not simply read off the phenomena. Any two objects, forces, or events that are construed as the same under one identifying description can be construed as different under another. Attributions of sameness, in other words, are description-dependent: something is the same under a certain description, or *as* a so-and-so of a particular sort. The onus is on Erikson to show how a neutral meta-language can refer to 'the same forces', without question-begging assumptions about the criteria used to establish the attribution of sameness and difference (Neu 1977).

Third, the phenomenon of therapeutic artifacts suggests that there are reasons for thinking that different psychotherapeutic systems *manufacture* psychological, behavioral, and phenomenological artifacts *differentially*. During the course of Eriksonian psychoanalysis, for example, certain aspects of the client's psychology, behavior, and phenomenology will conform to the theoretical postulates and clinical profiles typical of the Eriksonian version of psychoanalytic symptomatology, etiology, and nosology. Similarly, during the course of shamanist healing, certain aspects of the client's psychology, behavior, and phenomenology will conform to the theoretical postulates and clinical profiles typical of shamanism's symptomatology, etiology, and nosology. The question then is not whether different psychotherapeutic systems refer to the 'same forces', but whether they *can* refer to the 'same forces' in the first place, given the differential artifacts they each generate.

If the psychodynamic psychotherapies have the potential to generate in clients complexly-woven overlays of psychological, behavioral, and experiential artifacts that would not otherwise have existed outside the treatment, then Erikson's claim that psychotherapists of widely different theoretical orientations are dealing with the 'same forces' is doubtful. Over the course of treatment, a sufficiently dense layering of therapeutic artifact may be built up, with one artifact overlaid upon the other in an evolving and unnoticed series of accretions which masks whatever original layers served as their ground. Psychotherapy A will crystallize certain incipient behaviors or psychological states in such a way that they conform to the demands of the therapeutic theory of A (rather than vice versa), with the client's insights into these behaviors and psychological states appearing as *bona fide* discoveries of antecedently existing facts. But psychotherapy B would crystallize those same incipient states differently, thereby generating the conditions for different insights. Once stabilized under the form of psychotherapy A or B, neither insight can be described as picking out—from different angles, or with different terminologies—the 'same' psychological, behavioral, or phenomenological facts (as Erikson claims): instead, each one has changed the incipient states by overlaying them with alternative artifactual configurations. What Erikson construes as competing interpretations of the same underlying psychological forces (viz. pains and ambivalence) are in actuality interpretations of divergently configured artifactual overlays.

Thus the hypothetical ideal of comparing and contrasting competing psychotherapeutic systems by trying to determine how they would affect one and the same imaginary client in parallel treatments meets a number of logical obstacles (Farrell 1981; Corsini *et al.* 1991). Freud appeared to be aware of some of these. In addressing the issue of whether psychoanalysis is therapeutically effective, he is reported to have said jokingly that 'the best control is to treat the same person twice, once with analysis and once without, and then compare results' (Pfeffer 1959). In such an hypothetical scenario (one that is developed in Farrell 1981, and Corsini *et al.* 1991), client A would be treated concurrently in two parallel treatment modalities, classical Freudian psychoanalysis and psychotherapy Y, neither of which are allowed to interfere with the effects of the other. It would be possible then to examine the therapeutic benefits of the two approaches to A, with a view to determining which one was better suited to A's needs.[8] But if rival psychotherapies manufacture some of the very facts that partially confirm their respective theoretical explanations and clinical practices, and if they do so differentially, then the result would be two separate histories of differently configured artifacts, rather than one and the same person accessed by different treatment methods.

The Narrativist Objection

The main conceptual hypothesis explored in this work is the following: a) some therapeutic changes in psychodynamic psychotherapy may be functions of powerful placebos that rally the mind's natural healing powers, rather than functions of hypothesized characteristic factors of the treatment methods of the psychodynamic psychotherapies; b) one type of placebo that may be operative in psychodynamic psychotherapy is the explanatory fiction, found at work in psychodynamic interpretations and insights. As it was mentioned earlier, this hypothesis is bound to meet with skepticism. Some of the more empirically-based objections have already been addressed very briefly. Two of the most weighty conceptual objections to be raised at this stage of the argument are the following: i) what seems to count as insight or interpretation placebos are in fact therapeutically potent narratives, with their own unique and irreducible type of truth; and ii) there is no such thing as a psychological equivalent of a sugar pill, and hence no such thing as an insight or interpretation placebo, because the very attempt to transpose the concept of placebo from physical medicine to psychotherapy is misconceived. These objections will be addressed in turn.

One well-known approach that appears to supply the conceptual grounds needed to undermine the insight placebo hypothesis is narrativism. Even if psychodynamic interpretations and insights fail to accurately represent the facts of a client's psychology, behavior, and personality—that is, even if they are false or fictitious—they are still true in some other sense, and therefore not placebos. What other sense is this? They are true in the sense that they are coherent, plausible, and meaningful narratives. They display what might be called narrative truth (Spence 1982). If psychodynamic interpretations and insights are true in at least this one sense, then they cannot be the psychological equivalent of sugar pills. This approach to exploratory psychotherapy, which is defended by Spence (1982), Schafer (1981, 1992) and others in the narrativist and hermeneutic tradition (Guignon 1998; Hersch 2003), rests on the crucial assumption that there is more than one sense of truth. Spence, for example, argues that 'it was once accepted that psychotherapy worked by digging into the unconscious... and curing symptoms by exposing truth. Conflicting therapies disagreed about the meanings or factors behind symptoms, but all believed that only dealing with these 'real things' in their 'real places' could really cure. These metaphors are no longer valid' (Spence 1982: 203).

The narrativist approach to psychotherapy does not give up on the ideal of truth altogether, as the postmodern approach to psychotherapy appears to do (Held 1995, 2007; Erwin 1997). Rather, it sets up a double set of epistemic books, by distinguishing between different kinds of truth, different types of evidence, and different methods of getting at these different kinds of truth. Spence, for example, makes a sharp distinction between historical truth and narrative truth. Historical truth consists of the correspondence of an interpretation or insight with so-called 'extra-linguistic' matters of fact. This, he argues, is both an inappropriate and an unachievable model of truth in matters psychotherapeutic. Narrative truth, by contrast, consists of the internal coherence of the narrative in terms of which extra-linguistic facts are organized and given meaning in interpretations and insights. The narrative truth of an interpretation or insight is established by appealing to their internal coherence, the goodness of fit between the narrative and the clinical data, and the narrative's congruence with a consensually recognized knowledge base. Coherence is not merely a sign of truth, but is itself the condition of truth.

Spence argues that the truth of psychoanalytic (and by implication, psychodynamic) interpretations and insights emerges with the creation of an adaptive and internally coherent system of meaningful connections among the historical and psychological facts. This is a process involving the same kinds of imaginative selection and abstraction deployed by artists who experiment with materials with a view to constructing a unique synthetic whole. 'Meanings are not objectively there to be found, but are constructions of therapists' and clients' minds. The story of clients' lives, which develops in therapy, is not the real history, archaeologically reconstructed, but is one possible narrative: perhaps more orderly, detailed and coherent than the pretherapeutic one, but not necessarily more true' (Spence 1980: 100). Those interpretations and insights that are considered to be narratively true are flexible enough to accommodate factual errors, false memories, and psychologically incorrect descriptions—but these are inconveniences that are tolerated as relatively insignificant 'noise' with respect to the effort of psychotherapists and clients to create new meaningful narratives.

But how is it that insights and interpretations that float free of the facts of a client's psychology, behavior, and personality can still be therapeutically effective? Spence argues that the psychological problems from which clients suffer are caused primarily by a lack of intelligibility or meaning, rather than from the lack of objectively true accounts of the causes of their psychology and behaviors; treatment, therefore, consists primarily in the restoration of intelligibility or meaning. The view that psychological disorders are caused by the lack of intelligibility or meaning presupposes a weighty counterfactual principle of contrast: namely, without intelligibility and meaning, particularly in the form of narrative structuring, human experience would disintegrate into a degraded and incoherent state.

Like artists, psychotherapists and clients enjoy a certain degree of interpretive, editorial, and criteriological freedom in developing interpretations and insights that are considered to be narratively true. In order to relate the unknown to the known, and to supply order and structure where before there was none, free rein is given to imaginative editing, re-writing, narrative 'filling in', and the narrative 'smoothing over' of factual discrepancies. Spence claims that an interpretation that merits the title of narrative truth 'may bring about a positive effect not because it corresponds to a specific piece of the past but because it appears to relate the known to the unknown, to provide explanation in place of uncertainty... We have come to see that certain kinds of pragmatic statements can produce changes in behavior simply by virtue of being stated' (Spence 1980: 290). This would appear to explain the treatment effect illustrated in Mendel's example of the false interpretation.

There are a number of theoretical difficulties with the narrativist approach to psychotherapy (see Grünbaum 1984; Held 1995, 2007; Erwin 1997), and with narrativism as a general theoretical model (Jopling 2000; Strawson 2004), and these weaken its ability to mount an effective criticism of the insight placebo hypothesis. First, the narrativist approach under-determines the specific contents of psychotherapeutic narratives, and is therefore crucially vague on what makes it suited specifically to psychodynamic approaches to psychotherapy as opposed to any other approaches. In other words, if the only criteria governing the therapeutic admissibility of interpretations and insights are coherence and plausibility, then it is not clear what could serve to distinguish psychodynamic interpretations and insights from non-psychodynamic ones, if both equally satisfy the criteria of coherence and plausibility. Narrative coherence alone is not sufficient to distinguish one from another. What this means is that almost any narrative content could satisfy the criterion of coherence and be counted as narratively true: demonological and astrological narratives, existentialist or experientialist psychotherapy narratives, gestaltist or feminist psychotherapy narratives, and so on.

Second, it is not clear how the narrativist approach can supply clear grounds for upholding the distinction between *mere* story telling that satisfies the criterion of internal coherence, and *truth-tracking* story telling. The mere acquisition of therapeutically effective narrative insight, for instance, is not sufficient to establish the insight as truth-tracking: it may simply be a case of clients exercising a knack for formulating narratives that have a semblance of coherence and plausibility. The reverse is also possible: robust truth-tracking insight is compatible with narrative ineptitude. Moreover, a narrative insight that merely happens to be historically and psychologically true is not *ipso facto* equivalent to genuine insight. Clients in narrative psychotherapy may know enough about themselves to produce historically and psychologically plausible narratives, but they may not be genuinely insightful because their actions are jarringly mismatched to their narratives. There must be something more to insight than merely the production of internally coherent and plausible narratives.

The third problem with the narrativist strategy is that interpretations and insights that exchange contact with psychological and historical reality for narrative coherence are on an epistemic slippery slope. With every increase in interpretive, editorial, and criteriological freedom comes an increase in the empirical under-determination of interpretations and insights. This might look like an enviable degree of narrative freedom. But at the far end of the slippery slope, the impact of an unyielding historical, psychological, and behavioral reality that could supply external correction and intersubjective corroboration is hardly felt. At this far end of the slope there is little to stop psychotherapists and clients from developing coherent but historically revisionist interpretations and insights that serve the ends of lying, self-deception, or moral convenience. By renarrating the events of the past, and renarrating the story of the dynamics of their psychology, behavior, and personality, psychotherapists and clients would be in a position to correct fortune in the same way that Soviet-era historians corrected fortune by rewriting the history of the Soviet Union. The narrative approach to psychotherapy may thus have morally undesirable consequences (Held 1995), because it jeopardizes the distinction between a coherent and factually accurate narrative, and a coherent but systematically self-deceived narrative that is driven by personal preference, fantasy or moral convenience (Jopling 1996b, 2000).

The Identity Objection

Another objection to the insight placebo hypothesis is the following: the effort to transpose the concept of placebo and placebo controls in medical and pharmaceutical research to psychotherapy research is incoherent, and so the very idea that there is a psychological analog to the sugar pill or the saline injection is misconceived from the start. This is an important, and mainly conceptual, objection. To grasp its significance, however, some preliminary background is required.

Since its invention, the randomized double-blind controlled clinical trial has had such an enviable degree of success in helping researchers to determine the relative effectiveness of medications and medical procedures that it has emerged as the highest standard of medical evidence (Gold *et al.* 1937; Gold 1946, 1954; Shapiro and Shapiro 1997a; Kaptchuk 1998b). Its success was not lost on psychotherapy researchers, who found themselves faced with a plethora of 'unchallenged claims to profound and undifferentiated therapeutic benefit' (Parloff 1986a: 521), but had little in the way of objective standards of measurement to sort out and test these claims. Starting in the mid-1950s, a number of researchers (Meehl 1955; Rosenthal and Frank 1956; Paul 1966) issued a call to import the double-blind controlled clinical trial design into trials of psychotherapy effectiveness, with the goal of evaluating the comparative effectiveness of different psychological treatments for specific psychological disorders. This would, it was thought, maintain the same degree of methodological rigor as clinical trials in medical and pharmaceutical science. The call was well-heeded, and many hundreds of outcome studies have since endeavored to compare specific psychotherapeutic techniques with a placebo psychotherapy—that is, one that lacked the specific or characteristic therapeutic factors of the psychotherapy (i.e. those hypothesized to be the active therapeutic ingredients), but nonetheless contained enough of the non-specific or non-characteristic factors to serve as a credible placebo.

But what is a placebo psychotherapy in the first place? Is there really such a thing? What would it look like? Does the very idea of an equivalence or analogy between a physical placebo such as a sugar pill and a psychological placebo make sense? While there is little agreement on this vexed question, and little agreement on how to tackle it, a long tradition of psychotherapy research dating back to the 1950s has nonetheless forged ahead on the robust assumption that there *is* a workable equivalence; and, consequently, that psychotherapy placebos of one sort or another can serve as credible controls in clinical trials and outcome studies. No single placebo control has emerged from these outcome studies as the placebo of choice; nor has any consensus emerged among psychotherapy researchers on the range of items that could count as workable psychotherapeutic placebos. One of the notable results of proceeding on this assumption, then, is a large, conflicting, and ever-changing body of clinical and experimental data about therapeutic efficacy. Several well-known psychotherapy researchers, however, have called the putative equivalence between medical placebos and psychological placebos into question, and have argued that the use of placebo controls in psychotherapy outcome research is misconceived. Before examining their arguments, however, it is important to survey briefly some of the types of placebos used in placebo-controlled psychotherapy outcome studies, in order to know what it is precisely that the arguments are targeting.

One review of the literature provides a useful overview of some of the main types of psychotherapy placebo control in use in a large number of psychotherapy outcome studies (Horvath 1988): the classic medical placebo, the theoretically inert placebo, the component control placebo, and the alternate therapy control.[9] According to Horvath, one of the most commonly used placebos in psychotherapy outcome studies is the classic medical placebo, imported from medical and pharmaceutical clinical trials as a control against which an hypothesized active treatment is measured. The medication placebo (such as a lactose pill) is considered to be *therapeutically inert*, at least from the point of view of the psychotherapeutic theory that is being tested. Even medication placebos, however, may contain therapeutically active components that are not shared with the treatment undergoing testing.

Another type of placebo commonly used in psychotherapy outcome studies, according to Horvath, is the *theoretically inert* placebo. This is a placebo that has no hypothesized treatment value, and no hypothesized causal role, at least from the point of view of the therapeutic theory being tested. In outcome studies using theoretically inert placebos, the treatments and the placebos against which they are compared are designed in such a way that they contain relatively few components or procedures, thereby making investigation and replication easier. While the placebo may contain some components that are also present in the experimental treatment, they do not contain any of the postulated active components of the treatment in question: they are not, in other words, alternative forms of treatment. A closely related type of placebo that is commonly used in psychotherapy outcome studies is the *component control* placebo, which is designed to closely replicate the components of the experimental therapy, with the exception of the specific treatment component whose therapeutic activity is under investigation. Unlike theoretically inert placebos, the component control placebo contains several components that may be considered to be therapeutically active, at least from the point of view of other theories of therapy. In other words, they may be considered alternative forms of treatment. Finally, Horvath notes that some psychotherapy outcome studies use alternate forms of therapy as placebo controls, although it is not clear what is to be gained from calling these placebos.

A number of psychotherapy researchers, however, reject the very idea of a psychotherapy placebo, and with it the very idea that there is a useful equivalence or analogy between a physical placebo such as a sugar pill and a psychological placebo. This is a radical challenge, because it calls into question the very legitimacy of the fifty-year-long research tradition in psychotherapy, clinical psychology, and psychiatry that relies on placebo controls. The main argument the critics defend is that it is impossible to transpose—at least with any degree of plausibility and logical consistency—the concept of placebo from the field of medical and pharmaceutical research (where according to Parloff the concept is already quite 'convoluted') to psychotherapy outcome research (Bergin 1971; Parloff 1986a, 1986b; Borkovec and Sibrava 2005; Herbert and Gaudiano 2005; Kirsch 2005; Lambert 2005). If their arguments are valid, then comparisons of the efficacy of psychotherapy with psychotherapy placebo are not possible, because the very idea of a psychotherapy placebo is ill-conceived. There is, in other words, no such a thing as the psychotherapeutic equivalent of the sugar pill or the saline injection; nor, by implication, is there such a thing as an insight or interpretation placebo. It is not that sufficient material or social conditions are lacking that would somehow prevent the invention of such placebos; rather, the very idea is misconceived.[10]

Bergin (1971: 246) was one of the first to raise a version of this objection:

> It is evident that several factors may account for 'spontaneous remission' phenomena, that these factors have therapeutic efficacy, that many of them occur in psychotherapy as well as naturally, but that they are not necessarily unique to the formal therapy process. This means that subjects used as control groups or to establish base line percentages of improvement for comparisons with treatment cases are not really controls at all! They are the recipients of formal, informal, and self-help procedures which are often enough identical or similar to psychotherapy, so that they cannot be justifiably used for this purpose. Thus, we have found that not only is the spontaneous remission rate lower than expected, but also that it is probably caused to a considerable degree by actual therapy or therapy-like procedures.

Bergin's argument is that psychotherapy placebo controls are really alternative forms of psychotherapy treatment; they are neither theoretically nor therapeutically inert, and so are not in fact placebos in the traditional sense. Parloff (1986a, 1986b) advances a similar argument to support his view that the use of placebo controls in psychotherapy effectiveness studies is methodologically ill-conceived. He begins by noting that in clinical trials that compare the effectiveness of a drug or medical treatment with a placebo, the placebo must objectively lack the so-called 'specific components' that are hypothesized to be therapeutically effective in the treatment of a disease or disorder. This is the only way to obtain a clear idea of the efficacy of the experimental drug or treatment. But a strategy that 'dismantles' treatments in this way—that is, by separating out specific from nonspecific components, in order to exclude the specific components from the placebo, does not apply to psychotherapy. There are, he argues, several reasons for this.

First, because there is no consensus among the different schools of psychotherapy about what constitutes the specific components of psychotherapy, the distinction between specific and nonspecific collapses. What is considered a specific therapeutic component by one theory of psychotherapy is considered nonspecific or incidental by another; and vice versa. Thus there is no agreement over what constitutes an adequate placebo control against which any one psychotherapy can be tested for efficacy. What to one school of psychotherapy is an adequate placebo (because it lacks certain specific components), is to another school an active treatment with specific components: crudely, one school's placebo is another's psychotherapy. This situation, Parloff claims, is not found in controlled clinical trials in medicine and pharmacology, where there is a greater degree of consensus about the specific–nonspecific distinction. This means that the absence of any standardized placebo control against which psychotherapeutic treatments can be tested undermines the placebo challenge. 'Because each placebo must be carefully designed and described to contrast with the particular experimental treatment for which it is to serve as a control, the hope of developing a standard placebo applicable to all treatments loosely identified as psychotherapy cannot be realized... Any placebo whose rationale was so ingenious as to elicit and sustain a high degree of credibility in patients would not long be considered theoretically inert' (1986b: 83).

Disagreement over what constitutes specific and nonspecific components in psychotherapy is undoubtedly rife. This is in part because of the confusion generated by the ambiguity of the very terms in which Parloff frames the argument (see Chapter 4, Part ii). Parloff's term 'nonspecific' is confusing because it connotes indistinctness. As Grünbaum (1986) notes, however, the effects of placebos can be just as sharply defined and specific as the effects of nonplacebos; and they can be just as precisely described as the effects of nonplacebos.

This is not all. Parloff's requirement that there be a standard placebo control that is acceptable to all forms of psychotherapy is too stringent. Just as there are different types of placebos in pharmaceutical and medical research, so there are different types of placebos in psychotherapy research. Different psychotherapeutic schools test their effectiveness against placebos by designing context-specific placebos: that is, placebos that objectively lack *only* the characteristic factors that are hypothesized to be therapeutically effective by a particular treatment method. A placebo control to test the effectiveness of behavioral psychotherapy, for example, would be inappropriate as a control for psychodynamic psychotherapy.

Parloff's requirement for a standard or all-purpose placebo that ranges across all forms of psychotherapy sets the bar for placebo controls unrealistically high, because it fails to distinguish between different degrees of standardization. There is no reason to require that a placebo be standardized in every relevant respect—as if this alone can insure fair clinical comparisons. No such thing as a standardized placebo exists in pharmaceutical trials or medical trials. Take, for example, lactose pill placebos. These are often considered as exemplar placebos in pharmaceutical trials. But they are far from standardized in all relevant respects: treatment context, pill size, shape and color, dispensing instructions, follow-up, and placebo side effects vary from one trial to another. The only thing that remains constant is the fact that a lactose pill is prescribed. This is, at best, a bare-bones level of standardization. Now if this is the most that can be expected of pharmaceutical placebo controls, it is unreasonable to expect that a higher standard apply to psychotherapy placebo controls. Minimal levels of placebo standardization are all that is required in controlled psychotherapy trials. As Erwin (1997) suggests, a pill placebo plus client wait list plus minimal psychotherapist contact serves as a more or less credible and minimally standardized placebo that could be used to test the effectiveness of many different psychotherapies.

Another argument Parloff advances against the placebo challenge is that useful placebo controls cannot be designed for psychotherapy trials, because many of the specific and nonspecific components of psychotherapies are not operationally defined, but are rather 'attributed haphazardly to vague classes of therapist behaviors and attitudes' (1986b). 'In the absence of a distinctive, intelligible, and replicable description of the experimental treatment form, it is not possible to devise or select a useful placebo control'. This criticism is overstated. While operational definitions and clearly written treatment manuals may be lacking in many schools of psychotherapy, they are not the only way to identify the so-called 'specific' and 'nonspecific' components of a psychotherapy; nor are they always the most reliable way, given the decontextualized nature of operational definitions. Even in the absence of clear operational definitions and workable treatment manuals, the distinction between characteristic and incidental factors is passed down through research literature, case histories, training programs, and clinical traditions.

Finally, Parloff claims that the sheer difficulty of differentiating placebo controls from alternate forms of treatment undermines the placebo challenge, and vitiates any attempts to compare the efficacy of psychotherapy against placebos. 'If the placebo includes ingredients hypothesized by any formal psychosocial treatment as specific for the treatment of specified problems, then the intended placebo, when applied to the same problems, must be considered an alternative treatment form rather than a placebo' (1986b: 84). This problem, he claims, was faced by the authors of the large depression study commissioned by the National Institute of Mental Health, the *Treatment of Depression Collaborative Research Program* (Elkin *et al.* 1985). The study compared two forms of psychotherapy (cognitive behavior therapy and interpersonal therapy), an antidepressant drug (imipramine) plus clinical management, and a drug–placebo condition (pill placebo plus clinical management). The researchers found they were unable to design a placebo for psychotherapy that 'met the definitional requirements'. 'Placebo conditions proposed were judged to be either too fanciful, implausible, unethical, or simply an attenuated version of an existing form of treatment' (Parloff 1986b: 84). Parloff does not elaborate on this point or provide detailed examples of the failed placebo candidates.

This objection is mainly a conceptual one: the very concept of a psychotherapy placebo control is incoherent. To serve as an adequate placebo control, a placebo must be identical to the experimental treatment against which it is being compared in every significant way except one: namely, it must lack the so-called 'specific factors' of the experimental treatment, which are presumed to be active (and which are subjected to clinical testing for that activity). If the criterion of identity is not satisfied, then it is not possible to establish a fair comparison between the placebo control and the treatment, and to establish a condition of genuine blindness in participants and experimenters in randomized placebo-controlled trials. In psychotherapy, so the objection goes, there are no conditions under which the criterion of identity between placebo and experimental treatment can be satisfied (see also Greenwood 1996, 1997): whatever looks like it might serve as a placebo is either too fanciful, implausible, unethical—or itself a kind of treatment. If the idea of a psychotherapy placebo control is conceptually incoherent, then the ideas of an interpretation placebo and an insight placebo in psychodynamic psychotherapy are also incoherent.

To see the force of this objection, take as an example the placebo that might serve as the placebo control in a randomized controlled trial for a new treatment of diabetes. To ensure a fair comparison, and thus to obtain valid results about the effectiveness of the new experimental treatment, the placebo pills (which might contain lactose) should be identical to the pills of the new treatment in all relevant respects, except that they should not contain the characteristic factors of the new treatment that are presumed to be active. Thus the appearance, dosage, packaging, and conditions of prescription and follow-up should be the same for the pills containing the placebo and the pills containing the presumed active drug.

Suppose however, for the sake of illustration, that the placebo pills are (to take an unlikely example) black, triangular, large, and foul smelling; suppose also that the prescription information is unclear, and the dispensing physician is pessimistic. By contrast, the pills containing the experimental drug are white, round, small, and odorless; and the prescription information is clear, and the dispensing physician is optimistic. Obviously in such a case the placebo is unfairly disadvantaged, because it lacks therapeutic credibility. If it is true that the patient's knowledge, expectations or beliefs about a therapy affect the therapy outcome (Benedetti *et al.* 2003), then the results of this unlikely trial would be useless. Patients would easily guess the group to which they had been randomly assigned, and this unblinding would result in substantive confounds of the trial results. The group of patients receiving the placebo would likely show less improvement as a whole than the group of patients receiving the experimental treatment, because, having guessed that they had been assigned to the placebo, they would expect to do less well than those on the new drug (since they would believe that placebos are inert). On the other hand, the group receiving the experimental drug would show greater improvement over the placebo group not only because of the therapeutic efficacy of the experimental drug or treatment (if there is any), but because patients who correctly guessed that they had been assigned to the drug group would expect the drug to work. In both cases, positive and negative expectations would influence the scores on outcome measures, and give experimenters false impressions about the effectiveness of the experimental drug (see Kirsch 1985; Kirsch and Sapirstein 1998; Kirsch *et al.* 2002; Kirsch 2003).

In other words, with the breaking of the experimental blind, the patients assigned to the placebo group would not only have no expectations for improvement, but their negative expectations (dashed hopes, disappointment) would interfere with the final measurements of the outcome. Such a trial would show very little about the effectiveness of the new treatment. This example may be far-fetched, but it shows that placebos must be identical to the experimental treatments (against which they are compared) in every significant way except one.

According to the identity objection, the criterion of identity between experimental treatment and placebo control cannot be satisfied in psychotherapy under *any* conditions. To be an adequate placebo control in a clinical trial comparing the effectiveness of a psychotherapy against placebo, the psychotherapy placebo would have to be identical to the psychotherapy in all relevant respects except one: namely, it would have to lack the characteristic factors of the psychotherapeutic treatment that are presumed to be active. But no such placebo exists, because it is not possible to factor out (or 'dismantle') the presumed characteristic factors from the incidental factors (or, in slightly different terms, the active from the nonactive ingredients) in interventions as complexly configured as psychotherapy.

In a placebo-controlled clinical trial of short-term psychodynamic psychotherapy, for example, the placebo control would have to omit all those factors that are presumed to be the characteristic factors of the psychotherapy: it would have to omit, among other things, the main principles of the Standard View. This would include psychodynamic interpretations, which are presumed (according to most theories of psychodynamic psychotherapy) to be among the therapeutically active factors. The problem here is that a placebo control that was similar to the psychotherapy in every relevant respect except for its characteristic factors could still be considered a form of psychotherapy, albeit a degraded or impoverished form of psychotherapy; it would not be a true placebo. Thus, a psychotherapy placebo that excluded interpretations would still be a form of psychotherapy; and an interpretation that is considered to be a placebo in one psychotherapy may not be considered empty or inactive in another. It is therefore false—so the objection goes—to suggest that there is anything resembling the psychological equivalent of sugar pills in psychodynamic psychotherapy. What appears to be an insight placebo or an interpretation placebo is really a function of a methodologically degraded psychotherapeutic treatment, and not a real placebo. Thus—so the objection goes—there are no such things as insight placebos and interpretation placebos.

This is a weighty objection. The response to it involves a conceptual argument that addresses the nature of placebo controls.

First, when it is taken as a general criterion for placebo controls in clinical trials (and not only in the narrower subset of psychotherapy trials), the identity criterion trades on a crucial ambiguity: namely, it fails to specify clear boundaries about the range of items that must be identical between the experimental treatment and the placebo control. Whether identity is construed narrowly or broadly, no placebo could possibly satisfy the criterion. This ambiguity also undermines the more specific objection against psychotherapy placebos.

If the identity criterion is interpreted narrowly, then a placebo needs to be identical with all the *physical* aspects of the experimental treatment against which it is compared in order to ensure a fair comparison. But physical duplication down to the smallest detail is not achievable. However carefully duplicated placebos may be, there will always be slight physical differences between the experimental treatment (or its administration) and the placebo (or its administration): differences in color, shading, weight, size, taste, or packaging of the pills, or differences in the physical, behavioral, and verbal conditions involved in the administration of the pills. The fact that some of these differences may be unnoticeable to patients or experimenters is irrelevant, since the narrow interpretation requires only that the placebo be identical with *all* physical aspects of the experimental treatment. The narrow interpretation of the identity requirement is impossible to satisfy.

Suppose this narrow interpretation is dropped and replaced with a more relaxed interpretation: the placebo (and its administration) must physically resemble the experimental treatment in all *relevant observable* respects, in order to ensure a fair comparison. This too has the same result as the narrow interpretation of the identity criterion. Even when the color, shading, weight, size, taste, and packaging of the pills, as well as the administration of the pills, are identical in all relevant observable respects across both the experimental group and the placebo group, significant differences can arise with side effects, thus violating the identity criterion. Some placebos, for example, have side effects that differ significantly from the side effects of the experimental treatments for which they serve as controls; and some placebos have no detectable side effects at all. According to the identity objection, then, the placebos are not identical to the experimental treatment in all the *relevant observable* respects; thus the comparison is an unfair one, different only in degree, and not in kind, from the black, foul-smelling placebo pill scenario. (It is a well-known problem in randomized controlled trials that the observation of the presence or absence of side effects allows trial participants and experimenters to try to break the blind by guessing the condition to which they have been assigned).

The requirement that the side effects of placebos and experimental treatments be identical in all relevant observable respects in order to ensure a fair comparison is even more difficult to satisfy; and it illustrates clearly how placebos are much more akin to a multi-dimensional *process* than a simple, physically discrete pill. One response that takes the identity objection seriously might be to design placebos capable of mimicking the salient side effects of experimental treatments (as long as they have a relatively low risk of harm): for example, placebo pills that contain ingredients that cause common side effects such as sweating, insomnia, or mild tremors. Once again, however, the identity objection can still be driven home. Even successful artificial side effects that appear to ensure the identity of placebo with the experimental treatment run up against the individual differences of the underlying physiological and psychological conditions of the hosts who are exposed to the placebo: side effects, in other words, are not always uniform or predictable across patient populations. The underlying host conditions that complicate the appearance of side effects, and that make the identity requirement virtually impossible to satisfy, include the onset, course, symptoms, and duration of the host's disease or disorder, as well as variables such as the host's age, weight, height, medical history, gender, and general state of health. The receptivity and noticeability of side effects are also dependent upon a number of cultural, linguistic, and symbolic conditions that differentially define a situation as a meaningful treatment situation for different hosts. Depending on these variables, one and the same side-effect-mimicking placebo will result in some hosts experiencing noticeable side-effects, and others not experiencing them at all. These differences can be minimized in the selection of participants, but they cannot be eradicated altogether to ensure that the underlying psycho-physical conditions of the hosts are identical.

Thus, while placebos may be physically identical to experimental treatments in all relevant observable respects, and placebo side effects may be designed within certain limits to be physically and temporally similar to the side effects of experimental treatments, it is difficult to control for conditions in which the host's reception of artificial and active side effects is identical. At this point, it might be concluded that because the identity criterion can never be satisfied, there are no such things as adequate placebos that could guarantee fair comparisons of experimental treatments with placebo controls. But this conclusion does not follow. The more plausible conclusion is that the identity objection is on the wrong track. The requirement that the placebo be identical to the experimental treatment in order to ensure a fair comparison is too high, and if followed strictly would rule out many otherwise useful and informative placebos. It is doubtful whether any placebos in the recent history of randomized controlled trials would satisfy the identity criterion.

What is the proper response to the identity objection? The *sine qua non* of a fair comparison in a clinical trial is not the presumed *identity* between the placebo and the experimental treatment, but the relative therapeutic *credibility* of the placebo. According to a therapeutic credibility-based criterion, there must, minimally, be a similar level of treatment credibility between the placebo and the experimental treatment for which it serves as a control (Erwin 1997). That is, the placebo must be as credible *qua* treatment to trial participants as the experimental treatment for which it serves as a control, while lacking the characteristic factors of the experimental treatment—that is, those that are presumed to be active. The physical appearance of the placebo (e.g. dosage, packaging, and conditions of prescription and follow-up), or the objective side effects of placebos, are less important in ensuring a fair comparison with an experimental treatment, than the *belief conditions* surrounding the administration and reception of placebos. By implication, it is the *absence* of relative therapeutic credibility of a placebo that ensures an unfair comparison. It is not the fact that placebo pills that are black, triangular, large, and foul-smelling are not *identical* to the experimental treatment that makes the trial comparison an unfair one, but the fact that they are far *less credible* as treatments than other placebo pills.

Therapeutic credibility, unlike identity, is a matter of more or less rather than all or none. This criterion therefore tends to be more charitable toward psychotherapy placebos than the identity criterion; and thus it helps to defend against the identity objection. To serve as an adequate placebo control in a clinical trial comparing the effectiveness of a psychotherapy against placebo, a psychotherapy placebo would not need to be identical in all relevant respects but for the characteristic factors; instead, it would have to display a similar level of therapeutic credibility as the psychotherapy itself, while omitting the characteristic factors of the psychotherapy that are presumed to be active (Erwin 1997).

To see the relevance of the treatment credibility criterion to psychotherapy, consider the unpromising evidential value of a clinical trial that claims to show that a psychological treatment X is more effective than a placebo, when the placebo used in the trial was not therapeutically credible to the participants or patients who received it (Erwin 1997). For example, it is easy to show that psychotherapy X outperforms placebo in a clinical trial, if the placebo is incredible or implausible: for example, placing participants on long wait lists with no psychotherapist contact, or placing participants on wait lists that consist of minimal contact with inattentive psychotherapists, or supplying participants with bizarre therapeutic rationales, or giving participants placebos that make them worse within a specific time frame. As some psychotherapy researchers have observed, in the 1960s and 1970s there were a number of controlled studies that showed that systematic desensitization outperformed placebo—but then significant doubts were raised about the plausibility of the placebos used in the studies (Borkovec and Nau 1972; Nau *et al.* 1974; Erwin 1997). 'Ideally, a placebo should control for a number of factors that might plausibly explain improvement, such as psychotherapist attention, demand for improvement, and therapeutic rationale. At a minimum, it must be at least as credible to the patient as the therapy to which it is being compared. Many of the pseudo-therapies used in psychotherapy research have not met this condition. Although credibility of a particular procedure will vary somewhat with different clients and clinical problems, a pill placebo plus minimal therapist contact has been found to be a credible and useful placebo control in many situations' (Erwin 1997: 152).

What matters then is not that the psychotherapy placebo be identical in every respect to the experimental treatment, but that it serve as a credible alternative to the treatment for which it is a control, while lacking the characteristic factors of the experimental treatment that are presumed to be active. A credible interpretation placebo or insight placebo would be one that is believable to people, but still lacks the characteristic factors of the presumed active interpretation or insight: that is, it would be false or fictitious.

Chapter 6

Placebos, Deception, and Self-Deception

Patients' Awareness of Placebos

The main hypothesis defended in this work is a conceptual rather than an empirical one: namely, that some therapeutic changes in the psychodynamic psychotherapies are functions of powerful placebos that rally the mind's natural healing powers, rather than functions of the hypothesized characteristic factors of the treatment methods of psychodynamic psychotherapies. Two of these placebos are the insight placebo and the interpretation placebo. There may be other placebos at work, but these are not discussed here. If the hypothesis is conceptually and logically coherent, it still remains to be seen whether it has empirical support: that is, whether there *are* such things as insight placebos and interpretation placebos, and if there are, what their rate of incidence is, the client populations they affect, the conditions in which they arise, and their relation to other treatment and client variables.

But before this work can be done, the conceptual component and its surrounding conceptual network need to be sketched out in greater detail. For the sake of further refining the preliminary architecture of concepts, suppose that the core part of this hypothesis is valid: insight placebos and interpretation placebos *are* conceptually possible. That is, the very idea of insight placebos and interpretation placebos makes sense: they are not logical or conceptual contradictions. Suppose too, as a preliminary guide to empirical research on placebo effects in psychotherapy, that some of the placebo research from other medical and scientific disciplines can help to cast light on placebo effects in psychotherapy. There may be, for example, definite and measurable patterns of placebo responsiveness in the psychodynamic psychotherapies, complementing definite and measurable frequencies of responsiveness to specific psychodynamic factors—just as there are definite and measurable patterns of placebo responsiveness in many branches of clinical medicine. Following Beecher's rough estimate, it might be supposed—purely for the sake of illustration—that a specific remedy has roughly a 75–95% probability of being efficacious for a small number of disorders, while there is a rough overall placebo efficacy rate of 30–40% for the majority of disorders (Beecher 1955). Similar efficacy rates might hold true for psychodynamic psychotherapy: that is, roughly 30% of clients in psychodynamic psychotherapy might respond to placebos.

These suppositions raise the following questions. *If* there are psychodynamic placebos, then would clients who are placebo responders *know* that they are responding to placebos if they had not already been informed about them—or would they remain in the dark? Would the placebo response be less effective if they knew they were responding to placebos rather than to active treatments? Would clients who respond to insight and interpretation placebos, for example, know that these insights and interpretations are placebos, or would they mistakenly take them to be authentic or valid? Would the placebo response be less effective if clients knew they were responding to insight and interpretation placebos? More generally, is the placebo response incompatible with the knowledge or awareness of placebos?

To see the force of these questions, consider the analogy with placebo use in physical medicine. Typically, patients who respond to placebos do not know that they are responding to placebos: they believe, instead, that they are responding to active treatments. Often this is because the physicians who administer placebos have withheld vital information about the treatment, or have told patients that they are receiving active treatments (while knowing all along that the treatments are placebos); or they have misled their patients inadvertently by informing them mistakenly that they are receiving active treatments (when, unbeknownst to the physicians, they are placebos). The administration of placebos, in other words, often involves what might be called practices of intentional ignorance. (The ethics of giving placebos will be discussed in Chapter 7.) It seems, at least at a cursory glance, that either patients know that their response is a response to placebos, or they remain in the dark because they have been deceived, or they have had vital information withheld. And it would seem that if patients know that they have been given placebos, then the placebo response would be greatly weakened, or even neutralized.

If the analogy with physical medicine is valid, then it could be expected that a similar situation would be found in psychodynamic psychotherapy. If there are such things as psychodynamic placebos, then clients who respond to them often would not know that they are responding to placebos if they had not already been informed. They would believe that they have received an active treatment, especially if this is what they have been told by the psychotherapists who administer the treatment. Clients, then, would either be intentionally or inadvertently kept ignorant by their psychotherapists in the same way that patients in physical medicine are intentionally or inadvertently kept ignorant by their physicians. It would seem, further, that either they *know* that their response is a response to placebo, or they are in the dark. And it would seem that if patients know that they have been given placebos, then the placebo response would be greatly weakened, or neutralized.

But are things really as simple as this? In fact, they are not: the issue is considerably more complex than it appears to be on both sides of the analogy between physical medicine and psychological treatment. It is not always as simple a matter as patients either knowing or not knowing that they are responding to placebo: there are also intermediate states located between knowing and not knowing, some of which are quite complex and convoluted. Nor is it always as simple a matter as the placebo response being incompatible with the awareness or knowledge of placebos. In some complex cases, it will be seen, patients neither straightforwardly *know* that they are responding to placebo, nor straightforwardly remain ignorant or deceived about it; in some even more complex cases, patients believe that they are responding to an active treatment, and yet they somehow know that they are not.

Once again, the epistemic complexities are usefully illustrated with the analogs provided by placebo-responding patients in physical medicine. The following are four of several possible epistemic conditions corresponding to the placebo response, beginning with the most straightforward:

i) placebo-responding patients who do not know that they have been given placebo, and who believe mistakenly that they are responding to an active treatment;

ii) placebo-responding patients who know that they have been given placebo;

iii) placebo-responding patients who, on the basis of guesswork and inference, believe that they have been given placebo;

iv) placebo-responding patients who believe that they are responding to an active treatment, and yet at the same time somehow know that it is not an active treatment.

In greater detail, these conditions are as follows:

i) The most straightforward epistemic conditions characterizing placebo therapeutics in physical medicine involve placebo-responsive patients who do not know that they have been given placebos. Patients mistakenly believe that they are receiving an active treatment, and their beliefs and expectations are an integral component of their response to the treatment. Mistaken belief, and with it the network of affiliated epistemic and emotive conditions, such as heightened expectations for improvement, heightened credulity, and hope, represents one end-point of the epistemic spectrum of placebo responsiveness.

ii) At the opposite end of the spectrum are those epistemic conditions that occur when placebo-responsive patients are informed by their physicians that they are receiving placebo treatments. These cases, using so-called 'open' or 'non-hidden' placebos, are far less common than the former cases, and they have generated relatively little scientific inquiry. On the surface, it would seem that open placebos are self-defeating treatments, as they advertise their own conditions for disbelief. There are, naturally, patients who react with incredulity or discouragement to the information that they are receiving placebos. This tends to weaken or neutralize the placebo effect. But there is a subset of the open placebo patient group that includes patients who continue to demonstrate objective therapeutic improvement and symptom remission despite their knowledge that the treatment is 'only' a placebo. Somehow, the knowledge that they are receiving placebo does not undermine the placebo effect. In recent studies of placebo therapeutics, for instance, several cases of successful placebo therapy were reported in patients who were informed that they were receiving pharmacologically inert substances (Vogel *et al.* 1980; Brown 1994, 1998a, 1998b; Aulas and Rosner 2003). In another older study, 14 psychiatric outpatients with somatic symptoms were given a week-long trial of an open or non-hidden placebo (Park and Covi 1965). Thirteen of the patients experienced objective symptom relief, even when they were fully informed at the outset of the trial that they were receiving placebos. These cases, which will be discussed in detail in Chapter 7, appear to be examples of the placebo effect occurring without any of the practices of intentional ignorance by physicians. More empirical research is required to make sense of these results: the studies need to be replicated, the methodological designs need to be fine-tuned, and alternative explanations of therapeutic improvement need to be ruled out (e.g., self-limiting disorders, regression to the mean, reactivity of measurement (Bootzin and Caspi 2002), the Hawthorne effect (the effect of being under study on the persons being studied (Adair 1984; Last 1988)). Moreover, more basic conceptual and phenomenological research needs to be carried out to make sense of the belief states of patients who are exposed to open placebos (see de Sousa 1988).

iii) Between the two end points of knowing and not knowing about placebo administration are several less straightforward epistemic conditions. One of these involves placebo-responsive patients who come to *believe* (but still do not know) that their response to the treatment is a placebo response. Their beliefs are based on informed hunches, guesswork, or inference, but not on any objective information that they have been given placebos. Something like this response is seen in randomized controlled double-blind clinical trials. Typically, trial participants are informed that the treatments they are receiving are either placebos or active treatments, but they are not told which condition they have been assigned to: hence the so-called 'blind'. Still, it is not uncommon for participants to make guesses about the condition to which they have been blindly assigned, and this has a tendency to confound trial results.

There are at least three epistemic conditions corresponding to attempts to break the blind. First, some placebo recipients may guess incorrectly that they have been assigned to the active treatment condition after observing certain physiological changes in their condition, or certain side effects known to be associated with similar treatments already approved for use. This may cause heightened expectations for improvement, or heightened levels of credulity about the effectiveness of the (mistakenly identified) experimental treatment, which in turn may enhance the treatment effects seen in the placebo group. Second, some placebo recipients may guess that they have been assigned to the placebo condition after failing to observe the expected physiological changes or side effects. This may weaken the effect of the placebo treatment, since participants may abandon all expectations for improvement. Third, some placebo recipients who correctly guess that they have been assigned to the placebo control group may continue to experience measurable therapeutic changes and side effects that resemble those of the active treatment. That is, their belief that the changes they are experiencing are due to the placebo somehow does not hinder therapeutic progress, or undermine expectations for improvement. This response is not unlike that seen in open placebo studies. The main difference, however, is that in blinded conditions participants have had to make guesses or inferences about their response on the basis of limited information, whereas participants in the open placebo studies have been fully informed that they are receiving placebos.

iv) Another less straightforward epistemic condition in placebo therapeutics involves placebo-responsive patients who believe that they are responding to an active treatment, and yet at the same time know that it is not an active treatment. That is, they believe things about themselves (and their treatment responses) that they also know are false. For example (as seen in open placebo cases), some patients believe they are responding to an active treatment despite knowing that the treatment is a placebo; other patients believe they are responding to an active treatment despite having good grounds for regarding the treatment as a placebo. What could explain this? One hypothesis is that there may be some form of *self*-deception occurring in patients that compensates for the absence of *external* deception or information-withholding from the physicians who administer the placebo: that is, the patients hold beliefs ('the treatment is effective') that they also have good grounds for regarding as false ('the treatment cannot be effective because it is medically or pharmacologically inert'). Similarly, placebo recipients (in condition ii) who correctly guess that they have been assigned to the placebo control group and yet continue to experience measurable therapeutic changes and side effects may hold beliefs that they also have good grounds for regarding as false. Typically, conflicting beliefs such as these can occasion a kind of troublesome self-division.

Conditions iii) and iv) show that it is not always as simple a matter as patients either knowing or not knowing that they are responding to placebo: there are also complex intermediate states located between knowing and not knowing. The conditions also show that the placebo response is not always incompatible with the knowledge or awareness of placebos. Moreover, while intentional ignorance by physicians or clinicians is a common component of the placebo response, it is not found in all cases. In some cases, it may be that self-deception rather than deception by others is a component of the placebo response.

Return now to the other side of the analogy: that is, clients' awareness or lack of awareness of placebo responses in psychodynamic psychotherapy. If the analogy is valid, then there are a number of complex intermediate states between the two end points on the epistemic spectrum. It is not quite as simple a matter as either knowing or not knowing about the placebo response; nor is there a straightforward incompatibility between the placebo response and the patient's knowledge or awareness of placebos.

Corresponding to the analogs above, there are in psychodynamic psychotherapy at least four (and most likely several more) epistemic conditions pertaining to placebo-responding clients: i) clients who do not know they have been given psychodynamic placebos, and believe mistakenly that they are responding to an active psychodynamic treatment; ii) clients who know they have been given psychodynamic placebos; iii) clients who on the basis of guesswork and inference believe that they have been given psychodynamic placebos; and iv) clients who believe that they are responding to an active psychodynamic treatment, and yet at the same time somehow know that it is not an active treatment. Of primary interest here is epistemic condition iv), not only because it impugns some of the characteristic factors of psychodynamic psychotherapy, and some of the core components of the Standard View, but because the epistemic vagaries of this condition have received little or no hearing in the psychodynamic literature.

If the analogy with placebo responsiveness in physical medicine holds, then it can be supposed that there are some clients who are administered psychodynamic placebos who believe that they are responding to an active treatment, and yet somehow know that they are not. They have convinced themselves of something that they know is not the case. This seems to be counter-intuitive, even paradoxical. How could such a conflict between believing that *x* is the case and knowing that it is not be possible? How could anyone, especially someone engaged in therapeutic self-exploration, be so epistemically divided against themselves? What would such a conflict look like in actual clinical practice? Could some part of the placebo response be attributable to self-deception rather than to deception or intentional ignorance caused by another?

The following are schematic examples of how *some* clients in psychodynamic psychotherapy might come to believe that something is the case and yet somehow know that it is not. The first set of examples illustrates how the conflict might play out on a mainly cognitive level, and the second set illustrates how it might play out on a mainly affective level.

- Clients might have convinced themselves that their psychological explorations are authentic and truth-tracking, despite knowing that these explorations are context-sensitive, suggestion-prone, or epistemically problematic.

- Clients (in psychoanalytic psychotherapy) might have convinced themselves that the technique of free association is a valuable source of information about their unconscious, despite knowing about how psychotherapeutic suggestion, leading questions, doctrinal compliance, and other confounding factors can lead to artificial or contrived associations, and ultimately to a body of contaminated clinical evidence which could influence the psychodynamic interpretations they are given.

- Clients might be convinced that their treatment is effective, despite knowing that a number of outcome studies show that psychodynamic psychotherapy is, in general, no more effective than a placebo.

- Clients might believe that their psychotherapists are experts in matters of human psychology, despite knowing that a number of studies impugn these claims to expertise.

- Clients might believe that the psychodynamic interpretations of their dreams are valid, despite knowing that the interpretations are overly general (one-size-fits-all interpretations), exaggerated, or empirically impoverished.

- Clients might believe that the powerful feelings they have towards their psychotherapists are real re-enactments of ancient emotions, despite knowing that the feelings say more about the powerful relation that is occurring in the here-and-now between two adults.

Cognitive conflicts, or conflicts between beliefs and knowledge, are not the only relevant types of conflicts that can pit a person against him or herself: there are also conflicts between beliefs and belief-laden emotions. The following are examples of how some clients in psychodynamic psychotherapy might come to believe that something is the case and yet somehow *feel* that it is not.

- Clients might have convinced themselves that their psychological explorations are authentic and truth-tracking, despite experiencing high levels of anxiety around the possibility that they may be forced, artificial, or off-track.

- Clients (in psychoanalytic psychotherapy) might have convinced themselves that the technique of free association is a valuable source of information about their unconscious, despite strong feelings of ambivalence about its usefulness or relevance.

- Clients might have convinced themselves that their treatment is effective, despite strong feelings of futility about the treatment.

- Clients might have convinced themselves that their psychotherapists are experts in matters of human psychology, despite having lost confidence in their abilities.

- Clients might believe that the psychodynamic interpretations of their dreams are valid, despite feelings of despair about the accuracy, arbitrariness, or irrelevance of the interpretations.

These are highly simplified examples of the conflict between believing that something is the case and yet knowing that it is not. They are lacking in detail, content, and real-world fit. Consider now an example in greater detail that will remedy some of these shortcomings while at the same time addressing the issue of insight. Some clients might believe that psychodynamic interpretations and insights are authentic or valid, and yet somehow know that they are not authentic or valid. More specifically, they might believe things about their own psychology, emotions, behavior, childhood, or personality (beliefs acquired during the course of psychodynamic treatment) that they also somehow know are false. They might, for instance, be vaguely aware that the therapeutically-guided explorations that have led to their insights are contaminated by unwanted epistemic influences; or they might be vaguely aware that the psychodynamic interpretations to which they give their assent, and which they believe serve to illuminate important aspects of their personality and childhood, have poor evidentiary credentials. *If* this sort of thing occurs in psychodynamic psychotherapy, then it is clearly a case of insight gone awry. Having insights into oneself that one also knows are false is not really insight. What is it? It is self-deception. More precisely, it is self-deception under the guise of insight.

At this point, however, one sensible counter-argument to this suggestion might be the following: the very idea that psychodynamic clients can acquire insights about themselves that they also know are false does not make sense; it is conceptually incoherent. Insight is incompatible with self-deception, just as it is incompatible with illusion, blindness to self, self-misunderstanding, or self-ignorance; where insight is, there self-deception is not. The very point of psychodynamic psychotherapy is to track down and eradicate self-deception and self-ignorance in all their manifest and less than manifest guises. It is not possible that an enterprise so completely dedicated to self-exploration and insight could have such disastrously antithetical results. These are substantive conceptual claims that appeal, among other things, to the logical relations that structure the concepts of self-deception and insight. As conceptual claims, however, they cannot be taken at face value; without further conceptual analysis, they are far from obvious. It is neither self-evident nor *a priori* certain that insight is incompatible with or excludes self-deception.

Another counter-argument might be to dismiss these issues on empirical rather than logical grounds as either clinically implausible or clinically insignificant. It might be claimed, for example, that self-deception is, as a matter of fact, quite rare in psychodynamic psychotherapy, because of carefully applied psychodynamic methods and psychotherapist expertise. If it does occasionally occur, it can be attributed to breakdowns in clinical standards, sloppy therapeutic procedures, or poorly trained psychotherapists— rather than to any intrinsic flaws in the Standard View of psychodynamic psychotherapy.

It is worth remembering at this stage in the discussion that the leading questions about the relation between self-deception, deception, and placebos with which this chapter opened are mainly conceptual in nature. At issue are two claims, one wide and one narrow. The wide claim is that it is possible that patients in physical medicine or clients in psychotherapy believe that they are responding to active treatment while somehow knowing that they are not. The narrow claim, which is more directly relevant to the purposes at hand, is that it is possible that clients in psychodynamic psychotherapy believe things about themselves (and endorse insights) that they also somehow know are false. To dismiss the entire issue as clinically insignificant or implausible, without first exploring the conceptual territory, is tantamount to an *a priori* empiricism. Until the wide and narrow claims can be shown to be conceptually possible or impossible, appeal to evidence such as clinical data, clinical anecdote, or case histories is premature; so too is appeal to common sense. It is important, in other words, to have a clear idea about what precisely the wide and narrow claims mean. Once this groundwork is sketched out, empirical investigation can proceed, with a view to determining whether such phenomena exist, what their clinical profile looks like, their patterns of development, their variations, and their effects on therapeutic outcomes. Even if no evidence for their presence can be found, this does not rule out *a priori* the *possibility* of such phenomena occurring in physical medicine and exploratory psychotherapy.

Grünbaum's Critique of Freud

Grünbaum's (1984) well-known account of pseudo-insight in classical Freudian psychoanalysis serves as a good starting point for exploring the conceptual possibility of self-deception in exploratory psychotherapy. Grünbaum likens psychoanalytic suggestion to brainwashing (1984: 135). The analysand is indoctrinated in the psychoanalytic regimen, becomes an 'ideological disciple' of the therapeutic theory of psychoanalysis (1984: 137), and displays towards the analyst what Grünbaum, following Ehrenwald (1966), calls 'doctrinal acquiescence'. At a certain critical point in the treatment the analysand 'succumbs to proselytizing *suggestion*' (Grünbaum 1984: 130). On the other side of the equation, the analyst is always at risk of making suggestible analysands 'succumb' to 'fanciful *pseudo*insights persuasively endowed with the ring of verisimilitude' (Grünbaum 1984: 130), through the psychotherapeutic equivalent of indoctrination.

Wollheim dismisses Grünbaum's suggestion hypothesis on the basis of its relative simplicity and lack of detail: 'the situation is envisaged [by Grünbaum] in the following way: (one) the analyst makes his wishes known; (two) the patient complies' (Wollheim 1993: 111). This is a strawman criticism: it distorts and oversimplifies Grünbaum's critique of Freud. But it points, however obliquely, at a complex problem lurking in Grünbaum's account of analysand suggestibility as a central factor in the production of pseudo-insights, and in the production of contaminated clinical data: namely, that his account is based on a psychologically incomplete picture of the complex cognitive and emotional responses of analysands. Much more is happening in the analysand than meets the eye. Grünbaum's account of suggestion pictures analysands as passive victims of the suggestive influences of psychoanalysts, and suggestion as an insidious and undetectable force. More specifically, it pictures analysands as unaware of the presence of these suggestive forces, as blind to their own vulnerability to suggestion and doctrinal compliance, and as oblivious to the epistemic contamination to which their exploratory activities and insights are subjected. What befalls them, and results in pseudo-insights, is not of their own doing. But is this always the case?

There are two problems with Grünbaum's picture of suggestion in psychoanalysis. One concerns the nature and degree of therapeutic influence, and one concerns the experiences and the cognitive abilities of the analysands who are subjected to that influence. First, while the analogy of psychoanalysis with brainwashing has a superficial degree of plausibility, it is not necessary for making the case that Grünbaum intends. The analogy breaks down because it does not distinguish between the many varieties of psychological influence, some more subtle or pervasive than others. Because of its overwhelming intrusiveness, brainwashing is located at the far end of a continuum that measures degree of psychological influence. Closer to the middle of the continuum are several varieties of coercion (e.g. browbeating, hectoring, and double-binding); at the other end of the continuum are several varieties of persuasion (e.g. rhetorical influence, charisma, and character influence). Victims of brainwashing differ from analysands on a number of basic dimensions: i) analysands have chosen to undergo psychoanalysis, and are free to terminate it at any stage, unlike victims of brainwashing; ii) analysands are encouraged to reflect upon and interpret the changes they are undergoing, unlike victims of brainwashing, who may be unaware of the extent of their brainwashing; iii) analysands are encouraged to aspire to the goal of insight and greater personal autonomy, whereas victims of brainwashing are encouraged to accept uncritically the norms dictated by the agents of brainwashing; and iv) analysands continue with their everyday lives after the analytic hour has finished, whereas victims of brainwashing experience their everyday lives as irremediably altered.

The other problem with Grünbaum's picture concerns the analysand. It is too one-sided a picture. Therapeutic influence upon the analysand is reduced to: i) cases of straightforward duping, or other-deception, in which analysands are the victims of manipulative and suggestion-based deceptions; or ii) cases of inadvertent error and misinformation, in which analysands are innocently caught up in the elaborate mistakes of others (namely, misguided psychoanalysts led astray by false or self-confirming therapeutic theories). In both scenarios, it would be reasonable to consider analysands as partially or fully excused from any significant degree of *epistemic responsibility* for their mistaken views about the truth-value and authenticity of their newly-acquired insights. For example, victims of other-deception (such as lies) are not normally considered fully responsible for the consequences of those beliefs and actions that are the direct result of the deception, if, all other things being equal, they displayed a reasonable degree of epistemic responsibility in the conditions in which they were originally deceived. There are, clearly, degrees of excusability, reflecting on the one hand the level of epistemic responsibility displayed in each case, and on the other the complexity of the deception to which they fell victim. Those who engage in half-hearted efforts of corroboration and evaluation, and who show little epistemic caution, are more blameworthy than those who aim in their knowledge-seeking practices for rigor and comprehensiveness. Similarly, victims of inadvertent misinformation or error are normally excused for the consequences of those beliefs and actions which follow from their being misinformed, if they originally displayed a reasonable degree of epistemic responsibility and prudence. In both cases, the victims suffer from false beliefs, illusions, simple errors, and self-misattributions, but through no fault of their own. Their ignorance could be characterized as sincere, as they have had no hand in the deception brought upon them.

Grünbaum's picture suggests that analysands are innocent victims of other-deception or other-generated error: they are 'brainwashed', or they 'succumb' outright to 'proselytizing suggestion', or they are misled by mistaken but well-intentioned psychoanalysts. These constitute the class of what will be called *good faith* epistemic practices. Also included in this class are such states as outright error, misattribution, careless judgment, and unwarranted inference. But belief acquisition in suggestive contexts is more complex and variegated than this. Just as there is a class of good faith epistemic practices, so there is a class of *bad faith* epistemic practices. These include self-deception, willful ignorance, quasi-rational selective attention, and selective forgetting. What is required to improve on Grünbaum's account is an explanation that shows just how far being misled (in psychotherapy) goes beyond simply being *mistaken* about oneself, or being brainwashed: that is, an explanation that shows how it is possible that clients in the psychodynamic psychotherapies can believe things about themselves that they also know are false.

It would be naïve to claim that inadvertent other-generated errors *never* befall clients in the psychodynamic psychotherapies. As in all other healing disciplines, psychotherapists and psychoanalysts are vulnerable to making clinical errors, which are often visited upon their clients: inadvertent mis-diagnoses, misinterpretations, misprognoses, misapplied treatment methods, and misalliances are among the more noticeable of these mistakes. Some psychotherapeutic mistakes have humble origins: mishearing a client's remarks, failing to ask simple factual questions, inattention to symptoms, recording errors, and so on. Some mistakes have their origins in the design foibles of cognitive architecture: availability and representativeness biases, attributional errors, and faulty probabilistic judgments (Dawes *et al.* 1989; Dawes 1994). And some mistakes have unfortunate origins, such as blinding theoretical dogmatism, or narrow-minded prejudice against certain types of client. The mistakes range from the simple to the complex. Interpretations that are widely off the mark count as complex mistakes. So too do those cases in which psychotherapists practice with therapeutic theories that later are rejected as false, incomplete, or flawed. At the time of treatment, however, when psychotherapists believed that their theories were true, and believed that their interpretations referred to real entities or forces, their clients were inadvertently misled.

Clients whose therapeutic explorations, discoveries, and insights are influenced by misdiagnoses, misinterpretations, or psychological theories that are later rejected as false are led astray unintentionally. They are victims of other-generated error. Their insights are mistaken.

It would also be naïve to claim that practices of intentional deception and intentional ignorance *never* occur in the psychodynamic psychotherapies. In order to advance the progress of the therapy, or to protect what they perceive to be the best interests of their clients, psychotherapists may on some occasions deliberately deceive their clients about significant issues about which they know the truth, or withhold vital information about the nature of the treatment. Such was Janet's strategy with many of his patients, as well as Mendel's (1964) temporary but expedient strategy (see Chapter 5). Clients whose exploratory psychotherapy has been influenced by intentional misdiagnoses, misinterpretations, or psychological theories are also victims of other-deception. Their insights too are mistaken.

Clients who are the victims of inadvertent other-generated error, intentional deception, and intentional ignorance are mistaken in good faith. They hold in good faith what are in fact false beliefs about the etiology, symptomatology, and nosology of their disorders; more generally, they hold false beliefs about their psychological makeup, motivations, and behavior. At the same time, they are genuinely unaware of their own epistemic vulnerability, and their own epistemic and psychological suggestibility in the matter; and they are unaware of the epistemically unusual conditions under which they have acquired their beliefs and insights. If they have satisfied consensually endorsed epistemic norms about the nature, range, and relevance of therapeutic evidence, and consensually endorsed norms of practical reasoning and inductive inference in matters psychological, then they are no more epistemically responsible than those who in good faith have been unwittingly or duplicitously led to hold false beliefs about non-psychological states of affairs.

But while many clients in the psychodynamic psychotherapies may be exemplars of epistemic good faith, and may end up the unwitting victims of deception or inadvertent psychotherapist error, it is possible that some clients may be in epistemic *bad faith*. They are not straightforwardly mistaken about themselves; nor are they straightforwardly deceived or led astray by their psychotherapists about the validity of their insights; they are, rather, *self*-deceived. They have had a hand in the deceptions or errors that have led them astray. Self-deception in the psychodynamic psychotherapies occurs when clients come to believe things about themselves that they somehow know are not true: that is, when they come to acquire and endorse insights which they somehow know are false, such as pseudo-insights, or inexact, implausible, or over-simplified insights. This may be rare; it is even possible that it has never occurred. These are empirical claims that would need to be investigated. But before this begins, the idea itself needs to be analyzed.

Self-Deception

Self-deception comes in a variety of strange sizes and shapes, and in many cultural variations (Ames and Dissanayake 1996). It is also surrounded by many equally strange phenomena: willful ignorance, self-induced deception, weakness of will, wishful thinking, rationalization, inner contradiction of beliefs, willful manipulation of beliefs, false consciousness, self-blindness, and double-mindedness (Rorty 1975, 1988, 1994; Martin 1985; McLaughlin and Rorty 1988). Competing with the proliferation of phenomena is a proliferation of philosophical and psychological models of self-deception.[1] For reasons of economy, however, neither the various phenomena associated with self-deception, nor the various explanatory models of self-deception, will be discussed here.

The following examples from outside the domain of clinical psychology illustrate prototypical cases of self-deception. While lacking in detail and contextual nuance, both nonetheless display a minimal level of psychological realism.

- 'A specialist in the diagnosis of cancer, whose fascination for the obscure does not usually blind her to the obvious, Dr. Laetitia Androvna has begun to misdescribe and ignore symptoms [in herself] that the most junior premedical student would recognize as the unmistakable symptoms of the late stages of a currently incurable form of cancer. Normally introspective, given to consulting friends on important matters, she now uncharacteristically deflects their questions and attempts to discuss her condition. Nevertheless, also uncharacteristically, she is bringing her practical and financial affairs into order: though young and by no means affluent, she is drawing up a detailed will. Never a serious correspondent, reticent about matters of affection, she has taken to writing effusive letters to distant friends and relatives, intimating farewells, and urging them to visit soon... None of this uncharacteristic behavior is deliberately deceptive: she has not adopted a policy of stoic silence to spare her friends. On the surface of it, as far as she knows, she is hiding nothing. Of course her critical condition may explain the surfacing of submerged aspects of her personality'. (Rorty 1988: 11)

- M, a 45-year-old corporate lawyer and senior member of a large law firm, describes himself as a social drinker. Over the last two years M has graduated from one to three cocktails upon coming home from work, from one glass of wine to one half of a bottle of wine with dinner, and from one bottle of beer to three bottles before bedtime. At least twice a month at business functions, he drinks to the point where he becomes incoherent and has to be escorted home by friends. At work he has started to drink during the lunch hour, and his consumption has increased gradually to the point where his co-workers are embarrassed by his loud and sometimes inconsiderate behavior. They are afraid to comment upon it. M is known as a tough, skillful, and aggressive lawyer with a long series of legal successes. But he has displayed poor legal judgment recently, and has been assigned easier cases. He notices this, but blames it on a new senior member, whom he believes is intent on forcing M out of the firm. Once a healthy and active individual, M now notices his slowly deteriorating health (poor skin, muscle aches, constant digestion problems); but he blames these problems on getting old. M's wife repeatedly asks him to curtail his drinking, and suggests that he consider seeking professional help, but M reacts by flying into a rage. He sincerely believes that he is only a social drinker. He tries to convince her that his job and the corporate culture in which he is immersed require social drinking. He tells her that drinking helps him to steady his nerves and helps to give him the aggressive edge that he needs in such a competitive environment. M believes that he has his life under control, and he continues to drink heavily.

What do these examples show about self-deception? First, they show that self-deception has a more complex structure than other-deception. Self-deception is not simply a case of a person deceiving himself just as he deceives another. Other-deception is characterized by three conditions: i) the presence of at least two persons, the deceiver and the deceived; ii) the deceiver who is in possession of a truth which he or she hides from the deceived; and iii) the deceiver who intentionally deceives the other person about this truth. But this model of other-deception cannot be grafted onto self-deception, because it fails to capture a central fact about self-deception: namely, that the deceiver and the deceived are *one and the same person*. There is no separation of deceiver and deceived, as there is in the case of other-deception. But if there is no separation, then it seems unavoidable that as the deceiver, a person must somehow be aware of the truth of that with which he deceives himself; and, curiously, as the deceived, he must somehow not be aware of this truth, in order to be duped by it. It is as if the self-deceiver must somehow know the truth *in order* to conceal it more carefully. Someone who is self-deceived is deceiver and deceived, not at two different moments but at one and the same time, as one and the same person.

Second, both examples show that self-deception is not exclusively a *cognitive* phenomenon: that is, it is constituted not only by conflicts or major inconsistencies between beliefs, but also by conflicts between entire patterns of behavior, volition, and emotion. Third, both examples show that self-deception does not involve conscious deliberation and planning. The alcoholic, for example, does not make an explicit and carefully planned decision to deceive himself about the benign effects of excessive drinking. To do so would be as self-defeating as trying to tell oneself a joke: the very effort advertises its own conditions for disbelief. Fourth, both examples show that self-deception is not an accident that befalls its victims, like an unforeseen illness, but rather bears some of the characteristic marks of intentionality. It is a form of goal-directed behavior, because it accomplishes an end that strategically benefits the person in his role of deceiver: for example, avoiding owning up to the frightening implications of mortality, as in the case of the self-deceived cancer victim; or avoiding facing up to the damaging criticisms and disappointments of others, as in the case of the self-deceived alcoholic.

Fifth, both examples show that the self-deceiver's attempts to hold beliefs that they also know are false occasions a kind of self-division that interferes with cognitive and behavioral consistency. The cancer victim who believes that she is healthy, and at the same time tries to disregard the significance of incontrovertible medical evidence, fights a losing battle. She cannot identify wholeheartedly with the belief that she is healthy, and therefore act decisively upon it, because her belief is not characterized by the same degree of epistemic assurance and evidential warrant that characterizes veridical beliefs. Self-deceptive beliefs require ongoing and situation-specific *ad hoc* maneuvers simply to keep them in place: for example, evasions, fabrications, and fine-tuned rationalizations. This is what makes self-deception epistemically 'metastable'. Its successful operation can only be achieved by relaxing the epistemic norms that function in everyday contexts of ends-oriented critical thought—norms that typically would sift out anomalous epistemic situations and dubious evidence. The efforts expended by self-deceivers to overcome this epistemic metastability are futile. Genuine consistency of thought and action are not achievable. The cancer victim who on one level believes that she is healthy will, on another level—in her actions—undermine the grounds of her belief. She is not one with herself, in the sense that she pursues a course of action that flows naturally and spontaneously from her beliefs. She cannot act on her beliefs with the single-mindedness displayed by people who are not self-deceived.

Sixth, both examples show how self-deception forces upon self-deceivers complex alterations in knowing practices and epistemic criteria. Because their beliefs (e.g. 'I am healthy', and 'I am only a social drinker, I have everything under control') are not adequately warranted by the available evidence, which is scanty, off-target, or fragmentary, self-deceivers must somehow ignore the evidentiary discrepancies, or account for them with *ad hoc* rationalizing strategies. These strategies include: trying to develop new categories of evidence, such as quasi-warranted evidence, that falls midway between warranted and unwarranted evidence; trying to adapt to the practical consequences of living with beliefs that are not adequately supported by warranted evidence, as if this is the norm rather than the exception; trying to relax otherwise rigorous consensually endorsed evidentiary norms. The problem with these strategies is that they only serve to keep the original evidentiary problems in view, even if only indirectly.

Several highly schematic examples of self-deception in clinical contexts were mentioned in passing earlier: clients who have convinced themselves that their psychological explorations are authentic and truth-tracking, despite knowing that these explorations are context-sensitive, suggestion-prone, or epistemically problematic; clients who have convinced themselves that the technique of free association is a valuable source of information about their unconscious, despite strong feelings of ambivalence about its usefulness; and clients who have convinced themselves that their treatment is effective, despite strong feelings of futility about the treatment. The following two fictional cases, building on these schematic examples, as well as on the two previous prototypical cases, illustrate how it might be possible for clients in psychodynamic psychotherapy to believe things about themselves that they also know are false, or that they have good grounds for regarding as false.

♦ After approximately two hundred and fifty hours of psychoanalysis, M, a 62-year-old family physician, gradually comes to a series of deep realizations about how some of his main psychological problems (anxiety, social inhibition, lack of intimacy) are caused by powerful but previously unrecognized Oedipal entanglements reaching back to the time when he was a toddler and young boy. The deeper the analysis probes, the more he is surprised to learn not only about the strength of the hostility he felt toward his father when he was a child, and the strength of his desire for his mother, but the pervasive and insidious influence these feelings continue to exert over his emotional life. M's analyst endorses these realizations and is pleased to see that they agree closely with his own interpretations. The realizations make sense to M, and (as he phrases it) they 'feel right'. They are also accompanied by a series of intense memories of his childhood; and they are followed by noticeable progress in the analysis, signaled by the quantity and quality of associations and the intensity of the transference. In fact, however, M's realizations are pseudo-insights: that is, they are incorrect with respect to etiology, historical fact, the facts of subjective experience, and personality structure. The putative entanglements were not as powerful and sexually charged as he believes; the feelings of hostility toward his father were only one among many intense feelings he experienced at the time, and not as psychologically significant as he believes; and the details of time, place, and persons are incomplete and confused. M's current problems are in fact caused by undiagnosed neurophysiological factors in response to environmental stressors, rather than by the psychodynamic causes picked out by his insights and his analyst's interpretations. M is not completely unaware of the possibility of a different diagnosis. He has been vaguely aware of a pattern of odd neurophysiological symptoms, but, uncharacteristically, has not investigated them further, as he would normally do with any of his patients presenting with such symptoms. To complicate matters, a core cluster of M's most emotionally charged memories, occasioned by the analysis, are false memories, although he is unaware that they are false, and feels a certain degree of confidence in their accuracy. Despite the many unrecognized errors in memory and self-understanding, M feels that he has been helped by his insights, and that his relations with his children and wife have improved. At the same time, however, he finds himself occasionally entertaining doubts about the validity of his insights, and the cogency of the psychodynamic reasoning that has led him and his psychoanalyst to endorse them as veridical. During these fleeting moments, he knows—at least in an 'intellectual' sense, as he puts it—that the historical evidence of his early childhood desires and interpersonal relations is too fragmentary and incomplete to supply adequate confirmation (or disconfirmation) for his insights. Trained in the medical sciences, and much more aware than the average person about the role of placebo effects, he is vaguely uncomfortable about the speculative nature of his realizations, and the possibility that they may be placebo responses. He also knows—again, in an 'intellectual' sense, based on his professional experience—that he should not fully trust memories about events and feelings that occurred more than fifty years ago. While the analyst's reconstructions of the putative events and feelings are painted in the strongest and clearest colors, M is aware that his own memories of them were initially indistinct and malleable, and that it was only with the analyst's help that he could 'fully' remember the details. Independent evidence about his childhood (from siblings, diaries, photos, and other records), while inconclusive, tends to cast doubt on the veracity of his memories. M also has a vague sense that the way his analyst is offering reconstructions of these events tends to be dogmatic, and does not allow for the possibility that the putative Oedipal entanglements might not have occurred. Finally, there are occasions when he knows—again in an 'intellectual' sense—that the feelings he has toward his analyst are 'really' feelings about a flesh-and-blood man in the here and now, and not 'really' projections of ancient feelings onto a parent figure. He feels uncomfortable about all of these doubts, but he does nothing about them: he does not reflect upon them, or spell them out in greater detail, other than mentioning them to his analyst after another 30 hours of analysis had elapsed. The analyst tells him that these are most likely symptoms of unconscious resistance: he is afraid of the truth of his realization, and his neurotic illness is trying to reassert its hold over him the closer he is to conquering it. M continues to endorse the realizations as true, and continues to believe that he is continuing to make valid discoveries about his past, behaviors, emotions, and personality. He continues with the treatment, but the doubts do not vanish.

◆ After 60 hours of short-term psychodynamic psychotherapy (with an attachment theory orientation), S, a married 48-year-old social worker and mother of two children is genuinely surprised to learn that some of her problems with maintaining intimate relationships have their origin in her deepest childhood fears of abandonment. Much of her treatment focuses on issues of attachment and loss in her childhood, and to make these issues come alive she is encouraged to re-experience some of her childhood feelings. With the help of her psychotherapist, she regresses repeatedly during therapy to more primitive stages of experience. During these sessions she is flooded with terrors and panic states that are accompanied by vivid images of her parents having spats, images of being lost in crowds, memories of feeling neglected by her parents, and horrific fantasies of grisly car accidents in which her parents are victims. After a number of therapy sessions devoted to regressing, S starts to develop what she considers to be important insights into her past and present feelings. She comes to the realization that her mother was, for the most part, distant, preoccupied, and unaffectionate, and that her father was mostly absent in her early years, and a remote figure whose real feelings were never very clear to her. She also realizes that she was never truly understood by her parents, or taken seriously and listened to. During the regression sessions, she experiences vivid memories of events from her childhood that seem to offer evidence for these realizations. S thus feels confident in attributing many of her current psychological problems to the lack of emotional warmth, empathy, and acceptance she experienced in her early years. In fact, however, a significant number of S's insights are false or pseudo-insights; and a significant number are distortions, exaggerations, or gross over-simplifications of complex historical and interpersonal situations. Furthermore, many of S's memories are in fact false memories; that is, memories of events that never happened, or memories that are so distorted with respect to the historical facts that they bear only the flimsiest relation to them. Nonetheless, S feels she understands herself much better than before, and she notices improvement in some of her symptoms. The insights she acquires after reflecting upon these regressions and the memories they arouse are persuasive and meaningful to her. At the same time, however, S is vaguely aware that the methods used by her psychotherapist to encourage these regressions are disturbingly powerful and, as she phrases it, 'intrusive'. At times the thought occurs to her that her psychotherapist is too manipulative: she asks too many leading questions, uses too much body language to express silent criticism or support, and plays too many reward and punishment 'head games'. S feels she has a close, trusting, and empathic relationship with her psychotherapist, but she sometimes wonders whether she is paying too high a price for this: namely, being forced to see things the way her psychotherapist sees them, and say things her psychotherapist wants her to say. The thought has occurred to her more than once that some of her improvement is not due to the treatment but to the passage of time. But she does not act on these doubts; and she tries not to notice the unusual circumstances under which her insights were acquired and her memories triggered. A number of factors incline her to not attend to these doubts: the impending termination of the therapy, the costliness of the therapy, the reputation of the psychotherapist, the persuasive theoretical explanations, and pressure from her partner to continue with the therapy. With time the doubts fade, but they do not vanish.

These fictional examples are obviously contrived, convenient and oversimplified. As such, they cannot be decisive in settling questions about the existence or nonexistence of clinical phenomena; nor can they be decisive in settling conceptual questions. Still, they bear enough resemblances to the two prototypical cases of self-deception discussed earlier that they display a minimal degree of psychological realism. To this extent they are useful in showing what self-deception in psychodynamic psychotherapy *might* look like.

First, neither of these cases could be described as cases of other-deception. Neither clients' insights nor memories are the direct result of being duped, lied to, or brainwashed (as Grünbaum's model of suggestion-induced pseudo-insight holds). Neither the psychoanalyst nor the attachment-oriented psychotherapist deliberately practise benevolent therapeutic deception (as both Mendel and Pierre Janet did), with a view to furthering their own ends or the ends of the treatment. Neither knowingly prescribes psychodynamic placebos under conditions of deception. Neither could be considered to be charlatans, quacks, or con artists who knowingly promote bogus cures to gullible patients: rather, both are sincere, highly trained, and ethically responsible practitioners.

Second, in neither of these cases could the false insights and false memories of the clients be attributed to inadvertent error or misinformation. That is, neither client could be described as being led astray in epistemic good faith by a false theory, an inadvertent misdiagnosis, a misinterpretation, or a misapplied treatment method, thus rendering him or her *innocently* caught up in the theoretical or clinical mistakes of others. Nor does either of them fall prey to inadvertently prescribed placebos. While M's insight involves endorsing an explanation of the etiology of his symptoms that is in fact false, his error has not befallen him as somatic illnesses or accidents befall their victims; nor has he stumbled inadvertently into his error as he would if he were making calculating errors in a difficult problem in differential calculus. Rather, in endorsing the psychoanalytic explanation, he failed to display the degree of epistemic caution that would have been consistent with his other practical and professional activities, which are governed by adherence to consensually endorsed epistemic norms about evidence, practical reasoning, and inductive inference. M's error was avoidable: a cautious and earnest physician, he failed to apply even the most rudimentary principles of differential diagnosis to himself, and thereby misdiagnosed the neurophysiological causes of his problems. (For similar misdiagnoses in real case histories, see Shapiro *et al.* 1978).

Third, in neither case could the clients, when acquiring insights and memories, be described as the passive or unwitting victims of the suggestive influences of their psychotherapists, as Grünbaum's critique would hold. From their professional lives, both are familiar with the power of suggestion, and the varieties of coercion, manipulation, and persuasion at play in interpersonal contexts; M, in particular, is familiar from his own training in diagnostics with concepts such as placebo effects, nocebo effects, expectancy effects, and contaminated evidence. Both clients, in other words, have sufficient epistemic resources to make reasonable inferences about the potential for evidentiary contamination in their own treatments; more specifically, both are vaguely aware that their exploratory activities, insights, and memories may be vulnerable to these influences. But neither client makes a deliberate commitment to identify and evaluate the role of these influences. Their neglect of these second-order epistemic issues is so persistent and well-targeted, and so carefully compensated by persistent attention to the first-order psychodynamic issues that make up the content of their insights, that it could be described as a kind of selective inattention: that is, a skillful and precise failure to attend to otherwise salient issues, resulting in what *seems* (to others and to themselves) to be sincere failures of recognition (Baier 1996).

Neither client, in other words, matches adequately the description of epistemic good faith: they are not victims of inadvertent errors or mistakes when acquiring their insights, nor are they victims of other-deception. Instead, they have had a hand in the errors that have led them astray, and this has resulted in their holding beliefs about themselves that they also know are false or doubtful.

*

This chapter began with an important but speculative question which has attracted relatively little scientific inquiry and even less epistemic and conceptual analysis: Is the placebo response incompatible with the patient's knowledge or awareness of placebos? Do patients and experimental participants who are placebo responders *know* that they are responding to placebos if they have not already been informed about them—or do they remain in the dark, as willing or unwilling victims of strategies of intentional ignorance? Is the placebo response less effective if patients know they are responding to placebos rather than to active treatments? If the analogy between placebo treatments in medicine and placebo treatments in clinical psychology holds, then these questions are also relevant for psychodynamic psychotherapy: Do clients who respond to insight and interpretation placebos, for example, know that they are responding to placebos, or do they mistakenly take them to be authentic or valid? Is the placebo response less effective if they know they are responding to insight and interpretation placebos?

On the face of it, it seems obvious that either people *know* that their response to a treatment is a response to placebo, or they remain in the dark (because they have been deceived); and it seems that if people know that they have been given placebos, then there can be no placebo response. But the situation is much less obvious than meets the eye. It was argued that it is not always as simple a matter as patients either knowing or not knowing that they are responding to placebos. In some unusual cases, patients neither straightforwardly *know* that they are responding to placebo, nor straightforwardly remain ignorant or deceived by others about it; and in some cases, patients believe that they are responding to an active treatment, and yet they somehow know that they are not. They have convinced themselves of something that they know is not the case. Some part of the placebo response, in other words, could be attributable to self-deception rather than to deception from another.

Despite its counter-intuitive nature, something like this unusual situation might be found in the psychodynamic psychotherapies: it is, at least, a conceptual possibility. Some clients might believe that the interpretations and insights they have acquired are authentic, and yet somehow they know that they are little more than psychological sugar pills. They might, for example, have convinced themselves that their psychological explorations are truth-tracking, despite knowing that they are deeply context-sensitive, suggestion-prone, or vulnerable to bias. Or they might come to believe things about their psychology, behavior, or childhood during the course of the treatment that they also know are false, or are explanatory fictions, or have good grounds for rejecting.

What this means is that placebo-responsive clients in psychodynamic psychotherapy are not always victims of intentional or inadvertent deception, as Grünbaum's (1984) account of pseudo-insight in classical Freudian psycho-analysis suggests, and as some of the standard theories of placebo response hold. Clients are not always genuinely unaware of the presence of these suggestive forces, or blind to their own vulnerability to placebo effects, or sincerely oblivious to the epistemic contamination to which their exploratory activities are subjected. Some clients are in epistemic *bad faith*. They have had a hand in the deceptions or errors that have led them astray, believing things about themselves that they also somehow know are false. Their placebo responsiveness is in part a function of self-deception, a kind of lying to them-selves. This may not be too far-fetched: the placebo has been described as the lie that heals (Brody 1982). Self-deception may be the lie clients tell to them-selves to help to rally the mind's native healing powers.

Chapter 7

Open Placebos

The Ethics of Giving Placebos

◆ Thought experiment: The Psychotherapy Hoax. X, a well-respected psychodynamic psychotherapist, announces to the general public that he has
practised as a psychotherapist with the sole aim of debunking psychodynamic psychotherapy. His inspiration for the hoax is the Kwakiutl shaman
Quesalid (Lévi-Strauss 1963), who became a shaman in order to debunk
shamanism, which he regarded as shameful trickery and exploitation.
Initially trained in the logic, epistemology, and history of science, X is skeptical about the validity of psychodynamic treatment methods, which he
regards as little more than a hodgepodge of suggestion, psychobabble, and
credible placebos—'a sort of psychological theriac' he writes, quoting
Pierre Janet. X is also skeptical about the scientific value of psychodynamic
(and psychoanalytic) explanations of human behavior, which he argues are
based on irrevocably contaminated clinical evidence. He is also concerned,
on ethical grounds, about the duping and exploitation of clients, the
dangers of inducing in clients false memories, as well as beliefs in false or
spurious psychological explanations, and a number of other unwanted
practical and ethical consequences that happen when people are led to
believe false explanations of human behavior. Dismayed about the relative
weakness of theoretical arguments in the face of institutional inertia, blind
dogmatism, and the massive popular appeal of the talking cures,
X decides to test his theoretical convictions by putting them into practice.
After a successful period of training, during which his real motives remain
undetected, X opens a practice and begins to treat clients. He deliberately
deploys bogus treatment techniques with a view to eliciting placebo
responses. Part of his debunking strategy, for example, involves concocting
deliberately false psychodynamic interpretations—which he offers to
his clients in all sincerity as *bona fide* interpretations of their psychology
and behaviors. Another part of the strategy, which he learned
from social–psychological experiments about false personality profiles (the
so-called 'Barnum effect'), is to offer to his clients trivial one-size-fits-all
interpretations. Yet another part of his strategy is to encourage clients to

develop insights that accord with his professed theoretical orientation, but which, like his interpretations, he knows have little or no bearing on their actual psychology, behavior, and history: explanatory fictions. X's strategy thus targets some of the major principles of the Standard View of psychodynamic psychotherapy. He is not surprised when some of his treatments prove to be highly successful; nor is he surprised that none of his clients detect his debunking strategy. Over the course of ten years, X conceals his motives and assembles evidence that will dismantle the Standard View one piece at a time. At the ten-year anniversary of the opening of his practice, X finally makes the announcement. His revelation stuns the psychotherapeutic community, earns the outrage of many of his former clients, triggers a number of lawsuits alleging malpractice, and generates a vigorous debate about the effectiveness of the talking cures, the ethics of giving placebos, and the ethics of paternalist deception and practices of intentional ignorance. Some critics argue that he was practicing psychotherapy all along, despite his intentions; others argue that he was a swindler of the highest order; others argue that he has performed an invaluable service to science.

This is a cautionary tale. A hoax such as this is neither unthinkable nor impossible to perpetrate. But while it bears certain resemblances to the Quesalid case (Lévi-Strauss 1963), and to certain scandal-ridden hoaxes aimed at debunking well-known theoretical positions (e.g. the Sokal hoax (Sokal 1996; Sokal and Bricmont 1998)), no such hoax has yet occurred in psychotherapy. Nor is the probability of such a hoax occurring particularly high: careful training and screening methods, institutional oversight mechanisms, peer reviews, daunting legal and financial ramifications, and the sheer psychological and ethical challenges of deceiving so many people over so many years, would interfere with its perpetration. But what the tale lacks in verisimilitude it makes up for in other ways. Most notably, the tale raises important issues about the ethics of giving placebos in psychotherapy.

Suppose that the main conceptual hypothesis explored in this work is valid: a) some therapeutic changes in psychodynamic psychotherapy are a function of powerful placebos that rally the mind's natural healing powers, rather than a function of a set of specific active ingredients that is unique to the treatment methods of the psychodynamic psychotherapies; b) one type of placebo that is operative in psychodynamic psychotherapy is the explanatory psychological fiction, which is found at work in psychodynamic interpretations and insights. What follows from this? Can any substantive guidelines about the ethics of giving placebos in psychodynamic psychotherapy be generated, once it is assumed that the hypothesis is valid? Is it ethically permissible for psychotherapists to give psychodynamic placebos to clients? Is it permissible to dispense interpretation placebos and to encourage insight placebos, if psychotherapists who dispense them know that they are the psychological equivalent of sugar pills? Is this a case of deceiving clients, or withholding vital information from them, or deliberately keeping them in the dark? If so, do practices of intentional ignorance such as this constitute harm to clients? Does it violate the Hippocratic Oath 'First do no harm'? Are there instances in which some types of intentional ignorance could be ethically permissible, if they result in therapeutic improvement? Are psychodynamic placebos such as these as harmful as psychotherapeutically-induced false memories? Finally, is it any more ethically permissible to dispense psychodynamic placebos if clients are fully informed about them and consent to their use?

While the debate about the use of placebos in randomized controlled trials involving psychopharmaceutical agents is robust (Young and Annable 1996; Roberts *et al.* 2001; Young and Annable 2002; Kim 2003; Rich 2003), there is comparatively little debate about the ethics of giving placebos in clinical psychological contexts where no trials or experiments are involved. Many of the prominent handbooks, casebooks, and practical guides devoted to professional ethics for clinical psychologists contain only scattered references to the ethics of placebo therapeutics (Bersoff 1995; Koocher and Keith-Spiegel 1998; Pope *et al.* 2001; Fisher 2003; O'Donohue and Ferguson 2003); and some contain none at all. With few exceptions (Vogel *et al.* 1980; Brown 1994, 1998a, 1998b; Andrews 2001; Oh 2004), most psychologists and psychiatrists do not explicitly advocate the use of placebos to treat conditions that are known to be placebo-responsive, such as depression.

There are also few explicit guidelines about the ethics of giving placebos in the codes of ethics of major national and international psychological and psychiatric associations. This is an odd situation, given that some of the most common psychological disorders are known to be responsive to placebo therapeutics, and given that five of the top ten leading causes of disability are considered to be psychiatric or psychological in nature (namely, depression, alcohol abuse, bipolar mood disorder, schizophrenia, and obsessive compulsive disorder (World Health Organization 1997)). Placebo response rates in the treatment of mental illness have been found to be quite high, at least in a number of studies. In the treatment of major depressive disorder, for example, one study found a placebo response rate as high as 50% (Khan *et al.* 2000; see also Kirsch and Sapirstein 1988). In another study on the treatment of bipolar disorder, the placebo response rate was 34% (Keck *et al.* 2000). In another study on panic disorder, the placebo response was as high as 23–34% (Rosenberg *et al.* 1991). *If* there is scientific evidence that placebos are sometimes as effective in treating certain psychological disorders as active psychological interventions (such as psychopharmaceutical agents or psychotherapy), then it would be reasonable to expect the major psychological and psychiatric associations to formulate explicit clinical guidelines about the ethics of giving placebos. But this has not happened.

No explicit discussion of the ethics of giving placebos is found, for example, in the American Psychological Association's 'Ethical principles of psychologists and code of conduct' (1992). The code states only that 'psychologists seek to promote accuracy, honesty, and truthfulness in the science, teaching and practice of psychology. Psychologists do not steal, cheat, or engage in fraud, subterfuge, or intentional misrepresentation of fact'. This is unavailing for those psychologists trying to determine if placebo treatments are ethically permissible. The World Psychiatric Association's *Madrid declaration on ethical standards for psychiatric practice*, approved in 1996 and amended in 2002, also contains no explicit statements about the ethics of giving placebos in psychiatric practice, and few implicit suggestions.

Again, there is little explicit discussion about the ethics of giving placebos to psychiatric patients as part of a treatment strategy in the American Psychiatric Association's *Principles of medical ethics with annotations especially applicable to psychiatry* (2001). Addendum 1 of the *Principles* includes a number of general statements about informed consent, honesty, and deception, but none explicitly forbids or sanctions the use of placebos as psychiatric treatments. Take for example the following statements about what is ethically permissible in psychiatric practice: 'A psychiatrist shall not withhold information that the patient needs or reasonably could use to make informed treatment decisions, including options for treatment not provided by the psychiatrist;' 'A physician shall deal honestly with patients and colleagues, and strive to expose those physicians deficient in character or competence, or who engage in fraud or deception;' 'A physician shall be dedicated to providing competent medical service with compassion and respect for human dignity'; 'A psychiatrist's treatment plan shall be based upon clinical, scientific, or generally accepted standards of treatment. This applies to the treating and the reviewing psychiatrist'; and so on. None of these statements explicitly forbids the use of placebos; nor do they explicitly condone the use of placebos.

The one notable exception to this dearth of informed discussion on placebo treatment is found in the American Psychiatric Association's official handbook of ethics, *Ethics primer of the American Psychiatric Association* (2001). In the section entitled 'Ethics and forensic psychiatry', it is stated that placebo use is ethically permissible if the placebo is administered by a 'physician-scientist'. However, the handbook also states that placebo use is considered to be ethically impermissible if the placebo is administered by a psychiatrist acting in a doctor–patient relationship. The distinction between 'physician-scientist' and 'doctor' is vague, but on one charitable interpretation it can be taken to mean that placebo use is ethically permissible only in experimental contexts where the principle of informed consent has been satisfied: for example, randomized controlled trials of psychopharmaceutical agents. In all other clinical contexts, however, placebo therapeutics is considered to be ethically impermissible.

By contrast, the debate about the ethics of giving placebos in medicine is vigorous, multifaceted, and already well into its middle age. Because it sets such a high standard for ethical argument, a brief summary of the major features of the debate will serve to frame the discussion of the ethics of giving placebos in clinical psychology, psychotherapy, and psychiatry. The debate, which reaches back almost 200 years, tends to divide physicians and medical ethicists along utilitarian, deontological, and pragmatist lines. These divisions become even more variegated and vulnerable to empirically driven revision as scientific research into the nature of placebos grows, and as myths and misconceptions about them are discarded. The debate falls into one of two broad categories: the ethics of giving placebos in clinical treatment settings, and the ethics of using placebos in experimental or research settings such as clinical trials (with participants who have consented to be randomly assigned to either placebo or experimental conditions). The central question in both categories remains the same: is it ethically permissible to knowingly give placebos to patients or experimental participants? If so, under what conditions is it ethically permissible, and why? If not, then why not? These questions break down into more specific questions. In clinical treatment settings, is it ethically permissible to knowingly give placebos to patients while telling them that they are receiving active treatments? If this constitutes patient deception, then are there any conditions in which such deception is ethically permissible (e.g. when the relevant diseases or disorders are known to be responsive to placebos)? In experimental or research settings, is it ethically permissible to assign experiment participants in randomized clinical trials to placebo control groups if there are alternative methods of testing the effectiveness of new drugs or treatment procedures, or when proven treatments are already available from which the participants could benefit?

Animating the debate is a fundamental conflict over the relative weighting assigned to two of the most basic principles of medical ethics: namely, the principle of beneficence (and the closely related principle of nonmaleficence) and the principle of respect for autonomy (Veatch 1982; Beauchamp and McCullough 1984). The main issues concern: a) the interpretation of each of these broad principles in the highly specific and oftentimes ambiguous clinical or experimental settings in which placebos are dispensed; and b) determining which principle or set of principles takes precedence over the others, and why.

The principle of beneficence requires that 'one helps others further important and legitimate interests and abstains from injuring them' (Beauchamp and McCullough 1984: 27). When the positive component of this principle is applied to the specific question of the administration of placebos, one interpretation would hold that experimental research or clinical trials should always have comparison arms that provide interventions that are at least equal to the standard care available in the community (Roberts *et al.* 2001). According to this interpretation—and there are others—it would be ethically impermissible to give placebos to control groups if there are other proven treatments against which the experimental treatment can be compared. Participants who are assigned to control groups should always get the best medical care possible, rather than dummy pills or sham interventions.

The principle of beneficence requires physicians to provide positive benefits for others; but one component of the principle (nonmaleficence) requires physicians to prevent and remove harmful conditions for others. When this is applied to the administration of placebos in experimental settings, it could be interpreted as meaning that experimental research with new drugs or medical procedures should only involve the healthiest individuals possible, so that the potential for harm and exploitation of vulnerable human participants is minimized. According to this interpretation, it would be ethically impermissible to give placebos to vulnerable patient populations in trials and experiments of new medications or procedures: children, the mentally ill, or the severely ill.

The principle of respect for autonomy holds that physicians ought to regard others as rightfully self-governing in matters of their choice and action (Beauchamp and McCullough 1984:14). When this is applied to the particular case of placebo administration, one interpretation would hold that experimenters should be open and fully informative about all aspects of an experiment or trial. This would mean that the intentional ignorance (e.g. deception or information withholding) that is commonly associated with giving placebos is ethically impermissible.

Finally, there is the more narrow ethical principle of clinical equipoise: namely, that in order to allow for objectivity, investigators must be in a position of genuine uncertainty about which arm of the experiment or trial will be most helpful to patients (Freedman 1987). According to one interpretation, the use of a placebo is unacceptable in any situation where there is an effective available treatment.

Interpretations of these general principles, including specific interpretations of the principles in light of the issue of giving placebos, are enshrined in the codes of ethics of a number of major medical associations and national regulatory associations (U.S. Food and Drug Administration 2002; Canadian Institutes of Health Research 2004), as well as international medical associations (World Medical Association 2000; Council for International Organizations of Medical Science 2003). National and international medical codes of ethics evolve and devolve over time, but many of them still turn upon the dynamic and productive tension between the principle of respect for autonomy and the principle of beneficence.

One of the most important of these institutional documents is produced by the World Medical Association, an organization comprised of about 80 national medical associations (with some notable exceptions). The World Medical Association's *Declaration of Helsinki* (2000), which endeavors to set global standards for medically-related human rights and the protection of individuals in clinical trials and experimentation, has been revised five times since 1964. The section in the *Declaration* that concerns the ethics of giving placebos focuses mainly on the use of placebo controls in randomized controlled clinical trials; it says little about the therapeutic use of placebos in clinical settings that do not involve trials or experiments. Nor does it provide substantive arguments or reasons for its positions. The latest two revisions of the *Declaration* reveal a great deal about how placebos have been regarded in medical therapeutics. In 1996, Article II.3 of the fifth revision of the *Declaration* stated: 'The potential benefits, hazards, and discomfort of a new method should be weighed against the advantages of the best current diagnostic and therapeutic method. In any medical study, every patient (including those of a control group, if any) should be assured of the best proven diagnostic and therapeutic method. This does not exclude the use of inert placebo in studies where no proven diagnostic or therapeutic method exists'. In 2000, the sixth revision of the *Declaration* (World Medical Association 2000, Article 29) stated: 'The benefits, risks, burdens and effectiveness of a new method should be tested against those of the best current prophylactic, diagnostic, and therapeutic methods. This does not exclude the use of placebo, or no-treatment, in studies where no proven prophylactic, diagnostic or therapeutic method exists'. Noticeably, the term 'inert' was removed.

A 'Note of Clarification' was later added to this crucial paragraph by the World Medical Association General Assembly (World Medical Association 2002).

> The WMA hereby reaffirms its position that extreme care must be taken in making use of a placebo-controlled trial and that in general this methodology should only be used in the absence of existing proven therapy. However, a placebo-controlled trial may be ethically acceptable, even if proven therapy is available, under the following circumstances: Where for compelling and scientifically sound methodological reasons its use is necessary to determine the efficacy or safety of a prophylactic, diagnostic or

therapeutic method; or where a prophylactic, diagnostic or therapeutic method is being investigated for a minor condition and the patients who receive placebo will not be subject to any additional risk of serious or irreversible harm. All other provisions of the *Declaration of Helsinki* must be adhered to, especially the need for appropriate ethical and scientific review.

This adds little in the way of clarification; indeed, since it openly contradicts the original *Declaration* of 2000, it is confusing.

The 2000 *Declaration* is clear at least in what it proscribes: placebo controls should not be used in trials of treatments for drugs for life-threatening conditions (e.g. acute infectious diseases or cancer), when proven safe and effective treatments are otherwise available. This is an absolute ban: no exempting or excluding conditions of any sort are tolerated. The *Declaration* is also clear in what it considers ethically permissible: placebo controls can be used in clinical trials where there is no known effective treatment. The main disagreement surrounding the *Declaration* concerns the use of placebo controls in those clinical trials in which temporary deferral of treatment poses no long-term threat to a patient's health, *and* when there is a known effective therapy that is available. On this particular point, some medical ethicists have argued that placebo controls should never be used in any clinical trials if there are known effective therapies available (Rothman and Michels 1994, 2002). This is because it is unethical to deprive patients of the level of care that they would have received if they had not been participants in a clinical trial. In other words, every patient in every medical study should be assured of the best proven current diagnostic and therapeutic methods. Sir Austin Bradford Hill, one of the architects of the modern controlled clinical trial, states the position thus—and in doing so reveals a bias against the effectiveness of placebos: 'Is it ethical to use a placebo? The answer to this question will depend, I suggest, upon whether there is already available an orthodox treatment of proved or accepted value. If there is such an orthodox treatment the question will hardly arise, for the doctor will wish to know whether a new treatment is more, or less, effective than the old, not that it is more effective than nothing' (Hill 1963). Active controls—that is, already approved drugs—rather than placebo controls should always be used in clinical trials, when those active controls are known to be safe and effective. In the absence of proven effective treatments, however, Rothman and Michels allow that placebo controls are appropriate.

One of the obvious problems with this position, however, is that the safety and effectiveness of active controls cannot always be taken at face value. There is a crucial distinction between 'a treatment *known* to be effective, and one *thought* to be effective, *hoped* to be more effective, *believed* to be effective, or in widespread use without evidence of effectiveness' (Pocock 2002: 237).

Other medical ethicists have argued that the ethical permissibility of placebo controls in clinical trials depends entirely on the *consequences* to well-informed patients of omitting or delaying a known effective therapy (Lewis *et al.* 2002; Temple 2002); it does not depend on the intrinsic rightness or wrongness of the particular acts of deception or intentional ignorance involved in carrying out a blinded trial, or the intrinsic rightness or wrongness of withholding effective treatments. Temple, for example, argues that in some cases it is ethically permissible to use placebos in clinical trials if patients are fully informed of the consequences of their treatment, and if there is no immediate threat to their health or well-being. There is, he argues, no significant difference between the delay of treatment that might occur in placebo-controlled clinical trials, and the decision to delay or forego symptomatic treatment that informed patients make on a daily basis (e.g. deciding not to treat headache, dental pain, anxiety, social phobia, obsessive compulsive disorder, depression, allergies, and so on). 'It simply does not make sense to assert that it is unethical to *invite* a fully informed person to participate in a placebo-controlled study in which a symptomatic treatment will be deferred or omitted if no harm (perhaps including excessive discomfort) is involved. There is no impact on the patient's underlying health in such studies and patients are always free to leave a trial without penalty and receive standard treatment' (Temple 2002: 211). To bar patients from making such decisions, even when they have given their fully informed consent, is to fail to respect their autonomy.

Other problems concern the *Declaration*'s model of placebo. One of the obvious problems with the 1996 *Declaration* is its uncritical assumption that placebos are 'inert'. This is far from obvious, and far from a scientifically validated theory. In trying to address this, however, the 2000 revision errs in other ways. While it makes no reference to 'inert' placebos, it overlooks the fact that placebos in some cases *are* efficacious prophylactic, diagnostic or therapeutic methods.

Perhaps the most central issue in the debate within physical medicine, and the issue with the most relevance for the ethics of giving placebos in psychotherapy, concerns the role of intentional ignorance. According to one widely held but problematic assumption, placebo use invariably involves the deliberate deception of patients, the deliberate withholding of information, or the deliberate cultivation of ignorance in patients: placebos are 'the lies that heal'. The assumption is that physicians who treat patients with substances or interventions that they know are pharmacologically or medically 'inert', but who lead patients to believe otherwise, *must* be deceiving, misleading, or manipulating their patients. It is the patients' mistaken beliefs in the efficacy of the treatment that triggers the placebo effect, and these beliefs can *only* be maintained by means of deception or one of the mechanisms of intentional ignorance. Since patient deception is in general unethical, placebo use (as a specific instance of deception or manipulation) is unethical. This view of placebo therapeutics has been supported by a number of medical ethicists (Simmons 1978; Veatch 1982; Beauchamp and Childress 1983), and justified according to a number of broad ethical theories.

This is a persuasive view, but it is not without problems. It rests on an older model of the placebo effect that dates back to an era when the action of placebos was seen as mainly psychological. Placebos such as sugar pills were once dispensed in order to placate anxious or hypochondriacal patients, resulting in what Thomas Jefferson called a 'pious fraud' (Brody 1982: 113). This model is often associated with the pejorative view that giving placebos is little more than medical chicanery.

Despite the outdated model of placebo effect, the idea that giving placebos is unethical because it involves deceiving patients receives support from both deontological and utilitarian approaches to medical ethics. The deontological or duty-based approach to patient deception can be traced back to Kant's efforts to make truth-telling a universal duty. According to this approach, deception of any form (e.g. lying, or withholding or distorting vital information), or deliberately keeping patients in the dark or the half-light is wrong, independent of the good or bad consequences that follow from the deception: it is a violation of the autonomy and dignity of persons. In medical contexts, this means that the practices of intentional ignorance, even if they are benevolent and in the best interests of the patient, always undermines the patient's right to give consent to his or her own treatment. Even in cases where medical privilege allows partial disclosure or withholding of information that may interfere with successful treatment, the physician's action 'must be consistent with the full disclosure of facts necessary for informed consent' (Simmons 1978: 174).

According to the utilitarian approach, by contrast, practices of intentional ignorance such as patient deception are unethical because of the negative consequences that follow from them; in particular, placebo use would lead to a net increase in harms over benefits for patients, physicians, and the medical community at large. One of the most salient short-term negative consequences is the erosion of physician–patient trust that is likely to occur once the intentional ignorance is revealed. There are also many long-term negative consequences: public skepticism about the value of medicine (Cabot 1903, 1906; Brody 1982), the possibility of medical malpractice lawsuits, the tendency of deceptions to multiply and to involve the complicity of other parties, addiction to placebos, delays in diagnosis, and the potential for financial exploitation that comes from setting prescription fees for dummy pills (Brody 1982: 114; Waring and Glass 2006).

One of the most influential consequentialist defenses of the view that giving placebos is unethical is developed by Bok (1974, 1975, 2002). Bok does not deny that placebos can be potent treatments that may relieve suffering. But giving patients 'inert' treatments that they think are active is deceptive, and therefore unethical: 'the very manner in which [placebos] can relieve suffering seems to depend on keeping the patient in the dark... the circumstances in which a placebo is prescribed introduce an element of deception' (1972: 19). Bok argues that giving placebos violates the principle of informed consent: that is, the right of patients to have complete, understandable information on their diagnosis, treatment, and prognosis, and the right of patients to refuse treatment (even if this refusal is not in their best interests). Bok also identifies a number of broad unwanted social consequences of patient deception: giving placebos undermines medical authority, it leads to the breakdown of patient–doctor trust, and it can easily spread beyond its immediate domain to other areas of the patient–doctor relationship (the domino theory of deception). Placebo therapeutics, moreover, may have toxic side effects, may result in dependency or addiction, and may tempt physicians to move from prescribing pharmacologically inert placebos to pharmacologically active placebos. Bok concludes that 'honesty may not be the highest social value; at exceptional times, when survival is at stake, it may have to be set aside. To permit a widespread practice of deception, however, is to set the stage for abuses and growing mistrust' (Bok 1974: 23).

This is not the last word on the ethics of giving placebos.[1] Some medical ethicists defend the use of placebos in medical therapeutics, using varieties of utilitarian or deontological arguments (Gribbin 1981; Rawlinson 1985; Brown 1994, 1998a, 1998b). Again, the assumption is that placebo-giving involves some form of intentional ignorance, the most extreme variant of which is patient deception. The deontological defense of placebo use involves arguing that the moral rule against deception is outweighed by other rules (Brody 1982: 114). The utilitarian defense involves identifying all the positive consequences that follow from placebo use, and showing that on balance (according to some presumed utilitarian calculus of harms and benefits) they outweigh all the negative consequences of intentional ignorance. O'Neill (1989) argues that while the deception involved in giving placebos violates the principle of informed consent, 'some non-fundamental aspects of treatment to which consent has been given may have to include elements of deception...

Use of placebos or of reassuring but inaccurate accounts of expected pain might sometimes be non-fundamental but indispensable and so permissible deception'.

Rawlinson (1985), for example, argues that the practice of benevolent deception in placebo administration is ethically permissible in exceptional circumstances, but only if it is strictly regulated, and only if it is practiced properly ('in an attitude of reluctance, after weighing its costs'). She identifies five conditions that need to be satisfied before benevolent deception is justified: '1. That it can never be employed for the convenience of the health care team, but only for the therapeutic benefit of the patient. 2. That it be used only in cases where substantial evidence indicates that it is necessary. 3. That the physician be able to make the case for the necessity of the deception to any reasonable observer. 4. That the physician determines whether or not any physical or psychophysical condition for which the treatment is indicated would be masked by reliance on the placebo. 5. That the physician carefully considers the character and value system of the patient and the effect of such deception on his or her self-respect and attitude toward the physician' (1985: 415). Rawlinson argues (against Bok, among others) that to ban the administration of placebos on the basis of speculations about the remote effects of its abuse is 'unwise, unnecessary, and a flagrant denial of the substantial evidence in the history of medicine that it is sometimes therapeutically indicated and efficacious'.

The main problem with the majority of these discussions about the ethics of giving placebos—those critical of the practice *and* those in cautious support of it—is that they proceed on the assumption that giving placebos always involves some form of intentional ignorance, ranging from outright deception of patients, to keeping patients in the dark. It is assumed that physicians who treat patients with substances or interventions that they know are pharmacologically or medically 'inert', but who lead patients to believe otherwise, are deceiving or manipulating their patients; that it is the patients' mistaken beliefs in the efficacy of the treatment that triggers the placebo effect; and that these beliefs can only be maintained by deceptive, coercive, or less-than-transparent means. For the most part, this assumption goes unquestioned. But changes in the concept of placebo, and in the scientific understanding of the placebo effect, have given rise to new ways to look at this assumption, and thus new ways to tackle the ethical issues. If placebo use can be de-coupled from the practices of intentional ignorance, then some of the ethical problems with giving placebos simply vanish.

First, recent placebo research in neurobiology, pharmacology, ethnopharmacology, molecular biology, and medical anthropology suggests that placebos are more than sham or illusory treatments that work solely on the psychological states of patients. Placebos appear to have the power to unlock the body's biologically programmed capacity for self-healing, and to rally the body's internal pharmacopeia (Brody 1997; Harrington 1997; Kleinman *et al.* 2002; Moerman 2002a). But if placebos are neither unreal nor inert, and if they are sometimes effective in treating a wide variety of psychological and non-psychological disorders, then one of the presumed conditions for the practice of intentional ignorance is removed. Physicians have no need to keep patients in the dark about non-inert and non-illusory treatments.

Second, it is false to assume that *all* cases of placebo use involve intentional ignorance. There are at least two types of conditions in which open placebos (i.e. patients are informed that they are receiving placebos) can be administered successfully, and one type of condition in which the placebo response can be triggered *without* the use of placebos or patient deception (Park and Covi 1965; Vogel *et al.* 1980; Brody, 1982; Aulas and Rosner 2003).

Condition i) No deception or intentional ignorance is involved when placebos are given to participants in double-blind randomized controlled clinical trials of drugs or medical treatments, as long as the participants have been fully informed that they may be receiving either an active drug or a placebo, and as long as they consent with full understanding of the treatment consequences. In these cases, the principle of informed *and educated* consent is satisfied (Ingelfinger 1972), and the participants' autonomy has not been violated. Participants who show positive responses in the trials know that the therapeutic changes they are experiencing may be due either to placebos or to the drug, and yet this knowledge does not always weaken the effectiveness of the placebo.

Condition ii) No deception or intentional ignorance is involved, and the principle of informed educated consent is satisfied, when participants in *nonblind* or open clinical trials, or patients in clinical situations, are informed that they are receiving placebos. While this has not been the subject of much research, there is some clinical evidence to suggest that patients who are informed that they are receiving saline injections, sugar pills or other placebos sometimes continue to experience measurable objective symptom relief. In one study (Park and Covi 1965), the knowledge that they were receiving placebos rather than active medications did not hinder the patients' therapeutic progress. Rawlinson (1985: 410–11) suggests a method in which open placebos could be administered without triggering a self-defeating patient response: in cases where placebos may reasonably be expected to be useful, and where pharmacologically active agents are ineffective or contraindicated, 'a physician could simply report to a patient that the prescribed agent appears to be pharmacologically inert with respect to his or her disorder, but that, in fact, it has been shown to be therapeutically effective in other patients suffering from the condition'. A variant of this message is suggested by Brown (1994, 1998a, 1998b). To a patient suffering from high blood pressure, who appears to be a suitable candidate for placebo treatment, a physician could issue the following words: 'You have two options. One is to take a diuretic. It will probably bring your blood pressure down, but it does have some side effects. There are also other treatments that are less expensive and less likely to cause side effects and that help many people with your condition. Some people find that herbal tea twice a day is helpful; others find that taking these pills twice a day is helpful. These pills do not contain any drug. We don't know how the herbal tea or these pills work. They may trigger or stimulate your body's own healing processes. We do know that about 20 percent of the people with your type of high blood pressure get their blood pressure into the normal range using this approach. If you decide to try one of these treatments, I will check your progress every two weeks. If after six weeks your blood pressure is still high, we should consider the diuretic' (Brown 1998a: 95).

Condition iii) The use of the open placebo effect (which is to be distinguished from a placebo *per se*) is found in those medical encounters where physicians help to make patients' diseases intelligible, instill in patients a sense of caring and social support, and increase patients' sense of mastery (Brody 1982; Moerman 2002b). As no placebos are prescribed in these situations, no deception is involved. Instead, the highly charged symbolic and interpersonal elements of the physician–patient relationship are deliberately activated by the physician (see also Kirsch and Baker 1993). Therapeutic effects derive not from the patient's false beliefs about the efficacy of what is in fact an 'inert' treatment, but from the trust, confidence, and heightened expectations for healing that are occasioned by the interpersonal relationship with a healing authority.

The Ethics of Giving Open Placebos

There are a number of myths, untested assumptions, and misconceptions about open placebos (Condition ii, above):

- Open placebo treatment is unethical because patients are not receiving the best care available.
- Patients will not accept open placebo treatment.
- Placebo treatment will not be effective if both the patient and the clinician know that the placebo pill is pharmacologically inert. 'If a patient knows that a treatment is a placebo, then the treatment cannot be of benefit' (Lieberman and Dunlap 1979: 553).

◆ Therapeutic improvement with open placebos is transient, and is not as real or durable as the improvement that occurs with medically active treatments (Brown 1994).

None of these claims can be taken at face value, because none are supported by any substantive scientific evidence or substantive medical reasoning. With the exception of a handful of papers (Vogel *et al.* 1980; de Sousa 1988; Brown 1994, 1998a, 1998b; Aulas and Rosner 2003) and one older clinical trial (Park and Covi 1965), the collective effect of which is to cast doubt on these myths and misconceptions, there has been very little systematic research on the relative effectiveness or ineffectiveness of open placebos in medical and psychological treatments; and there has been very little conceptual, epistemological, methodological, and phenomenological analysis of open placebos. The nature, mechanism, function, and frequency of open placebo responses, in other words, remains a medical mystery. Why? It is not because of the relative scarcity of open placebos; they are not rare, esoteric, or exotic. There are many trial participants who experience open placebo responses, or variants of them, in randomized controlled trials: that is, participants who believe that the therapeutic changes they are experiencing are caused by a placebo rather than an active drug, and yet who continue to experience therapeutic changes. And yet it is not these placebo recipients who are the focus of the vast bulk of experimental research in randomized controlled trials. Placebo responses (in both the non-open and open conditions) are not investigated in their own right. As Kirsch and Sapirstein (1998) observe, 'although almost everyone controls for placebo effects, almost no one evaluates them'. The assumption is that the placebo group is useful only because it supplies baseline data that can be factored out to determine the real treatment effect. Harrington also remarks that 'on the one hand, we acknowledge the power and ubiquity of placebo responses by our requirement that all new drugs be tested in double-blind placebo-controlled situations; however, we then define those same responses as the 'non-specific noise' in the treatment to be subtracted out of the picture. We often fail to notice that these factors are not inherently nonspecific but are only so because insufficient energy and attention has been spent on specifying them' (Harrington 1997: 1–2).

Without further scientific investigation, open placebos can no more be dismissed as self-defeating or self-neutralizing treatments than placebos administered under conditions of deception or intentional ignorance can be dismissed as sham or unreal treatments. Given that most discussions of the ethics of giving placebos are founded on the problematic assumption that giving placebos involves the cultivation of some form of intentional ignorance in patients, ranging from outright deception to the withholding of vital information, the systematic investigation of open placebos is potentially important for the development of new approaches to the ethics of giving placebos, and for new approaches to the challenges of harnessing the placebo effect for clinical and experimental purposes. It may be that for a certain percentage of the patient population with any given disease or disorder, open placebos will help to unlock the body's biologically programmed capacity for self-healing as effectively as placebos administered under conditions of intentional ignorance or deception (de Sousa 1988; Brown 1994, 1998a, 1998b; Talbot 2000; Bok 2002: 63).

So little is known about open placebos and the open placebo response that investigation needs to proceed on a number of parallel fronts:

- The definition of open placebo.
- The conditions of open placebo administration.
- The logic of patient belief.
- The nature of experimental design to elicit open placebo responses.
- The neurobiology of open placebo response.
- The phenomenology of patient response to open placebos.
- The ethics of giving open placebos.
- The harnessing of the open placebo response in clinical trials.

The following are hypotheses only.

The Logic of Belief: Some Hypotheses

When patients (or clients in psychotherapy) are fully informed that the treatment they will be receiving is a placebo, how will they respond? What beliefs will they hold about their treatment? What will their feelings be? Perhaps the most obvious answer is that the information that they are receiving placebos would lead either to heightened incredulity, confusion, disappointment, or lowered expectations—all counter-therapeutic responses that suggest that the treatment strategy of giving open placebos is ultimately self-defeating. But this answer is entirely speculative: no empirical studies and no conceptual or phenomenological analyses, have shown this to be the case. Empirical studies need to be conducted to determine how patients respond to open placebos, the conditions under which they respond, and the rate of frequency of response. Some hypotheses for future investigation are in order here.

While incredulity and disappointment may be common responses to open placebo treatments, they are far from the *only* responses. The open placebo studies (Park and Covi 1965; Vogel *et al.* 1980; Brown 1994, 1998a, 1998b; Aulas and Rosner 2003) suggest that some patients continue to experience measurable therapeutic changes, even when fully informed that their treatments consist of placebos. How is this possible? What beliefs do such patients hold about their treatment? Are their beliefs consistent and coherent, or are they somehow conflicted or contradictory? What, in other words, is the *logic* of their belief states?

The following are some hypothetical explanations of the logic of belief. Each of these needs to be investigated empirically and analyzed conceptually. It is hypothesized that open placebo responders may be:

 i) self-deceived about the treatments they are receiving;

 ii) practicing a form of self-willed belief;

 iii) selectively inattentive to aspects of the treatments;

 iv) feigning that the treatments are effective;

 v) engaged in a willing suspension of disbelief.

Hypothesis i) Self-deception. It is hypothesized that some patients who respond to open placebos in physical medicine or psychological treatments are self-deceived: that is, they believe that something is the case (the placebo works, or might work), but at the same time, somehow, they know that it is not the case (the placebo does not, cannot, or probably will not work). To maintain these two conflicting beliefs, they must deny, ignore, or distort the counter-evidence that could subvert their belief that the placebo works; and they must distort reasonable evaluations of the available evidence, by disregarding them or rationalizing away the implications.

Hypothesis ii) Self-willed belief. It is hypothesized that some patients who respond to open placebos may experience therapeutic progress because they intentionally make themselves believe that placebos are effective treatments, despite the fact that they once believed otherwise. Thus they go through the motions of taking pills, following their doctor's or psychotherapist's advice, and behaving *as if* their symptoms are improving—and this 'as if' stance is itself conducive to therapeutic improvement. Self-willed belief is not a rare phenomenon. The seventeenth-century philosopher and mathematician Blaise Pascal (1966) advocated a similar practice of intentional self-manipulation to religious nonbelievers: 'Kneel and you shall believe'. Pascal thought that his famous wager argument would convince nonbelievers of the importance of believing in God and becoming devout Christians; but as mere arguments were insufficient to make them hold beliefs that they once rejected, something else was required. Pascal described the process of how to come to believe as a kind of intentional behavioral self-manipulation: go to church, take holy water, participate in masses and confession, and do everything *as if* you already believe. 'That will make you believe quite naturally, and will make you more docile' (Pascal 1966: fragment 418). Pascal's point is that by going through the outward motions often enough, nonbelievers can intentionally make themselves accept beliefs that they once regarded as false or incoherent. A similar regimentation of thought and action may work with openly administered placebos.

Hypothesis iii) Selective inattention. It is hypothesized that some patients who respond favorably to open placebos may do so because they are selectively inattentive to different facets of placebo treatment, or to the information that they are receiving placebos. Selective inattention is not accidental or random: it consists of persistent, skillful, and often precise failures to attend to otherwise salient facts (e.g. the pill is only a sugar pill, the interpretation is only a placebo interpretation), resulting in what appear to be sincere failures of recognition. This is often compensated by persistent attention to other facts, or by the cultivation of uncharacteristically narrow focusing (Baier 1996). Thus patients who know that they are receiving placebos may downplay salient facts about their therapeutic progress, while focusing intently on a narrow range of other facts. But for this to be possible, they must first somehow recognize as salient the very facts that must not be focused upon (e.g. it is only a sugar pill): that is, they must first notice what they will not notice. Selective inattention is often systematic in approach, sensitively configured to the emotional or interpersonal demand characteristics of the situation, and responsive to patterns of reasoning and observation. To maintain it with any viable degree of consistency requires that patients not notice their uncharacteristic inattentiveness and strategic deflections.

Hypothesis iv) Feigning. It is hypothesized that some patients who respond favorably to open placebos may do so because they have adopted a feigning stance: that is, they feign that placebos are *bona fide* medical or psychological interventions on the same order as active medications, while remaining aware that they are placebos.

Hypothesis v) Willing suspension of disbelief. It is hypothesized that some patients who respond favorably to open placebos may do so because they intentionally suspend their disbelief or doubt, in much the same way that readers of fiction willingly suspend their disbelief (Coleridge 1907; Prentice *et al.* 1997; Prentice and Gerrig 1999). Park and Covi (1965), for example, reported that many of the patients who were informed that they would be treated with placebos refused to believe it: they continued to believe that their treatments were effective nonplacebic treatments, even when they knew that they were placebos. The willing suspension of disbelief is found in many nonmedical contexts, where people believe things that they know are fictional or unreal. Identifying with movie characters and literary characters involves the temporary suspension of disbelief; so too does the continued use of products or services that are known not to work (e.g. pushing a pedestrian crosswalk button at a traffic intersection, while knowing that it is broken or disconnected from the traffic light grid).

Experimental Design with Open Placebos: Hypothesis

Future research on harnessing open placebo responses for clinical and experimental purposes faces a number of challenges. One of these is to design experiments, clinical trials, and studies that measure the range, frequency, and conditions of the open placebo response, and to compare these with the range, frequency, and conditions of the non-open placebo response. As with randomized controlled trials using placebos, this experimental design must take into account such confounding variables as Hawthorne effects, self-limiting disorders, observer bias, and regression to the mean.

Another challenge is to investigate whether it is logically and methodologically feasible to harness the open placebo response in controlled clinical trials that rely primarily upon the non-open response (i.e. placebos in double-blind procedures). The standard two-arm design of clinical trials (with the random assignment of participants either to an experimental drug or medical procedure, or to a placebo) might be improved with the addition of multiple arms, one of which includes openly administered placebos. The goal of multiple arm clinical trials involving both hidden and open placebos would be the same as the standard two-arm trial: namely, to test the efficacy of the experimental drug or procedure against placebo (both open and non-open), and against the natural history of the disease or disorder.

The Administration of Open Placebos: Hypothesis

It is hypothesized that the effectiveness of open placebos in clinical studies and clinical treatment situations will depend largely on the conditions under which placebos are given to patients, as well as the knowledge, beliefs, or opinions that patients have about open placebos. If, as a number of placebo researchers have observed (Moerman 2002; Benedetti *et al.* 2003; Kirsch 2003), the patient's knowledge of therapy affects the therapy outcome, then it follows that the ways in which patients become knowledgeable about their therapy will also affect therapy outcome: how they know matters as much as what they know. In other words, corresponding to the various methods of open placebo administration, to the various methods of conveying the relevant information to patients, and to the various ways of gaining informed and educated consent (Ingelfinger 1972), are various kinds of knowledge, belief, and opinion. Patients for instance may be informed by an expert (e.g., a physician, clinical trial director) or by an adjunct (e.g., a nurse, a laboratory associate) that their treatments involve placebos, and each of these informants may display different levels of concern, optimism, and authoritativeness; patients may be informed that their treatments involve placebos, with or without comprehensive explanations of their treatment, and with or without comprehensive debriefing sessions after the placebo treatment; and patients may be given different descriptions of placebos and their side effects (e.g., "the pill is pharmacologically inert," "the pill contains no medicine," "the pill is pharmacologically inert but has proven in some previous cases to have positive effects," and so on). Patients may be *informed* about the role of placebos, without being *educated* about how they work, what they are, or what the risks are (Ingelfinger 1972). Each of these methods of informing patients may generate different kinds of knowledge or belief, and each may serve to enhance or weaken patients' expectations about treatment. A survey of the various methods of placebo administration in randomized controlled clinical trials could serve as a workable analog for the design of various methods of open placebo administration (see Marlatt and Rohsenow 1980; Kirsch and Sapirstein 1998; Benedetti *et al.* 2003; Kirsch 2003).

It is further hypothesized that many of the physical factors that make a difference to the placebo response when placebos are administered under conditions of deception or intentional ignorance will also make a difference to the open placebo response: for instance, the size, shape, and color of placebo pills (Moerman 2002a), the dosage amounts and timing of doses, the physical severity of the placebo (e.g. placebo injections versus placebo pills), and the warnings about side effects.

Vogel *et al.* (1980) discuss the complexities of open placebo administration in clinical practice using the imaginary case of a post-myocardial infarction patient who is recovering in hospital, but is at increased risk for arrhythmias because of his uncontrolled anxiety. If the patient cannot be prescribed antianxiety medications because he is too anxious about addiction or dependence, and because he fears loss of control, then prescription of a placebo may be indicated. 'If the patient asks exactly what the drug is, the physician can answer, 'If you permit, I would rather not tell you exactly what it is until after we see whether it works'. Or the physician can say 'It is a treatment—a placebo—which, although chemically without known activity, may relieve anxiety or pain, perhaps in some way similar to the effects of suggestion or hypnosis' (Vogel *et al.* 1980: 107). This strategy holds significant therapeutic potential 'if the physician–patient relationship has been carefully and correctly established'.

The Neurobiology of Open Placebo Response: Hypothesis

It is hypothesized that there are distinct and disorder-specific neurobiological patterns of open placebo response, just as there are distinct and disorder-specific neurobiological patterns of placebo response under conditions of intentional ignorance or deception; and it is hypothesized that these two classes of patterns may diverge significantly. For example, the neurobiology and neurochemistry of placebo analgesia may vary depending upon whether the placebo is administered openly or under conditions of intentional ignorance or deception.

Review of an Open Placebo Study

In the early-Beecher heyday of placebo research, Park and Covi (1965) designed an open placebo study to test the hypothesis that disclosure of the inert content of pills does not counteract therapeutic improvement. The study, which has not been replicated, is not without design flaws: it contains, for instance, a small patient sample, questionable symptom matches and comorbidity profiles between patients, an overly short treatment course, no wash-out period for potentially confounding psychoactive medications taken by patients, and no control groups (e.g. a no-treatment group). Moreover, it relied on now-outdated psychological assessment measures and diagnostic criteria. Despite these drawbacks, the study still serves as a rough model for the design of future studies of open placebos. It also serves as a test case for discussions about the ethics of giving open placebos in clinical situations involving non-life-threatening diseases or disorders.

Park and Covi's study followed 15 newly-admitted adult outpatients at an urban psychiatric clinic. Diagnosed as 'neurotic', the patients presented with symptoms of moderate to high anxiety. Their ages ranged from 19 to 67 years, and the mean age of the sample was 35 years. During the study the patients were seen twice. The first visit consisted of a complete psychological evaluation lasting one hour, followed by a short meeting during which the placebo was prescribed, and their informed consent to placebo treatment was secured. The second visit took place one week later and involved two assessment interviews. Patients were assigned to one of two psychiatrists, who carried out the interviews and assessments. Interviews were recorded on tape.

Because of the potential for confusion or doubt, the prescription of placebo in the first visit followed a carefully designed script: 'Mr. Doe, at the intake conference we discussed your problems and your condition, and it was decided to consider further the possibility and the need of treatment for you before we make a final recommendation next week. Meanwhile, we have a week between now and your next appointment, and we would like to do something to give you some relief from your symptoms. Many different kinds of tranquilizers and similar pills have been used for conditions such as yours, and many of them have helped. Many people with your kind of condition have also been helped by what are sometimes called sugar pills, and we feel that a so-called sugar pill may help you, too. Do you know what a sugar pill is? A sugar pill is a pill with no medicine in it at all. I think this pill will help you as it has helped so many others. Are you willing to try this pill?' (Park and Covi 1965:337) Some patients expressed doubts about the purpose of the treatment, but only one patient was clearly reluctant to take the pills.

Patients were then given a one-week supply of pink capsules in a small bottle with an official label bearing the name 'The Johns Hopkins Hospital'. They were instructed to take one pill three times daily, to complete the full course of pills, and to discontinue any other psychoactive medications. The statement that the pills had helped many other patients with similar conditions was then repeated, to counteract any lingering doubts patients held about the effectiveness of their pink pills.

The second visit one week later consisted of a brief interview with the alternate psychiatrist, during which symptoms, symptom remission, and options for further treatment were discussed. Several psychological measures were used to assess therapeutic improvement, including measures for overall change, doctor and patient symptom checklists, target symptoms, and pathology.

Fourteen of the 15 patients completed the study. At the end of the study eight patients still believed that the pills were placebos, and six had come to believe that they contained an active drug. Patients in the latter group arrived at that conclusion after noticing side effects and therapeutic improvements which, they inferred, could not possibly be due to a sugar pill. Thirteen patients showed improvement on the symptom checklist; all 14 patients improved on the target symptoms measures; 13 patients improved on the patient overall change measures; and 12 patients improved on the pathology measures. 'In summary, there is very strong statistical evidence, on the basis of both doctor and patient ratings, that the completing patients as a group felt considerably improved. Eleven patients were rated as improved on all five measures. One patient was improved on all measures except for the Pathology Score, for which there was no change' (Park and Covi 1965: 338).

Park and Covi noted that the most important finding of the study was that improvement occurred in patients who believed that placebos had been administered 'in spite of such belief'. There was no difference in improvement ratings between the eight patients who believed the pills were placebos and the six patients who had come to believe that the pills contained an active drug. Only three of the patients had absolutely no doubts that the pills contained an inactive ingredient; the three other patients who believed that the pills were placebos, but who were not 'absolutely certain' about it, thought that they might have contained a 'special sugar' of some sort.

Nine of the 14 patients believed that the pills were the major factor in their improvement. Five of the six patients who believed that the pills probably contained medicine attributed their improvement to the pills, and four of the eight patients who believed the pills probably contained placebo attributed the major improvements to the pills. Of the six patients who believed that the pills contained active medication, three experienced side effects, which they attributed to the pills. None of the eight patients who believed the pills contained only placebos experienced side effects.

The Park and Covi study included a number of informative descriptions of the reactions of some of the patients to the news that the pills were placebos.

- ◆ Patient A was a 20-year-old married female described as suffering from irritability, crying spells, a history of suicidal gestures, and feelings of inadequacy. She expressed no concerns or doubts when informed that the pills were placebos containing no medicine, and remained firmly convinced that the pills contained no medicine. At the follow-up visit she said that she had found the pills had been more helpful than Nervine, a psychoactive medication she had once taken. She believed the sugar pill was the effective agent in her treatment, remarking that when it had been prescribed she had assumed without question that it would help 'ease her mind'. Patient A wanted to continue therapy with the same physician, and continue taking the placebo pills.

- ◆ Patient C was a 28-year-old married female described as suffering from extreme tension, shortness of breath, trembling, crying spells, insomnia, suicidal thoughts, and poor appetite. Because of fears of harmful side effects and the possibility of addiction, she was reluctant to take any medications. She agreed to the treatment only when she understood that the pills were inactive. While she had no doubts that the pills were placebos, and experienced no side effects, she still attributed her considerable improvement to the pills. In the follow-up visit she remarked that if patients take pills in the right frame of mind, they may feel improved because the pills offer 'moral support'. She added that she had found the doctor reassuring; and that 'I think I had a lot to do with it...By knowing myself that I had to control myself to keep myself in the right frame of mind'.

- Patient T was a 45-year-old divorced male, described as rigid and influence-resistant, and as suffering from insomnia, loss of appetite, weight loss, restlessness, feelings of despair, death wishes, obsessive thoughts, and various somatic symptoms. By the time of the follow-up visit he was convinced that the pills contained medicine: his first words at the meeting were 'It wasn't sugar, it was medicine!' Patient T experienced definite symptom reduction (e.g. fewer obsessive thoughts, and a new pattern of thinking about his inter-personal problems), as well as physiological side effects which he attributed to the pills (e.g. dry mouth, butterflies in his stomach). Patient T also had a strong positive reaction to the doctor, whom he felt was optimistic and confi-dent yet not authoritative or paternalistic. He felt that the doctor had told him he was receiving a placebo so that he would think that he was really helping himself, when actually the drug was the therapeutic agent.

- Patient U was a 24-year-old married female, described as suffering from insomnia, anorexia, irritability, tension, and depression. She had worked for a pharmacy as well as a pharmaceutical company, and was unreservedly skeptical when informed about the placebo in the first meeting. She asked whether the doctor thought patients could be helped just by the idea of taking pills, and suggested to him that it might have been better if she had not been informed. Her first words at the follow-up visit were 'They are not sugar pills—because they worked'. Patient U also reported that the pills were more effective than several other psychoactive medications she had taken for her symptoms on previous occasions. She was keen to continue with the treatment.

- Patient F expressed some confusion about the contents of the pills, asking if the sugar pills worked in some way as a treatment for diabetes. Although the doctor tried to explain to her that the pills contained no active ingredients, she still expressed concern that the pills would make her feel drowsy. At the follow-up visit she claimed to be feeling better than she had in the last twenty years, and stated that she believed that the pills contained only placebo. She felt the treatment had been effective because she had been told so many times that she would improve.

- Patient H was a 28-year-old married man, described as rigid and lacking in insight, and as suffering from irritability and anger. He stated categorically in the first visit that placebos would not work. In the follow-up visit he stated that the pills had not helped, and then with further interviewing became aware that he had experienced some reduction in his symptoms. He offered two explanations for his symptom reduction: either he had helped himself, or the pills may have contained a mild tranquilizer. In other words, if the pills were placebos, they did not help him, and if they were tranquilizers, they did. He noted that taking the pills served to remind him to work on his problems and to change himself.

◆ Patient S was a 32-year-old woman with Raynaud's disease, described as suffering from tension, anxiety, and apprehension. When placebo was prescribed, she expressed doubts about its effectiveness: 'Why would it help, because for people, each time they take a pill, it's a symbol or something of someone caring about you, thinking about you three or four times a day?' In the second visit she attributed her improvement to the pills, which she said did not contain medicine in the usual sense, although they might have contained 'something like a liniment'. In further discussion she indicated that the prescription of pills that contained no medication made her aware that she could help herself.

A number of factors could explain the effectiveness of open placebo treatments in each of these cases. Some of the more obvious of these factors are: expectation, motivation and self-help, interpersonal dynamics, symbolic healing, and selective inattention.

i) Open placebo treatments may be effective because they rally patients' expectations of getting better. Patients who are informed that they are receiving placebos tend to improve because they expect to improve, after having been told that the treatment (even if it is a placebo treatment) has proven to be effective in similar cases.

ii) Open placebo treatments may be effective because they encourage patient self-help. Pills with nothing in them force patients to the realization that they must help themselves.

iii) Open placebo treatments may be effective because they highlight more clearly than conventional treatments the interpersonal dynamics of the doctor–patient relationship. Patients tend to improve because of their interactions with a confident, caring, and optimistic professional, even if he or she is dispensing placebos.

iv) Open placebo treatments are effective because the very act of taking pills, regardless of pharmaceutical content, serves as a potent symbolic reminder to patients to attend to their problems and to change their behaviors.

v) Open placebo treatments are effective because patients hold the general belief that a situation that is defined as a treatment situation will help, regardless of its specific details. This requires in patients a kind of selective inattention to the treatment details, or a willing suspension of disbelief.

These are not the only factors that could explain the effectiveness of open placebo treatments. Any studies of open placebos must also avoid the types of mistaken inferences that Beecher and others made about placebos administered under conditions of deception or ignorance. Beecher, as it was seen earlier, overlooked the effects of a number of possible confounding agents, each of which could give the false impression of a placebo effect. The very same factors could also be confounded with open placebo responses. These factors include the natural course of the disease or disorder (including spontaneous improvement, fluctuation of symptoms, regression to the mean, habituation), additional treatment, observer bias, time effects (e.g. improved investigator skills from one measurement to the next, seasonal changes, and decreases in 'white coat hypertension' in patients), irrelevant response variables, subsiding toxic effects of previous medications, and patient bias (including 'answers of politeness' and experimental subordination, and conditioned answers) (Kiene 1993a, 1993b; Ernst and Resch 1995; Kienle and Kiene 1997; Kaptchuk 1998a, 1998b). To control adequately for some of these factors, such as the natural course of the disease or disorder, studies of open placebo treatments would need to assign one group of patients to the no-treatment condition, and another to the open placebo condition. The true open placebo effect would be determined by subtracting the effects observed in the no-treatment control from those observed in the open placebo condition. Without a no-treatment control group, in other words, there is no way to know with any certainty that the improvement displayed by the patients in the study was caused by the placebo they had been prescribed, or was simply the natural history of the disorders from which they suffered.

The Ethics of Giving Placebos in Psychotherapy

+ Thought experiment: The Psychotherapy Hoax, Version 2. (The story to this point is the same as in Version 1; see page 227). After a successful period of training, during which his real motives remain undetected, X opens a practice and begins to treat clients. The techniques he uses are explicitly designed to elicit placebo responses from his clients. But because he has ethical reservations about the intentional ignorance and deception that is commonly associated with giving placebos, he uses only open placebos: that is, he informs his clients that the treatments consist of psychotherapeutic placebos, which he explains are the psychological equivalent of sugar pills. He also educates them about the placebo effect. The inspiration for this treatment, he claims, is the pioneering Park and Covi (1965) study. Part of X's treatment, for example, involves concocting nearly vacuous but plausible psychodynamic interpretations—which he offers to his clients with the qualification that they are explanatorily empty. Another part of his treatment involves encouraging clients to develop insights into their psychology, behavior, and personality that accord with his own nearly vacuous theoretical orientation, but which, like his interpretations, carry the proviso that they are insight placebos. Another part of his treatment is to place would-be clients on a lengthy wait list with minimal psychotherapist contact, in order to have a no-treatment control group with which to compare the placebo treatments. X's debunking strategy targets each of the major principles of the Standard View of psychodynamic psychotherapy. Some of his treatments are unsuccessful: a certain number of his clients do not react well to the news that the treatments, including the interpretations and insights, are 'only' placebos. Some of these clients do not react favorably to the news that they are not 'really' engaged in the exploration of the psyche, or acquiring real insight, or 'getting in touch' with an 'inner' or 'core' or 'authentic' self, as they had assumed was the proper task of psychodynamic psychotherapy. The news that they are engaged in making up therapeutically beneficial explanatory fictions that function as placebos is counter-therapeutic. Curiously, however, a clinically significant number of X's treatments are successful. Over the course of ten years, X assembles empirical evidence that undermines the Standard View one piece at a time.

To test his hypothesis about the role of placebo effects in psychodynamic psychotherapy, X also designs and conducts several clinical studies comparing the brief psychodynamic psychotherapy in which he was trained with a variety of psychotherapy placebos, both deceptive and open. His inspiration for this is the Strupp (1979) study with depressed college students who were assigned either to untrained but empathetic college professors or to trained clinical psychologists. Because X's studies are part of an elaborate hoax, and because they involve client deception, they are not presented for approval before any Ethics Review Boards; nor do they receive research funding. In one study, for example, X used a five-arm design, with 100 participants who were diagnosed with moderate depression (using a battery of well-known depression inventories, check lists, and diagnostic manuals). The treatment group received genuine brief psychodynamic psychotherapy for 12 weeks. In the three control groups, participants were given sham psychotherapy. Actors were trained to display psychotherapist behaviors such as empathy, therapeutic note-taking, and therapeutic questioning. The actors were also trained to offer to clients trivial one-size-fits-all psychodynamic interpretations based on a prepared script, and trained to encourage clients to develop insights without checking for accuracy, precision, or truth-value. In group 1, the participants were given the psychodynamic treatment and informed that they were in the *verum* group (i.e., receiving the active treatment). In group 2, the participants were given the psychodynamic treatment and informed that they were in the placebo group. In group 3, the participants were given the placebo treatment and informed that it was a placebo treatment. In group 4, the participants were given the placebo treatment and informed that it was the active treatment. In group 5, the participants received no treatment at all, and the natural history of the disorder was observed. X found that the group receiving psychotherapy did not significantly outperform the groups receiving placebo on most of the major clinical outcome measures, but each placebo group outperformed the no-treatment control group by a clinically and statistically significant margin. Concerned about the identity objection (viz., that the control groups receive a degraded form of psychotherapy rather than a proper placebo), X also experimented with different placebo controls: a personal diary with daily 30-minute writing assignments about important emotional issues (Pennebaker 1997: 162), and lactose pills plus minimal psychotherapist contact. The results with each of the different placebo controls supported the general conclusion that the groups receiving psychotherapy did not significantly outperform the groups receiving placebo on most of the major clinical outcome measures.

At the ten-year anniversary of the opening of his practice, X reveals to the general public that he has been practicing a kind of open placebo therapy. He publishes a number of case histories, and the results of his clinical studies. His revelation stuns the psychotherapeutic community, but it does not earn the outrage of many of his former clients, nor does it trigger any lawsuits from clients. After a lengthy investigation, he is dismissed from the College of Psychologists and loses his accreditation. The hoax generates a vigorous but short-lived debate about the effectiveness of psychotherapy, the ethics of giving placebos, and the concept of open placebos. It has little effect on the general public's perception of psychotherapy, merits little more than a footnote in psychotherapy textbooks, and is relegated to the museum of curious hoaxes.

Suppose that the main conceptual hypothesis that is explored in this work is valid. Suppose further that empirical studies are later designed that show that the hypothesis has robust empirical support: that is, placebo responses are shown to occur with a certain determinate rate of frequency, with certain types of psychological disorders, in some of the psychodynamic psychotherapies. Suppose still further that empirical studies are designed that show that among these placebos are interpretation placebos and insight placebos, also occurring with a certain determinate rate of frequency.

What is the upshot of all this? Is it *unethical* for psychotherapists to give placebos to clients? If psychodynamic placebos are effective treatment options, as they appear to have been in the case histories described by Janet, Mendel, and Frank, and as they are imagined to have been in the thought experiments above, then are there any compelling ethical considerations for why they should *not* be used? What harm could there be to clients if placebos are therapeutically effective? Is this a case in which the therapeutic ends justify the treatment means? These questions can be rephrased both more formally and more generally: Is it ethically permissible for psychotherapists, clinical psychologists, and psychiatrists to knowingly administer psychological placebos without first informing and educating clients about them, and without gaining their consent? Does the use of psychological placebos without the fully informed and educated consent of clients constitute an infringement of their autonomy? Does it constitute a failure of the psychotherapist's duty to care, or an erosion of the psychotherapist's obligation of undivided loyalty to the interests of clients? Could it be construed as a kind of harm to clients? Finally, are psychotherapists guilty of making fraudulent claims (about, among other things, the nature and truth value of psychological explanations, including insights and interpretations) if they do not make full public disclosure and proper representation about the potential or actual role of psychological placebos?

These are difficult questions, and the efforts to address them are not helped by the dearth of literature in clinical psychology, psychotherapy, and psychiatry about the ethics of giving placebos. To render the discussion slightly more manageable, therefore, the questions will be reframed as questions specifically about psychodynamic placebos, and even more specifically as questions about insight placebos and interpretation placebos.

The *prima facie* ethical case *for* placebo use in psychodynamic psychotherapy is based on weighing the consequences of placebo therapeutics against the consequences of treatment practices that are benevolent but rely upon client deception or some form of intentional ignorance. If psychological placebos do in fact have the potential to trigger the mind's native self-healing capacities (as their bodily analogs appear to do in physical medicine), and if the level of effectiveness of psychological placebos in the treatment of certain disorders is statistically and clinically significant, then (the argument holds) they are, in certain conditions, ethically permissible, because the net beneficial therapeutic consequences of placebos administered under conditions of deception or intentional ignorance would, in general, outweigh the net harms (following from benevolent paternalist deception, or client ignorance). This does not license the unrestricted use of psychological placebos in all treatment contexts. Placebo use must be strictly regulated and carefully practiced. To protect clients, certain treatment conditions would first have to be satisfied, with the ultimate goal of administering the right interpretation placebos or insight placebos at the right time, in the right circumstances, to the right placebo-responsive clients, and with the right safety precautions and follow-up measures. Rawlinson's five conditions (1985: 415), modified for psychotherapeutic contexts, help to supply broad guidelines here. Psychological placebos should be used: i) only for the client's sake, and not for the sake of psychotherapist convenience; ii) only when there is strong evidence that they are therapeutically necessary; iii) only when the case for deception or intentional ignorance can be made to reasonable observers; iv) only when the treatment would not lead to reliance on the placebos; and v) only after the psychotherapist has a good understanding of the client's character and value system, and the effect that deception or intentional ignorance will have on the client's self-respect and attitude toward the psychotherapist.

In addition to symptom remission, the net benefits to be gained from non-open placebo therapeutics in psychodynamic psychotherapy include: stimulating clients' hopes or expectations for recovery, providing a degree of intelligibility for previously unintelligible symptoms, giving clients rich cognitive tools and habits of reflective thought that can be helpful after the termination of treatment, and protecting clients from some of the harsher side effects of conventional treatments.

Janet states the position succinctly: '[My] belief is that the patient wants a doctor who will cure; that the doctor's professional duty is to give any remedy that will be useful, and to prescribe it in the way in which it will do most good. Now, I think bread pills are medically indicated in certain cases, and that they will act far more powerfully if I deck them out with impressive names. When I prescribe such a formidable placebo, I believe that I am fulfilling my professional duty, and that I am keeping with my real though tacit undertaking with my patient; and I am quite sure that if he gets well he will bear me no grudge' (Janet 1925, 1: 338).

Not surprisingly, this is far from the end of the story. There are also several strong *prima facie* ethical considerations weighing against the use of psychodynamic placebos. Together, they constitute a compelling argument against the *unrestricted* use of psychodynamic placebos (even when the five conditions are satisfied).

First, if psychodynamic placebos are used intentionally or inadvertently during the course of treatment without the fully informed and educated consent of clients, then clients have been deceived, misled or kept in the dark about their treatment options and the nature of their treatment (e.g. the characteristic and incidental factors of the treatment). Even if this is followed by therapeutic improvement, and clients 'bear no grudges' about the intentional ignorance, it still counts as a violation of the principle of respect for autonomy. Clients deserve to make their own decisions about which courses of treatment to pursue, rather than to have the decision made for them by others claiming to know what is best for them; and they deserve to know if their treatments are effective because they involves placebos rather than the alleged characteristic factors of the treatment.

The use of intentional or inadvertent placebos also has a number of well-known negative consequences (Bok 1975, 1976, 2002): the potential for erosion of psychotherapist–client trust once the deception or intentional ignorance is revealed (notwithstanding Janet's optimism about forgiving patients), the potential for malpractice lawsuits, the tendency of deceptions (or other strategies of intentional ignorance) to multiply and to involve the complicity of other parties, and the possibility for financial exploitation of clients. There are also concerns about the social responsibility of psychotherapists who administer placebos deceptively or under conditions of intentional ignorance, and then proceed to charge clients, state-supported health care providers, or private third-party health care providers for the full cost of their services.

Second, psychotherapists who intentionally or inadvertently use psychodynamic placebos without clients' awareness or consent are at risk of making false or unsubstantiated epistemic claims about the accuracy and truth value of psychodynamic insights, interpretations, and explanations. Earlier, in the brief survey of contemporary psychodynamic positions on insight (Chapter 2), it was noted that one of the central themes common to many psychodynamic psychotherapies is that the insights acquired in psychodynamic psychotherapy are authentic and true. The survey revealed little awareness among psychodynamic theorists of the epistemic complexities of psychodynamic insights and interpretations, coupled with high levels of epistemic confidence and theoretical self-assurance about their authenticity. Messer and Warren, Arlow, and Kottler and Brown, to take just three from the survey, credit the acquisition of psychodynamic insight with such things as the conquest of neurosis, conflict resolution, and maturation (Messer and Warren 1995: 93); the ability to seek fulfillment, liberating self-transformation, self-actualization, and the happiness of others (Arlow 1995: 16-17); and true psychological growth and lasting change (Kottler and Brown 1999: 28). These are lofty claims. But in cases where psychotherapists have intentionally or inadvertently used insight or interpretation placebos with some degree of success, and without clients' awareness or consent, such claims are seriously misleading. Whether they are no more than innocent theoretical mistakes committed by epistemically naïve psychodynamic theorists, or symptomatic of narrow theoretical dogmatism, imprudent oversalesmanship, or epistemic irresponsibility, they are all at risk of falling into the same class of overconfident boasts identified by John Ayrton Paris: 'boasted remedies' that are one day destined to 'fall into disrepute, and in their turn serve only as a humiliating memorial of the credulity and infatuation of the physicians who recommended and prescribed them' (Paris 1843: 4–5).

Clients not only deserve an honest and accurate assessment of their psychotherapists' putative expertise; they also deserve to know if the treatments (or 'boasted remedies') they have in fact received are the treatments that they were promised they were going to receive, or that they formally agreed upon in binding contractual agreements. With such an intensely personal and consequential issue as insight, clients deserve to know whether they are really experiencing liberating self-transformation, true psychological growth, or lasting change *because* of their insights—or whether something quite different is occurring. They deserve to know if their exploratory efforts have really succeeded. Concomitantly, psychotherapists have a duty to describe their practices and therapeutic outcomes honestly, without exaggerations about therapeutic effectiveness or epistemic purity. Given the epistemic problems with the theory and practice of psychodynamic psychotherapy, it is reasonable to require psychotherapists to qualify the claims of the Standard View with explicit epistemic cautions about the role of suggestion, placebo and expectancy effects, evidentiary contamination, psychodynamic artifacts, common factors, the Barnum effect, and other factors that could interfere with clients trying to acquire self-knowledge, or trying to 'get in touch' with an 'inner' or 'core' or 'authentic' self. It is also reasonable to require psychodynamic psychotherapists to advertise more mundane benefits for their treatments.

Third, psychological treatments that intentionally or inadvertently lead to pseudo-insights and insight placebos can have personal, interpersonal, and social consequences as ethically calamitous as those sometimes triggered by false memories. As a general rule, people who are significantly misled about the real nature and causes of their behaviors, psychology, emotions and personality, and yet who believe on the contrary that they enjoy significant levels of insight and self-knowledge, are more at risk of engaging in actions that are imprudent or selfish than those people who are not so misled (Jopling 2000). It is often other people—family, friends, associates, caregivers—who are most hurt by the false or inaccurate self-understandings that inform a person's actions and interpersonal attitudes (Jopling 1996b). The more pervasive a person's self-misunderstanding or self-deception, the more his or her awareness of other people is diminished, and with this narrowing, fewer possibilities for interpersonal conduct and moral responsiveness are presented as viable options (Jopling 2000).

Finally, there is something ethically troubling about psychological treatments that have the potential to lead some people further away from the truth (about, for instance, the real nature and causes of their behaviors, psychology, personality, or past), while giving them the illusion or strong conviction that they are getting closer to it. The fact that some clients may experience significant therapeutic improvement following non-open psychodynamic placebos may offer *prima facie* support for the claim that the therapeutic ends justify the treatment means—but these ends do not come without a price. What is it? Socrates supplies the outlines of an answer here. Few things, Socrates argued, could be more damaging to the health of the soul and the well-being of persons than their claiming to know something, when in fact they do not know. This is a special kind of self-ignorance: namely, ignorance of oneself as a *knower* who is charged with the task of knowing self, world, and others as accurately and responsibly as possible.

Socrates' point, reiterated throughout the Platonic dialogues, is that people who do not examine themselves *insofar as they are knowers* are typically unaware of the extent of their ignorance and knowledge, and their capacities and limitations for knowledge acquisition. They are unable to distinguish what they really know from what they seem to know, or feel they know, or have strong convictions about knowing. This kind of intellectual pride is as much a moral error as an intellectual error. Its symptoms include unbounded self-assurance, glib sagacity, false rhetoric, and as Hacking claims in the context of one kind of psychological treatment that leads to false memories, 'glib patter that simulates an understanding of [one]self' (1995: 266). Intellectual pride is antithetical to such virtues as self-control and self-direction, as well as to something as simple as care for the soul. It is also the opposite of wisdom, which, according to the Socratic model at least, consists in the honest recognition of one's own ignorance. If the hypothesis about insight placebos is valid, then similar intellectual errors may occur in the psychodynamic psychotherapies. That is, the treatments may leave clients claiming to know things about themselves, when in fact they do not know. Their claims to knowledge may count as yet one more instantiation of the general truth that there are many more ways to be wrong, confused, ignorant, or deceived about things as complexly configured as one's behavior, personality, psychological make-up, developmental history, and psychological pathology than there are ways to be correct.

In light of these *prima facie* ethical considerations, some general conclusions can be formulated about the ethics of giving placebos in psychodynamic psychology. These conclusions are also sufficiently generalizable to apply to the use of psychological placebos in a number of non-psychodynamic forms of psychotherapy, clinical psychology, and psychiatry, particularly those that accord some degree of therapeutic importance to insight. The most general conclusions are the following:

◆ It is unethical to give psychodynamic placebos if it involves deceiving clients or withholding vital information about their treatment.

◆ Psychodynamic placebos should not be given to clients suffering from severe or life-threatening psychological conditions (such as psychoses or suicidal depression), irreversible fatal diseases, or conditions of serious morbidity.

◆ Psychodynamic placebos should not be used when there is the potential of irreversible harm to clients.

◆ Psychodynamic placebos should not be used in the treatment of vulnerable clients or clients who are too incapacitated to give fully informed and educated consent.

◆ Psychodynamic placebos should not be used when there is the potential for psychologically dangerous side effects.

Conclusions as wide-ranging as these might give the impression that it is *always* wrong to use placebos in psychodynamic psychotherapy. But this is based on the assumption, shared by many medical ethicists, that placebos are always given under conditions of deception or intentional ignorance. This assumption, as was seen above, is false. There are at least two treatment contexts in which giving placebos in psychodynamic psychotherapy satisfies these guidelines, does not involve deception or intentional ignorance, and falls within the range of ethically permissible treatments:

i) It is ethically permissible to use psychodynamic placebos when clients are fully informed that their treatments involve placebos (such as insight and interpretation placebos), and when they give educated consent to the treatment. The analog to this is found in physical medicine, in Conditions i–iii. This approach has the virtue of satisfying the principle of informed and educated consent; and it respects clients' rights to make fully informed decisions about their treatment.

ii) It is ethically permissible to trigger placebo responses in psychotherapy if no deception or intentional ignorance is involved (Condition iii). Placebo responses may be triggered when interpretations and insights help to make clients' symptoms intelligible, and help to increase their sense of mastery—*and* clients have not been deceived, misinformed, or misled about the truth-value of the relevant interpretations and insights. The principle of informed and educated consent is satisfied when clients are informed that interpretations and insights may be placebos that trigger placebo responses, and when they are sufficiently educated about the treatment.

To protect clients from potential harm, several treatment conditions must also be satisfied (in addition to Rawlinson's conditions i, ii, iv and v).

- Psychodynamic placebos (like all placebos) should be administered only with careful and regular monitoring of clients throughout the placebo period, to ensure the safety of placebo treatment.

- Psychodynamic placebos should be used only in conditions in which a temporary deferral of treatment would pose no long-term threat to the psychological health or well-being of clients.

- Psychodynamic placebos should be used only with an 'early escape' mechanism that allows clients to opt out of treatments when psychological symptoms reach a pre-defined level of intensity (Temple 2002).

The main objection to the claim that it is ethically permissible to give psychodynamic placebos in certain highly specific treatment contexts is that open placebos are ineffective, self-neutralizing, or counter-therapeutic; and that the withholding or delaying of proven effective treatments that is an inevitable consequence of placebo use will needlessly prolong suffering. The very knowledge that treatment consists of placebos—so the objection goes—undermines the treatment: no one can improve knowing that they are taking a 'mere' sugar pill, or the psychological analog of a sugar pill. As has already been suggested, however, this misconception about open placebos does not fare well in light of the available (though slim) clinical evidence, which suggests that open placebos enjoy a degree of clinical success (Park and Covi 1965; Vogel *et al.* 1980; Brown 1994, 1998a, 1998b; Aulas and Rosner 2003). While the specific mechanisms by which open placebo treatments operate are not yet known, what is clear from these studies is that treatment success depends to a large extent upon the manner in which clients are informed about their treatment options, the manner in which client consent is gained, and the manner in which the placebos are administered. Careful rationales of the placebo treatment, accompanied by psychotherapist confidence, optimism, and teaching, appear to be essential to counteract clients' doubts or hesitation about open placebo treatments.

How would this approach have worked in Frank's case history (Frank and Frank 1991: 205–210), which was discussed in Chapter 2? As will be recalled, at an early stage of the treatment, and with only a limited amount of clinical evidence from which to make reliable inferences about the causal role of past events, Frank offered a simple psychodynamic interpretation of the causes of his client's symptoms: namely, that abandonment by her parents at an early age had caused the client to fear trusting other people, including her husband; and that these traumatic childhood events were directly linked to her current symptoms. Despite its simplicity and lack of individuating detail, the interpretation 'went off like a gong', triggered in the client a series of insights, and occasioned (or was at least followed by) positive therapeutic changes.

In his description of the case history, it will be recalled, Frank does not claim that the interpretation was psychologically and historically true; nor does he claim that his client's subsequent insights were true. His claims were considerably more modest and cautious: the interpretation was 'plausible' and 'reassuring'; it enabled his client to 'relabel' her feelings as normal; it allowed her 'to construct a more optimistic apologia'; and it 'enhanced her sense of mastery' (Frank and Frank 1991: 207). Still, it can be inferred from the case description that Frank's presentation of the interpretation to the client was confident and authoritative, and not weighted down with any significant epistemic qualifications: that is, it can be inferred with a reasonable degree of certainty that he did not explicitly inform the client that the interpretation might be psychologically or historically false, or a plausible explanatory fiction. It can also be inferred from the case description that Frank did not temper his client's newly acquired insights with any explicit epistemic cautions. What does this mean? It means that it is likely that the client was left with the impression that Frank's interpretation was psychologically and historically true, that her insights were valid, and that the process of psychological exploration during the psychotherapy was authentic. There is little doubt that this is not a case of intentional deception; that is, Frank did not deliberately deceive his client, lie to her about her past (as Janet might have done), deliberately concoct a false interpretation (as Mendel did), or deliberately supply her with an arbitrary interpretation (as both Mendel and X did). At the same time, however, it is likely that Frank knowingly withheld from the client a number of significant epistemic qualifications about the interpretation—which he acknowledged after the fact (see Frank and Frank 1991: 210 on 'correct' interpretations). If this is the case, then she was not fully informed or educated about the treatment and its potential for triggering the placebo effect; and so her consent to treatment was based, in part, on incomplete information.

If, instead, Frank had explicitly informed the client in advance that his interpretation and her subsequent insights may be explanatory fictions that function like placebos in unlocking the mind's self-healing powers, and if he had informed her that they cannot be taken at face value as instances of genuine self-knowledge, then he would have satisfied in large part the principle of informed and educated consent as well as the principle of autonomy. These educative epistemic reminders may take the following form, which is based loosely on Brown's open placebo administration script (Brown 1994, 1998a, 1998b):

> You have two options at this point in the treatment. One is to continue with the exploratory therapy. This will probably help to reduce your symptoms, but it may take a long time. The other treatment option may prove to be less time consuming, less expensive, and less likely to cause side effects. It has helped some clients in psychotherapy with problems similar to yours. It involves working with psychodynamic explanations, interpretations, and insights concerning your psychology, history, behaviors, feelings and personality that are not literally true, but more like explanatory fictions. It involves making no claims to the psychological and historical truth when exploring your problems and your past. When we work with these interpretations and insights, we are working with the psychological equivalent of sugar pills. They are not however fanciful, arbitrary, or silly; but nor can we say that they are true. Some clients have found this approach to be helpful, and have found their symptoms to remit; others have not. We do not yet know how this approach works. False or fictional interpretations of your behaviors, history, and psychology may serve to rally your mind's own healing processes in ways that we do not yet fully understand—but the closest analog we have is the case of sugar pills and placebo surgeries that somehow rally the body's natural healing processes for certain kinds of diseases. What we do know, however, is that a clinically significant percentage of people with psychological problems that are similar to yours experience therapeutic gains using this approach, just as a significant percentage of people with physical diseases experience therapeutic gains when given sugar pills or false surgeries. If you decide to try this approach, I will check your progress every two weeks. If, after four weeks, your symptoms are still troubling you, we will consider reverting to the conventional treatment strategy; if your symptoms increase at any time in the next six weeks to a level of intensity that we will agree upon prior to the treatment, then we will also revert to the conventional treatment strategy. You are also free to opt out of this treatment strategy at any time. Now if you agree with this approach, I would like to proceed with the following interpretation of your symptoms…

This is a relatively streamlined way of presenting some basic epistemic warnings to clients about the vagaries of psychodynamic insights and interpretations. On the other hand, these educative epistemic reminders may take a more robust and historically self-aware form, beginning, for example, with John Ayrton Paris' warning about the 'boasted remedies of the present day' whose destiny is to end up as 'humiliating memorials of the credulity and infatuation of the physicians who recommended and prescribed them'; followed by some simple historical observations about the astonishing transience of explanatory theories and research paradigms in the medical, behavioral, and psychological sciences; followed then by cautionary remarks about the countless ways there are to be wrong, confused, ignorant or deceived about one's psychology, behavior, and personality; and concluding with a Socratic warning about the errors of claiming to know when one does not know.

Notes

Chapter One

1   The idea that some psychological disorders follow a natural history also receives limited support from studies in the cross-cultural prevalence of serious mental disorders such as schizophrenia: the so-called pathogenicity versus pathoplasticity debate (Waxler 1977; Torrey 1980, 1987; Leff 1986; Sartorius *et al.* 1986; Jablensky 1987). On one of the many sides of the debate is the view that sociocultural factors influence only the incidental aspects of disorders (namely, course and outcome), but not their incidence or defining form. On one of the other sides is the view that sociocultural factors influence both the incidence of the disorder and its incidental aspects (Lin and Kleinman 1988). The former position receives support from a series of influential studies conducted by the World Health Organization on psychotic individuals in nine cities (Prague, London, Moscow, Washington D.C., Aarhus, Agra, Cali, Ibadan, and Tapei) (Jablensky 1987). It was found that in all nine cities, patients displayed a nuclear set of features that included first rank symptoms of schizophrenia. Moreover, in no setting were any of these features particularly rare. If some psychological disorders follow a natural history and tend to be self-limiting, then it seems likely that evidence of this history would be found in diverse societies. Untreated depression in Agra, India would follow roughly the same onset, course, duration, and symptom remission as untreated depression in Washington, D.C., despite divergent sociocultural factors in the etiology and pathogenesis of depression. Moreover, untreated depression would be no less common in developing than in developed societies. However, while the evidence from the pathogenicity–pathoplasticity controversy about schizophrenia helps to illuminate the question of the natural history of psychological disorders, it does not settle it. Because the controversy is far from over, and because the disorders are markedly different, the evidence can be considered suggestive at best. There may be wide-ranging cross-cultural commonalities in certain psychological disorders, but this alone does not prove that they follow a natural history.

2   Erwin (1996b: 53; see also Erwin and Siegel 1989) characterizes the differential principle as follows: 'Evidence E confirms a hypothesis H *only if* it does so differentially [by providing] at least some reason for believing that H is true and does not provide equal (or better) reason for believing some rival hypothesis that is at least as plausible.'

Chapter Two

1   Freud writes: 'In every case the news that reaches your consciousness is incomplete and often not to be relied on. Often enough, too, it happens that you get news of events only when they are over and when you can no longer do anything to change them. Even if you are not ill, who can tell all that is stirring in your mind of which you know nothing or are falsely informed? You behave like an absolute ruler who is content with the information supplied him by his highest officials and never goes among the people to hear their voice. Turn your eyes inward, look into your own depths, learn first to know

yourself!' (SE 17: 143). References to *The standard edition of the complete psychological works of Sigmund Freud* are abbreviated in the text as SE.

2   Freud described the process as follows: 'We wish to make the ego the matter of our enquiry, our very own ego. But is that possible? After all, the ego is in its very essence a subject; how can it be made into an object? Well, there is no doubt that it can be. The ego can take itself as an object, can treat itself like other objects, can observe itself, criticize itself, and do Heaven knows what with itself. In this, one part of the ego is setting itself over against the rest. So the ego can be split; it splits itself during a number of its functions—temporarily at least. Its parts can come together again afterwards' (SE 22: 58).

3   Thus Erikson (1958: 75) suggests that the 'proof' of an interpretation 'lies in the way in which the communication between therapist and patient keeps moving, leading to new and surprising insights and to the patient's greater assumption of responsibility for himself.'

4   Freud's evocative description of the power of analytic insight might suggest this. He writes that 'when the riddle [the psychoneuroses] present is solved and the solution accepted by the patients, these diseases cease to be able to exist. There is hardly anything like this in medicine, though in fairy tales you hear of evil spirits whose power is broken as soon as you can tell them their name—the name which they have kept secret' (SE 11: 148).

5   The lead author Jerome Frank was the treating psychotherapist in this case history, rather than Julia Frank, who was added as second author in the most recent (1991) edition of *Persuasion and Healing*. The case history appears intact in the earlier single author editions of *Persuasion and Healing*.

Chapter Three

1   Campbell (1978: 19–29) claims that any symptom relief ensuing from an unconscious 'misalliance' between the analyst and analysand (i.e. one that is based on suggestive interpretations) will be transient, since the patient will be left vulnerable to later stresses (cited in Grünbaum 1984: 134). Thomä (1977; cited in Grünbaum 1984: 134) claims that patient skepticism will counteract any suggestive influences of the interpretations, especially when the analysand has hostile feelings towards the analyst.

2   In addition to these theoretical criticisms, the principle of therapeutic specificity has met with criticism from the clinical angle. It has been argued that psychotherapies defending the principle tend to polarize the field of mental health care, because they interfere with integrative research aimed at developing a unified approach to psychotherapy (Marmor 1980). It has also been argued that those psychotherapies defending the principle may be anti-therapeutic, because they interfere with the development of more comprehensive accounts of client problems (Lesse 1980).

3   Torrey (1986: 17–34) calls this the 'Rumpelstiltskin principle', after the fairy tale in which the good queen broke the evil dwarf's power over her by guessing his name. Clients gain a sense of control when they are provided with a conceptual system that identifies and classifies experiences that had once seemed inexplicable.

4   Named after the carnival operator P.T. Barnum, whose carnivals offered something for everyone.

5   Nietzsche, for instance, argued that untruth, and the will to ignorance, are fundamental conditions of human life. Included in the list of adaptive and life-enhancing qualities are illusion, ignorance, deception, blind stupidity, and crude over-simplification.

The unqualified commitment to truth is destructive of the blind momentum of life: 'It is not enough that you understand in what ignorance humans as well as animals live; you must also have and acquire the will to ignorance. You need to grasp that without this kind of ignorance life itself would be impossible, that it is a condition under which alone the living thing can preserve itself and prosper: a great, firm dome of ignorance must encompass you' (Nietzsche 1968: p. 609; Nietzsche 1886/1966: 188). The plays of Henrik Ibsen and Eugene O'Neill (1946) also illustrate these Nietzschean themes, and show how life for the average person can be tolerable only with a veil of comforting and self-serving illusions—pipe-dreams and 'life-lies'—filtering out life's harsher elements (Jopling 1996b). Without these psychological crutches, most people would not be able to function normally and maintain adaptive self-regarding attitudes. The plays of Ibsen and O'Neill thus focus upon a recurrent theme: when pipe-dreams and life-lies are burst, in the name of an honest confrontation with reality, tragedy inevitably follows. Too much self-knowledge is psychologically destabilizing.

6　One experiment that illustrates the impoverished empirical content of psychodynamic interpretations focused on a 54-year-old female schizophrenic patient who dragged a broom around a hospital ward for close to one year (Allyon *et al.* 1965). Two psychiatrists were asked to observe the patient's behaviors through a one-way window and then interpret the meaning of her 'symptoms'. One psychiatrist argued that the broom represented an essential perceptual element in the patient's field of consciousness, and that her behavior resembled that of a small child who refused to give up a favorite toy. The other argued that her behavior was a ritualistic or magical procedure, and that the broom was for her a child that gives her love, a phallic symbol, and the scepter of an omnipotent queen. Both interpretations were widely off the mark. In fact, the patient dragged the broom around because she was behaviorally conditioned to do so. Allyon *et al.* had instructed the hospital attendants to give the patient a cigarette and a broom, and to reward her every fifteen minutes if she continued to hold the broom. Through behavioral conditioning, she dragged the broom around the hospital 40% of the time for about one year, after which time the behavior was extinguished.

Chapter Five

1　The 'Hawthorne effect' is a methodological effect that occurs when people are made aware that they are participating in an experiment, or are made aware of the hypothesis being tested in the experiment, or receive special attention because they are in an experiment—conditions that could result in improvements in performance which would not otherwise have occurred (Adair 1984; Last 1988). This jeopardizes the external validity of the experiment, because the findings may not be generalizable to situations other than those in which the particular researchers and experimental participants are present. The 'experimenter effect' occurs when an experimental treatment is effective or ineffective mainly because of the particular experimenter who administers the treatment, rather than because of the treatment itself. 'Treatment effects' also jeopardize attempts to generalize to conditions in which different experimenters administer the relevant treatment. Again the 'novelty effect' occurs when new or unusual experimental treatments are effective simply because they are different from the treatments that participants normally receive. Again the experimental results have poor generalizability, because the effectiveness of the treatments tends to diminish as the novelty wears off. The 'disruption effect' occurs when experimental treatments disrupt the normal routine of participants. While they may be initially ineffective, participants might eventually assimilate the treatments into their routine, and thereby make them more effective than they were at first. The results of the initial tryout are therefore not generalizable to a condition of continued use. 'Pretest sensitization' occurs when an initial test or measure that is given to participants to establish a baseline state prior to the actual experiment interacts with the actual experimental condition or treatment that follows it. The pretest inadvertently sensitizes the participants to the objects or themes that are the focus of the experiment, thereby improving their performance in post-test scores over groups that did not receive the pretest. If the experiment is conducted without a pretest, different results are obtained. 'Post-test sensitization' occurs when the results of a social science experiment depend upon the administration of a post-test. A post-test may cause certain aspects of the treatment or experiment to catalyze or be activated after the experiment. If the experiment is conducted without a post-test, different results are obtained. 'Experimenter bias' occurs when researchers' positive or negative expectations about the outcomes of their experiments are inadvertently transmitted to participants in such a way that the participants' behaviors during the experiment are affected (Rosenthal 1976). This results in experimental findings that may not be generalizable to situations other than those in which the particular researchers and participants are present. The classic experiment illustrating the effects of experimenter bias is Rosenthal's 'maze-bright' and 'maze-dull' rats (Rosenthal and Fode 1963).

2   See Blanck and Blanck (1974: 320–2) for a case history illustrating many of the primary elements of directive therapeutic intervention, yet resulting in the patient's refusing to accept the therapist's interpretations.

3   Symptom artifacts may also occur in psychopharmacological treatments. With the marketing of new generations of psychoactive drugs, it is not uncommon for new psychological disorders to be 'discovered'—and new disorders to be experienced by patients—that require treatment by those very drugs (Healey 1997, 2004; Healy and Doogan 1996). New diagnostic profiles, psychological tests, etiologies, and treatment interventions go hand in hand with new populations of patients, presenting with new symptoms. This is a case of diagnostic bracket creep: the expansion of categories of psychopathology into everyday behaviors, in such a way that what were once considered to be normal responses to the hardships of life come to be reconceptualized as disorders that merit treatment interventions. The growth of normalizing psychotechnologies is a culturally parochial phenomenon. Just as the perception of one's nose as too big, or one's wrinkles as too ugly, can only be made in a culture that treats these features as correctable flaws, so the perception of certain psychological states or behaviors as undesirable can only be made in a culture that treats those states as abnormal and correctable. With diagnostic bracket creep comes symptom artifacts—that is, psychological states or behaviors that occur only in the interaction of clients with the psychological intervention, psychological terminology, or psychological diagnosis. The symptoms appear to be natural, and independent of volition and intention. But they would not exist as such without the diagnostic categories under which they are identified and discriminated one from another.

4   Some evidence for this can be found in attribution theory and labeling theory in social psychology and sociology. Labeling certain behaviors as disordered or deviant serves to define those behaviors, and alters them in ways they would not otherwise have been altered. The labeling functions as a kind of baptism, with the people labeled coming to identify with their labels, and engaging in behaviors that tend to confirm the label.

Just as labels have the power to produce behavioral artifacts, so diagnoses can produce symptom artifacts.

5   Hacking's (1995) history of multiple personality disorder provides one account of how symptom artifacts arise as a result of the 'looping effects' of human kind terms. The rapid growth of psychiatric and psychological classification schemes from the mid-nineteenth century onwards, Hacking argues, is responsible for the rise in self-confirming etiologies. Psychiatric classification schemes typically sort human behaviors into broad kinds, such as multiple personality disorder, child abuse, homosexuality, abnormalcy, autism, and alcoholism (Hacking 1986, 1994, 1995, 1998, 1999). These have the appearance of objective and well-defined categories, not unlike natural kinds, and they seem to make lawlike generalizations and predictions possible. In the sciences of memory and the sciences of deviancy, kind terms serve not only to sort peoples, behaviors, conditions, and experiences, but to influence the very things they putatively sort. They have odd 'looping effects', which are not found in the kind terms of the natural sciences. Classifying people as X changes them from what they were before, such that they behave differently. For example, prior to the 1880s, Hacking claims, there were no such people as multiples. 'When did multiple personality come into being? Late in the afternoon of the 27th of July, 1885' (Hacking 1995: 171). Prior to that point—prior to the creation of the relevant conceptual and description space, and the creation of the relevant psychiatric, forensic, statistical, clinical, and criminological practices—there were no such people as multiples. After that point, not only did new symptoms, behaviors, and experiences come to be; a new way of being a person opened up hand in hand with the new modes of description and the new classifications. But as new classifications bring with them changes in the self-conceptions and in the behaviors of the people classified, these changes in their turn demand revisions to the initial classifications, which in turn induces further looping-related changes, and so on. Some accounts of the etiology of psychological disorders are therefore self-sustaining and self-confirming, and lead to the production of symptom artifacts that are experienced as real by the patients who are diagnosed under that particular etiological system. Their symptoms appear to be natural, and independent of personal volition and intention. What has happened, however, is that patients have been supplied with a persuasive etiological model that reorganizes their conception of the past. New etiological models do not *create* the past; rather, they become 'disseminated as a way of thinking of what it was like to be a child and to grow up. There is no canonical way to think of our own past. In the endless quest for order and structure, we grasp at whatever picture is floating by and put our past into its frame' (1996: 88–89). In this way the process of multiple therapy 'concretizes a story into a fact' (1996: 90). 'We should not think of multiplicity as being strictly caused by child abuse. It is rather that the multiple finds or sees the cause of her condition in what she comes to remember about her childhood, and is thereby helped. This is passed off as a specific etiology, but what is happening is more extraordinary than that. It is a way of explaining oneself, not by recovering the past, but by redescribing it, rethinking it, refeeling it' (1996: 94–5).

6   Stendhal's novel *The Charterhouse of Parma* contains a vivid account of how inchoate and unarticulated feelings of love can acquire different shapes, depending upon how they are socially identified and described.

7   Schachter and Singer's (1962) famous experiment showed how experimental participants' interpretations of their emotional states could be influenced when they were supplied with false information from an external source (such as another person);

and that participants' emotional states are poorly introspectable, because the physiological evidence and experiential markers for many emotions are insufficient to distinguish them one from another. They concluded from this that people in general tend to experience vaguely undifferentiated emotional states, which then come to be identified and labeled indirectly on the basis of externally disambiguating information.

8 See Farrell's thought experiment (1981: 101–28); see also Naftulin *et al.* (1975). See also Corsini *et al*'s (1991) account of a fictional client who is exposed to five kinds of psychotherapy for the same set of psychological problems: Adlerian therapy, person-centered therapy, rational–emotive therapy, behavior therapy, and eclectic therapy. While Corsini *et al.* assume that the client is treated concurrently rather than consecutively in the different treatment modalities, they do not consider the epistemic problems raised by the problem of therapy-generated artifacts.

9 Horvath's review surveyed two leading journals for all published psychotherapy outcome studies that used placebo controls: namely, the *Journal of Consulting Psychology* for the years 1964 and 1965, and specific volumes of the *Journal of Consulting and Clinical Psychology* for the years 1969, 1970, 1974, 1975, 1979, 1980, 1984, and 1985. The result was a total of 39 psychotherapy outcome studies that used placebo controls in one guise or another. The criteria for inclusion in the review were relatively simple: the condition or group against which a particular psychotherapy was being tested for effectiveness was considered by the authors of the studies either as a placebo or 'attention placebo' treatment, or as a control condition for nonspecific therapeutic variables. Studies that used no-treatment control conditions were not included. One drawback with these criteria is that they allow the inclusion of studies in which authors supply little or no rationale for their choices of placebo.

10 Kirsch's (2005) defense of a version of the identity argument leads him to conclude that evaluating the efficacy of psychotherapy by controlling for placebo factors should be abandoned altogether. Kirsch defines the placebo as a sham treatment, and explains the placebo effect as that which is produced by the self-confirming nature of response expectancies (i.e. expectancies that are directly self-confirming because they tend to produce the anticipated experience (Kirsch (1985, 2005; Kirsch and Rosadino 1993; Montgomery and Kirsch 1988).

The first problem Kirsch identifies with the attempt to import the placebo model into psychotherapy research is a practical one: namely, it is practically impossible to design a placebo that is both identical in appearance to the active treatment (against which the placebo is being compared) and devoid of relevant active ingredients. This match-and-replace strategy is relatively unproblematic in medical research: placebos are typically identical in appearance to the experimental drug or procedure against which they are compared, but the latter's hypothesized physically active properties are omitted from the placebo. Nonetheless, the placebos have all of the relevant psychological characteristics of the experimental drug or procedure, thereby ensuring a fair comparison. The match-and-replace strategy, however, does not work in psychotherapy research, because psychological treatments have no physical properties that can be singled out and omitted. All of the relevant properties that would need to be replaced are themselves psychological. But this creates a problem: 'If a psychological treatment contained the same psychological properties as the real treatment (i.e. if the therapist used the same words and procedures), it would no longer be a placebo or a control condition of any other kind. Instead, it would be the treatment. As a result, procedures used as placebos in psychotherapy research are usually very different from the psychotherapies to which they are being compared' (Kirsch 2005: 796). These placebos include such things as listening to stories, reading books, attending language classes, viewing films, participating in 'bull' sessions, playing with puzzles, sitting quietly with a silent therapist, and discussing current events (Kirsch 796). None of these ensure a fair comparison or a fair control; none look like a real placebo.

The second problem Kirsch identifies with importing the placebo model into psychological research is a conceptual one. It makes no sense, he argues, to extend the placebo concept from medical research to the psychotherapeutic setting, if the aim is to control for the psychological effects of administering a treatment and to determine whether the physical properties of a treatment have any effect, because psychotherapies do not have physically active properties at all: their entire substance is words, or meanings, and not physical states. There is no point trying to control for the psychological effects of a treatment if the treatment is a psychological one in the first place. 'There is a problem with identifying psychotherapy with the placebo effect. A placebo is something that is sham, fake, inert, empty. Psychotherapy is none of these. In this sense, it is different from medical placebos, and it does not deserve the pejorative connotations associated with the term' (Kirsch 2005: 797). Kirsch therefore doubts a very basic distinction: namely, that some psychotherapies are shams, fake, or inert, and some are not. By implication, he doubts that there is a valid distinction to be drawn between sham, fake or inert components of a psychotherapy, and bona fide components. The very concept of a sham psychotherapy is, Kirsch claims, questionable: it could not be a treatment that is ineffective, because placebos can be effective. Nor could it be a treatment whose effects are nonspecific, because the effects of placebos are often no less specific than any other psychologically produced effects. And if the effects of a psychological treatment are due entirely to expectancy, it does not follow that the treatment does not work.

Kirsch concludes—paradoxically—that the terms placebo and psychotherapy are synonyms, and that the phrase placebo psychotherapy is an oxymoron. Because it has no physically active ingredients, psychotherapy can be considered a placebo by definition (hence the two terms are synonymous). At the same time, the phrase placebo psychotherapy can be considered an oxymoron, because of the practical and conceptual impossibilities blocking the way to designing placebo controls for psychotherapy outcome research.

Even if Kirsch's problematically sharp distinction between physical and psychological properties is overlooked, the problem with the argument is that it construes every property of every psychological treatment (placebo or not) as on a par with every other—so much so that 'it does not matter what those [psychologically] active ingredients are' (Kirsch 2005: 800). But this lumps together indiscriminately the characteristic and incidental factors of psychological treatments, thereby ruling out the very possibility of designing psychological placebos that omit the characteristic factors of a treatment. 'In principle, these [hope, faith, response expectancy] are no different from any other psychological factor than [sic] can alleviate distress' (Kirsch 2005: 800). But the psychological factors at play in psychotherapies are not all of a piece; they differ from one another in terms of relative causal powers, mechanisms of action, patient receptivity, epistemic status, degree of credibility, and theoretical centrality, among other things. Sorting out these factors is a central problem in psychotherapy research. Without knowing which causal factors lead to therapeutic improvement and which do not, and the relative degrees of efficacy of these causal factors, psychological treatments are reduced to inscrutable black box procedures, and the scientific validation of competing psychological explanations of therapeutic change is rendered irrelevant. In psychodynamic psychotherapy, for instance, it matters for diagnostic, theoretical, epistemic, and ethical reasons whether a treatment works by means of suggestion or by means of the excavation of actual psychological pathogens. More specifically, it matters (for similar reasons) whether an interpretation is a sham interpretation (such as a one-size-fits-all interpretation, or an explanatory fiction) or a bona fide interpretation.

Chapter Six

1 Some of the more well-known *philosophical* models of self-deception have been defended by Demos, Audi, Rorty, Sartre, and Fingarette (see Mele 1997 for a recent review):

a) Self-deception involves believing both p and not-p at the same time (Demos 1960). This split is possible because there are two kinds of awareness: simple awareness and awareness without noticing. Someone who is self-deceived is simply aware of his belief that p, without noticing his belief. It is this failure to notice or to attend to this belief that allows him to believe that not-p.

b) Self-deception involves believing both p and not-p, but one of these beliefs is unconscious (though not in the psychoanalytic sense) (Audi 1982). Someone is self-deceived about p if he unconsciously knows that not-p, but sincerely avows that p; and, he has at least one want that explains why his belief that not-p is unconscious, and why he is disposed to disavow his belief that not-p.

c) Self-deception occurs when there is a failure of integration between the various systems that make up the mind (Rorty 1988). If minds are loosely configured systems of quasi-autonomous cognitive, motivational, and mnemonic subsystems, without any central processing agent (or Cartesian theatre), then it is possible for one subsystem to believe p while another subsystem believes not-p.

d) Self-deception is an alienation of the self from itself, and an evasion of the task of *being* oneself: it is a kind of bad faith (Sartre 1969). It occurs when people play off their free agency against their facticity, leading to an inner division that interferes with personal agency and the acceptance of responsibility for self. Bad faith is a strategy that allows people to hide from themselves the hard existential truth that they are radically free, unsupported by any metaphysical foundation that might relieve them of the burden of continual self-definition. People in bad faith behave as if they are determinate and externally-determined entities like other entities in the world, and therefore without any significant latitude of choice as to what will constitute their identity and will.

e) Self-deception is the disavowal of a well-established engagement (e.g. binge drinking), which takes the form of refusing to identify oneself as the person engaging in certain behaviors and responses to others and the world (Fingarette 1969). Disavowal creates an inner split, because it entails avoiding becoming explicitly conscious of, or 'spelling out', the nature of these engagements. With the development of finely discriminating and situation-specific patterns of disavowal comes diminished control over the disavowed engagement, which is pursued increasingly in isolation from avowed aspects of one's personality.

Chapter Seven

1 Much of the discussion about the ethics of giving placebos proceeds as if cultural, social, and anthropological differences in the practice of medicine do not exist. Prescinding from

these differences is a reasonable way of increasing the degree of objectivity of moral argument, and thereby a way of reaching moral conclusions that are less vulnerable to charges of social bias and ethnocentrism. But it can also leave out too much. Medical anthropology offers a strikingly different perspective on the ethics of giving placebos from that of contemporary Western medical ethics. In the medical practices of some non-Western cultures, as well as in the history of Western medicine up to the late nineteenth century, the principle of respect for patient autonomy, and the principle of informed consent, has played only a limited role compared to the practices of benevolent paternalism. Few cultures have cherished personal autonomy as a moral ideal that embodies the highest vision of what it is to be a human being as much as cultures in the contemporary Western world; similarly, few have valued transparency and honesty as moral ideals that ought to be aspired to in all medical relationships. From the perspective of contemporary Western medical ethics, shamans, religious healers, and doctors in non-Western cultures would be viewed as engaging in unethical practices because of their use of deceptive, paternalistic, and less-than-transparent treatment methods to increase the effectiveness of their treatments. But this assessment is foreign to the perspective of patients within these cultures. If medical practices in some non-Western cultures were suddenly to be governed by these two principles—and, as a result, placebo use sharply curtailed—treatment effectiveness might drop precipitously: but this is a matter of speculation rather than of fact.

References

Adair, J.G. (1984). The Hawthorne effect: A reconsideration of the methodological artifact. *Journal of Applied Psychology*, **69**, 334–345.

Ader, R.A. and Cohen, N. (1975). Behaviorally conditioned immunosuppression. *Psychosomatic Medicine*, **37**, 333–340.

Ader, R.A. (1997). The role of conditioning in pharmacotherapy. In A. Harrington, ed. *The placebo effect: An interdisciplinary exploration* (pp.138–165). Harvard University Press, Cambridge, Mass.

Albee, G.W. (1990). The futility of psychotherapy. *Journal of Mind and Behavior*, **11**, 369–384.

Alexander, F. and French, T.M. (1946). *Psychoanalytic therapy: Principles and applications.* Ronald Press, New York.

Allyon, T., Haughton, E. and Hughes, H. (1965). Interpretation of symptoms: Fact or fiction. *Behavior Research and Therapy*, **3**, 1–7.

Amanzio, M., Pollo, A., Maggi, G., and Benedetti, F. (2001). Response variability to analgesics: A role for non-specific activation of endogenous opioids. *Pain*, **90**, 205–215.

American Psychiatric Association (2001). *The principles of medical ethics, with annotations especially applicable to psychiatry (including November 2003 amendments).* American Psychiatric Association: Washington, D.C. Available on the World Wide Web at: http://www.psych.org/psych_pract/ethics/ppaethics.cfm

American Psychological Association (2002). *Ethical principles of psychologists and code of conduct.* American Psychological Association: Washington, D.C.

Andrews, G., Sanderson, K. and Slade, T. (2000). Why does the burden of disease persist? Relating the burden of anxiety and depression to effectiveness of treatment. *Bulletin of the World Health Organization*, **78**, 446–454.

Andrews, G. (2001). Placebo response in depression: Bane of research, boon to therapy. *British Journal of Psychiatry*, **178**, 192–194.

Arkes, H.R. (1981). Impediments to accurate clinical judgment and possible ways to minimize their impact. *Journal of Consulting and Clinical Psychology*, **49**, 323–330.

Arlow, J. (1995). Psychoanalysis. In R.V. Corsini and D. Wedding, eds., *Current psychotherapies* (5th ed.) pp. 15-50. F.E. Peacock, Itasca, Illinois.

Audi, R. (1982). Self-deception, action, and willing. *Erkenntnis*, **18**, 133–158.

Aulas, J.J. and Rosner, I. (2003). Efficacy of a nonblind placebo prescription. *L'Encéphale: Revue de psychiatrie clinique, biologique, et therapeutique*, **29**: 68–71.

Baier, A. (1996). The vital but dangerous art of ignoring: Selective attention and self-deception. In R.T. Ames and W. Dissanayake, eds. *Self and deception: A cross-cultural philosophical enquiry*, SUNY, Press Albany, New York. pp. 53–72.

Basch, M. (1980). *Doing psychotherapy.* Basic Books, New York.

Bateman, A., Brown, D. and Pedder, J. (2000). *Introduction to psychotherapy: An outline of psychodynamic principles and practice*, 3rd ed. Routledge, London.

Baudouin, C. (1920). *Suggestion and autosuggestion* (E. Paul and C. Paul, trans.). George Allen and Unwin, London.

Beauchamp, T. and Childress, J.F. (1983). *Principles of biomedical ethics*. 2nd ed. Oxford University Press, New York.

Beauchamp, T. and McCullough, L.B. (1984). *Medical ethics: The moral responsibilities of physicians*. Prentice Hall, Englewood Cliffs, N.J.

Beecher, H. (1955). The powerful placebo. *Journal of the American Medical Association*, **159**, 1602–1606.

Beecher, H. (1959). *Quantitative effects of drugs*. Oxford University Press, New York.

Benedetti, F., Maggi, G., Lopiano, L., *et al.* (2003). Open versus hidden medical treatments: The patient's knowledge about a therapy affects the therapy outcome. *Prevention and Treatment*, **6**, Article 1. Available on the World Wide Web at: http://journals.apa.org/prevention/volume6/pre0060001a.html

Benedetti, F., Mayberg, H.S., Wager, T.D., *et al.* (2005). Neurobiological mechanisms of the placebo effect. *Journal of Neuroscience*, **25** (45), 10390–10402.

Bergin, A.E. (1971). The evaluation of therapeutic outcomes. In A.E. Bergin and S. Garfield eds. *Handbook of psychotherapy and behavior change*, Wiley and Sons, New York pp.217–270.

Bergin, A.E. and Lambert, M. (1978). The evaluation of therapeutic outcomes. In S. Garfield and A. Bergin, eds. *Handbook of psychotherapy and behavior change: An empirical analysis*, 2nd ed., J. Wiley, New York. pp.139–189.

Berkeley, G. (1710/1982). *A treatise concerning the principles of human knowledge*. Hackett, Indianapolis.

Bersoff, D.N. (1995). *Ethical conflicts in psychology*. American Psychological Association, Washington, D.C.

Beyerstein, B. (2001). Fringe psychotherapies: The public at risk. *The Scientific Review of Alternative Medicine*, **5**, 70–79.

Blanck, G. and Blanck, R. (1974). *Ego psychology: Theory and practice*. Columbia University Press, New York.

Boas, F. (1930). The religion of the Kwakiutl Indians. *Columbia University Contributions to Anthropology*, Vol. 10. Columbia University Press, New York.

Bok, S. (1974). The ethics of giving placebos. *Scientific American*, **231**, 17–23.

Bok, S. (1975). Paternalistic deception in medicine and rational choice: The use of placebos. In M. Black, ed. *Problems of choice and decision*, Cornell University Press, Ithaca, New York. pp.73–107.

Bok, S. (2002). Ethical issues in the use of placebos in medical practice and clinical trials. In H.A. Guess, A. Kleinman, J.W. Kusek and L. Engel, eds. *The science of the placebo: Toward an interdisciplinary research agenda*, BMJ, London. pp.53–74.

Bootzin, R.R. and Caspi, O. (2003). Explanatory mechanisms for placebo effects: cognition, personality and social learning. In H.A. Guess, A. Kleinman, J.W. Kusek, and L. Engel, eds. *The science of the placebo: Toward an interdisciplinary research agenda*, BMJ, London. pp.108–132.

Borch-Jacobsen, M. (1996). *Remembering Anna O: A century of mystification*. K. Olson with X. Callhan, trans. Routledge, New York.

Borkovec, T. and Nau, S. (1972). Credibility of analog therapy rationales. *Journal of Behavior Therapy and Experimental Psychology*, **3**, 257–260.

Borkovec, T. D. and Sibrava, N.J. (2005). Problems with the use of placebo conditions in psychotherapy research, suggested alternatives and some strategies for the pursuit of the placebo phenomenon. *Journal of Clinical Psychology*, **61**, 805–818.

Bowers, K.S. and Farvolden, P. (1996). Revisiting a century-old Freudian slip: From suggestion disavowed to the truth repressed. *Psychological Bulletin*, **119**, 355–380.

Braithwaite, A. and Cooper, P. (1981). Analgesic effects of branding in treatment of headaches. *British Medical Journal (Clinical Research Edition)*, **282**, Guilford Press.1576–1578.

Brody, H. (1980). *Placebos and the philosophy of medicine*. University of Chicago Press, Chicago.

Brody, H. (1982). The lie that heals: The ethics of giving placebos. *Annals of Internal Medicine*, **97**, 112–118.

Brody, H. (1985). Placebo effect: An examination of Grünbaum's definition. In L. White, B. Tursky, and G.E. Schwartz, eds. *Placebo: Theory, research, and mechanisms*, Guilford Press, New York. pp. 37–58.

Brody, H. (1986). The placebo response. Part 1: Exploring the myths. Part 2: Use in clinical practice. *Drug Therapy*, **16**, 106–131.

Brody, H. (1997). The doctor as therapeutic agent: A placebo effect research agenda. In A. Harrington, ed. *The placebo effect: An interdisciplinary exploration*, Harvard University Press, Cambridge, Mass. pp. 77–92.

Brody, H. and Waters, D.B. (1980). Diagnosis is treatment. *Journal of Family Practice*, **10**, 445–449.

Brown, W.A. (1994). Placebo as a treatment for depression. *Neuropsychopharmacology*, **10**, 265–269.

Brown, W.A. (1998a). The placebo effect. *Scientific American* (January), 90–95.

Brown, W.A. (1998b). Harnessing the placebo effect. *Hospital Practice* (July), 107–116.

Burton, R. (1628/1955). *The anatomy of melancholy*. F. Dell and P.J. Smith, eds. Tudor, New York.

Cabot, R.C. (1903). The use of truth and falsehood in medicine: An experimental study. *American Medicine 5*, 344–349.

Cabot, R.C. (1906). The physician's responsibility for the nostrum evil. *Journal of the American Medical Association*, **47**, 982–983.

Calestro, K.M. (1972). Psychotherapy, faith healing, and suggestion. *International Journal of Psychiatry*, **10**, 83–113.

Campbell, L.A. (1978). The role of suggestion in the psychoanalytic therapies. *International Journal of Psychoanalytic Psychotherapy*, **7**, 1–22.

Canadian Institutes of Health Research (2004). *Final report of the national placebo working committee on the appropriate use of placebos in clinical trials in Canada*. Available on the World Wide Web at: http://www.cihr-irsc.gc.ca/e/25139.html

Cardena, E. and Kirsch, I. (2000). What is so special about the placebo effect? *Advances in Mind-Body Medicine*, **16**, 16–18.

Castonguay, L.G. and Hill, C.E., eds. (2007). *Insight in psychotherapy*. American Psychological Association, Washington, D.C.

Chandler, M.J. and Holliday, S. (1990). Wisdom in a post-apocalyptic age. In R. Sternberg, ed. *Wisdom: Its nature, origins, and development*, Cambridge University Press, New York. pp.121–141.

Cioffi, F. (1998). *Freud and the question of pseudoscience*. Open Court, La Salle, Ill.

Coleridge, S.T. (1907). *Biographia Literaria*. Oxford University Press, Oxford.

Conferences on Therapy (1946). *New York State Journal of Medicine*, 1718–1727.

Connolly, M.B., Crits-Christoph, P., Shelton, C., *et al.* (1999). The reliability and validity of a measure of self-understanding of interpersonal patterns. *Journal of Counselling Psychology*, **46**, 472–482.

Conway, M. (1997). *Recovered memories and false memories*. Oxford University Press, New York.

Corsini, R.J. and Wedding, D., eds. (1995). *Current psychotherapies*, 5th ed. F.E. Peacock, Itasca, Illinois.

Corsini, R.J. and contributors (1991). *Five therapists and one client*. F.E. Peacock, Itasca, Illinois.

Council for International Organizations of Medical Science (2002). *International Ethical Guidelines for Biomedical Research involving Human Participants*. Geneva. Available on the World Wide Web at: http://www.cioms.ch/frame_guidelines_nov_2002.htm.

Crews, F. (1990). *The memory wars: Freud's legacy in dispute*. New York Review of Books, New York.

Critelli, J.W. and Newman, K.F. (1984). The placebo: Conceptual analysis of a construct in transition. *American Psychologist*, **39**, 32–39.

Crits-Christoph, P. (1984). *The development of a measure of self-understanding of core relationship themes*. Paper presented at an NIMH workshop on methodologic challenges in psychodynamic research, Washington D.C.

Crits-Christoph, P. and Luborsky, L. (1990). The measurement of self-understanding. In L. Luborsky and P. Crits-Christoph, *Understanding transference: The Core Conflictual Relationship Theme method*. Basic Books, New York.

Damasio, A. (2003). *Looking for Spinoza: Joy, sorrow, and the feeling brain*. Harcourt, Orlando.

Davis, C.E. (1976). The effect of regression to the mean in epidemiologic and clinical studies. *American Journal of Epidemiology*, **5**, 493–498.

Davis, C.E. (2002). Regression to the mean or placebo effect? In H.A. Guess, A. Kleinman, J.W. Kusek, and L. Engel, eds. *The science of the placebo: Toward an interdisciplinary research agenda*, BMJ, London. pp.158–166.

Dawes, R. (1988). *Rational choice in an uncertain world*. Harcourt Brace Jovanovitch, San Diego.

Dawes, R. (1994). *House of cards: Psychology and psychotherapy built on myth*. Free Press, New York.

Dawes, R., Faust, D, and Meehl, P.E. (1989). Clinical versus actuarial judgment. *Science*, **243**, 1668–1674.

Demos, R. (1960). Lying to oneself. *Journal of Philosophy*, **57**, 588–595.

Dennett, D.C. (1991). *Consciousness explained*. Little Brown, Boston.

de Sousa, R. (1988). Emotion and self-deception. In B.P. McLaughlin and A.O. Rorty, eds., *Perspectives on self-deception*, University of California Press, Los Angeles. pp. 324–341.

Dickson, D.H. and Kelly, I.W. (1985). The Barnum effect in personality assessment: A review of the literature. *Psychological Reports*, **57**, 367–382.

Dmitruk, V.M., Collins, R.W. and Clinger, D.L. (1973). The Barnum effect and acceptance of negative personal evaluation. *Journal of Consulting and Clinical Psychology*, **41**, 192–194.

Dostoevsky, F. (1880/1981). *The brothers Karamazov*. A.H. MacAndrew, trans. Bantam Books, New York.

Dryden, W. and Mytton, J. (1999). *Four approaches to counselling and psychotherapy*. Routledge, New York.

Eagle, M. (1993). Enactments, transference, and symptomatic cure. *Psychoanalytic Dialogues*, **3**, 93–110.

Ehrenwald, J. (1966). *Psychotherapy: Myth and method. An integrative approach*. Grune and Stratton, New York.

Eissler, K.R. (1969). Irreverent remarks about the present and future of psychoanalysis. *International Journal of Psycho-Analysis*, **50**, 461–471.

Elkin, I., Parloff, M.B., Hadley, S. and Autry, J.H. (1985). NIMH treatment of depression collaborative research program. *Archives of General Psychiatry*, **42**, 305–316.

Ellenberger, H. (1970). *The discovery of the unconscious: The history and evolution of dynamic psychiatry*. Basic Books, New York.

Erikson, E. (1958). *Insight and responsibility*. Norton, New York.

Ernst, E. and Resch, K.L. (1995). Concept of true and perceived placebo effects. *British Medical Journal*, **311**, 551–553.

Erwin, E. (1985). Holistic therapies: What works? In D. Stalker and C. Glymour, eds., *Examining holistic medicine*, Prometheus Books, Buffalo. pp. 245–272.

Erwin, E. (1993). Philosophers on Freudianism. In J. Earman, A.I. Janis, G.J. Massey, and N. Rescher, eds., *Philosophical problems of the internal and external worlds: Essays on the philosophy of Adolf Grünbaum*, University of Pittsburgh Press/Universitätsverlag Konstanz, Pittsburgh. pp.409–459.

Erwin, E. (1994). The effectiveness of psychotherapy: Epistemological issues. In G. Graham and G. Lynn Stevens, eds., *Philosophical psychopathology*, MIT, Cambridge, Mass. pp. 261–284.

Erwin, E. (1996a). *A final accounting: Philosophical and empirical issues in Freudian psychology*. MIT, Cambridge, Mass.

Erwin, E. (1996b). The evaluation of psychotherapy: A reply to Greenwood. *Philosophy of Science*, **63**, 642–651.

Erwin, E. (1997). *Philosophy and psychotherapy: Razing the troubles of the brain*. Sage, Thousand Oaks, Ca.

Erwin, E. and Siegel, H. (1989). Is confirmation differential? *British Journal for the Philosophy of Science*, **40**, 105–119.

Evans, D. (2003). *Placebo: The belief effect*. HarperCollins, London.

Eysenck, H. ed. (1960). *Behaviour therapy and the neuroses*. Pergamon, New York.

Eysenck, H. (1965). The effects of psychotherapy. *International Journal of Psychiatry*, **1**, 97–168.

Eysenck, H. (1969). *The effects of psychotherapy*. Science House, New York.

Eysenck, H. (1985). *Decline and fall of the Freudian empire*. Penguin, London.

Eysenck, H. (1994). The outcome problem in psychotherapy: What have we learned? *Behavior Research and Therapy*, **32 (5)**, 477–495.

Faden, R.R. and Beauchamp, T.L. (1986). *A history and theory of informed consent*. Oxford University Press, Oxford.

Farrell, B.A. (1981). *The standing of psychoanalysis*. Oxford University Press, Oxford.

Faust, D. (1986). Research on human judgement and its application to clinical practice. *Professional Psychology: Research and Practice*, 17, 420–430.

Festinger, L. (1957). *A theory of cognitive dissonance*. Row, Peterson and Co., Evanston, Ill.

Fields, H.L. and Price, D.D. (1997). Toward a neurobiology of placebo analgesia. In A. Harrington, ed., *The placebo effect: An interdisciplinary exploration*, Harvard University Press, Cambridge, Mass. pp. 93–116.

Fine, A. and Forbes, M. (1986). Grünbaum on Freud: Three grounds for dissent. *Behavioral and Brain Sciences*, 9, 237–238.

Fingarette, H. (1969). *Self-deception*. Routledge and Kegan Paul, London.

Fish, S. (1986). Withholding the missing portion: Power, meaning, and persuasion in Freud's 'The Wolf Man'. *Times Literary Supplement*, August 29, 935A–938A.

Fisher, C.B. (2003). *Decoding the ethics code: A practical guide for psychologists*. Sage, Thousand Oaks, Ca.

Fisher, S. and Greenberg, L.P. (1977). *The scientific credibility of Freud's theory and therapy*. Basic Books, New York.

Flanagan, O. (1991). *Varieties of moral personality: Ethics and psychological realism*. Harvard University Press, Cambridge, Mass.

Frank, J.D. (1983). The placebo is psychotherapy. *Behavioral and Brain Sciences*, 6, 291–292.

Frank, J.D. and Frank, J.B. (1991). *Persuasion and healing* (3rd ed). Johns Hopkins University Press, Baltimore.

Frank, J.D. (1989). Non-specific aspects of treatment: The view of a psychotherapist. In M. Shepherd and N. Sartorius, eds., *Non-specific aspects of treatment*, pp. 95–114. H. Huber, Toronto.

Freedman, B. (1987). Equipoise and the ethics of clinical research. *New England Journal of Medicine*, 317(3), 141–145.

Freud, S. (1933). *New introductory lectures*. W.H.J. Sprott, trans. Norton, New York.

Freud, S. (1953–1974). *The standard edition of the complete psychological works of Sigmund Freud*. J. Strachey, ed. and trans. Hogarth Press, London.

Freud, S. (1954). *The origins of psychoanalysis*. E. Mosbacher and J. Strachey, trans. Basic Books, New York.

Freud, S. (1963a). *An outline of psychoanalysis*. J. Strachey, trans. Norton, New York.

Freud, S. (1963b). *Dora: An analysis of a case of hysteria*. P. Rieff, ed. Collier, New York.

Fromm, E. (1970). *The crisis of psychoanalysis*. Fawcett, Greenwich, Conn.

Frosch, J. (1990). *Psychodynamic psychiatry: Theory and practice*, vol. 3. International Universities Press, Madison, WI.

Gabbard, G.O. (1994). *Psychodynamic psychiatry in clinical practice: The DSM-IV edition*. American Psychiatric Press, Washington, DC.

Garb, H. (1989). Clinical judgment, clinical training, and professional experience. *Psychological Bulletin*, 105, 387–396.

Garb, H. (1996). The representativeness and past-behavior heuristics in clinical judgment. *Professional psychology: Research and practice*, 27, 272–277.

Garb, H. (1998). *Studying the clinician: Judgment research and psychological assessment*. American Psychological Association, Washington D.C.

Garb, H. and Boyle, P. (2003). Understanding why some clinicians use pseudoscientific methods: Findings from research on clinical judgment. In S.O. Lilienfeld, S.J. Lynn and J.M. Lohr, eds. *Science and pseudoscience in clinical psychology*. Guilford Press, New York. pp.17–38.

Gaylin, W. (2000). *Talk is not enough: How psychotherapy really works*. Little Brown, Boston.

Galton, F. (1886). Regression toward mediocrity in hereditary stature. *Journal of the Anthropological Institute*, 15, 246–263.

Garrison, F.H. (1921). *An introduction to the history of medicine* (3rd ed.) Saunders, Philadelphia.

Geertz, C. (1983). *Local knowledge: Further essays in interpretive anthropology*. Basic Books, New York.

Gheorghiu, V.A., Netter, P., Eysenck, H.J. and Rosenthal, R., eds., in collaboration with Fiedler K., Edmonston Jr. W.E., Lundy, R.M. and Sheehan, P.W. (1989). *Suggestion and suggestibility: Theory and research*. Springer-Verlag, Berlin.

Gheorghiu, V.A. (1989). The development of research on suggestibility. In V.A. Gheorghiu, P. Netter, H.J. Eysenck and R. Rosenthal, eds., in collaboration with K. Fiedler, W.E. Edmonston Jr., R.M. Lundy and P.W. Sheehan, *Suggestion and suggestibility: Theory and research*, Springer Verlag, Berlin. pp. 3–55.

Gibbons, F. and Hormuth, S.E. (1981). Motivational factors in placebo responsivity. *Psychopharmacology Bulletin*, 17, 77–79.

Gill, C. (1985). Ancient psychotherapy. *Journal of the History of Ideas*, 46, 307–325.

Glaser, S.R. (1979). Rhetoric and psychotherapy. In M.J. Mahoney, ed. *Psychotherapy process: Current issues and future directions*. Plenum Press, New York. pp. 313–333.

Gliedman, L.H., Gantt, W.H. and Teitlebaum, H.A. (1957). Some implications of conditional reflex studies for placebo research. *American Journal of Psychiatry*, 113, 1103–1107.

Glover, E. (1931). The therapeutic effect of inexact interpretation: A contribution to the theory of suggestion. *International Journal of Psycho-Analysis*, 12, 397–411.

Gold, H., Kwit, N.T. and Otto, H. (1937). The xanthines (theobromine and aminophylline) in the treatment of cardiac pain. *Journal of the American Medical Association*, 108, 2173–79.

Gold, H. (1946). Cornell conferences on therapy: The use of placebos in therapy. *New York State Journal of Medicine*, 46, 1718–27.

Gold, H. (1954). How to evaluate a new drug. *American Journal of Medicine*, 12, 619–20.

Gorski, A. and Spier, R., eds. (2004). *Placebos: Ethics and health care research*. Special edition of *Science and Engineering Ethics*, 10, no.1.

Greenberg, G. (2003). Is it Prozac? Or Placebo? *Mother Jones* (November/December), pp.78–81.

Greenberg, G. (2007). Manufacturing depression: A journey into the economy of melancholy. *Harpers* (May), pp. 35–46.

Greenwood, J. (1996). Freud's 'Tally' argument, placebo control treatments, and the evaluation of psychotherapy. *Philosophy of Science*, 63, 605–621.

Greenwood, J. (1997). Placebo control treatments and the evaluation of psychotherapy: A reply to Grünbaum and Erwin. *Philosophy of Science*, 64, 497–510.

Gribbin, M. (1981). Placebos: The cheapest medicine in the world. *New Scientist*, 89, 64–65.

Grove, W.M. and Meehl, P.E. (1996). Comparative efficiency of informal (subjective, impressionistic) and formal (mechanical, algorithmic) prediction procedures: The clinical–statistical controversy. *Psychology, Public Policy, and Law*, 2, 293–323.

Grünbaum, A. (1977). How scientific is psychoanalysis? In R. Stern, L.S. Horowitz and J. Lynes, eds. *Science and psychotherapy*. Haven Press, New York. pp. 219–254.

Grünbaum, A. (1984). *The foundations of psychoanalysis: A philosophical critique*. University of California Press, Berkeley, CA.

Grünbaum, A. (1986). The placebo concept in medicine and psychiatry. *Psychological Medicine*, 16, 19–38.

Grünbaum, A. (1993). *Validation in the clinical theory of psychoanalysis: A study in the philosophy of psychoanalysis*. International Universities Press, Madison, Conn.

Grünbaum, A. (1996). Empirical evaluations of theoretical explanations of psychotherapeutic efficacy: A reply to Greenwood. *Philosophy of Science*, 63, 605–621.

Guess, H.A., Kleinman, A., Kusek, J.W. and Engel, L., eds. (2002). *The science of the placebo: Toward an interdisciplinary research agenda*. BMJ, London.

Guignon, C. (1998). Narrative explanation in psychotherapy. *American Behavioral Scientist*, 41, 558–577.

Hadot, P. (1995). *Philosophy as a way of life*. A.I. Davidson, ed., and M. Chase, trans. Blackwell, Oxford.

Hacking, I. (1986). Making up people. In T.C. Heller, M. Sosa and D. Wellerby, eds. *Reconstructing individualism: Autonomy, individuality, and the self*, Stanford University Press, Stanford, CA. pp. 222–236.

Hacking, I. (1994). The looping effects of human kinds. In D. Sperber and A.J. Premack, eds. *Causal cognition*, Oxford University Press, Oxford. pp. 351–383.

Hacking, I. (1995). *Rewriting the soul: Multiple personality and the sciences of memory*. Princeton University Press, Princeton.

Hacking, I. (1998). *Mad travelers: Reflections on the reality of transient mental illnesses*. University of Virginia Press, Charlottesville, Virginia.

Hacking, I. (1999). *The social construction of what?* Harvard University Press, Cambridge, Mass.

Hahn, R.A. and Kleinman, A. (1983). Belief as pathogen, belief as medicine: 'Voodoo death' and the 'placebo phenomenon' in anthropological perspective. *Medical Anthropology Quarterly*, 4, 16–19.

Hahn, R.A. (1997). The nocebo phenomenon: Scope and foundations. In A. Harrington, ed. *The placebo effect: An interdisciplinary exploration*, Harvard University Press, Cambridge, Mass. pp. 56–76.

Hall, C.S. (1963). Strangers in dreams: An experimental confirmation of the Oedipus complex. *Journal of Personality*, 3, 336–345.

Harrington, A., ed. (1997). *The placebo effect: An interdisciplinary exploration*. Harvard University Press, Cambridge, Mass.

Harrington, A. (2002). Seeing the placebo effect: Historical legacies and present opportunities. In H.A. Guess, A. Kleinman, J.W. Kusek and L. Engel, eds. *The science of the placebo: Toward an interdisciplinary research agenda*, BMJ, London. pp. 35–52.

Healy, D. (1997). *The antidepressant era*. Harvard University Press, Cambridge, Mass.

Healy, D. (2004). *Let them eat Prozac: The unhealthy relationship between the pharmaceutical industry and depression*. New York University Press, New York.

Healy, D. and Doogan D.P., eds. (1996). *Psychotropic drug development: Social, economic, and pharmacological aspects.* Chapman and Hall Medical, New York.

Heine, R.W. (1953). A comparison of patients' reports on psychotherapeutic experience with psycho-analytic, non-directive, and Adlerian therapists. *American Journal of Psychotherapy,* 7, 16–23.

Held, B. (1995). *Back to reality: A critique of post-modern theory in therapy.* Norton, New York.

Held, B. (2007). *Psychology's interpretive turn: The search for truth and agency in theoretical and philosophical psychology.* American Psychological Association, Washington, D.C.

Herbert, J.D. and Gaudiano, B.A. (2005). Moving from empirically supported treatment lists to practice guidelines in psychotherapy: The role of the placebo concept. *Journal of Clinical Psychology,* 61, 893–908.

Hersch, E. L. (2003). *From philosophy to psychotherapy: A phenomenological model for psychology, psychiatry and psychoanalysis.* University of Toronto Press, Toronto.

Hill, A.B. (1963). Medical ethics and controlled trials. *British Medical Journal,* 1, 1043–1049.

Hill, C., Castonguay, L.G., Angus, L., *et al.* (2007). Insight in psychotherapy: Definitions, processes, consequences, and research directions. In L.G. Castonguay and C. Hill, *Insight in psychotherapy,* American Psychological Association, Washington, D.C. pp. 441–454.

Hines, T. (1988). *Pseudoscience and the paranormal.* Prometheus Books, New York.

Hippocrates (1979). *Decorum.* In *Hippocrates,* vol. 2, W.H.S. Jones, trans. Harvard University Press, Cambridge, Mass.

Hollender, M.H. and Ford, C.V. (1990). *Dynamic psychotherapy: An introductory approach.* American Psychiatric Press, Washington, D.C.

Holmes, O.W. (1883). *Medical essays.* Houghton Mifflin, Boston.

Horvath, P. (1988). Placebos and common factors in two decades of psychotherapy research. *Psychological Bulletin,* 104, 214–225.

Hume, D. (1748/1998). *An enquiry concerning human understanding.* Open Court, La Salle, IL.

Humphrey, N. (2002). Great expectations: The evolutionary psychology of faith healing and the placebo effect. In *The mind made flesh.* Oxford University Press, New York.

Hunsley, J. and Di Guilio, G. (2002). Dodo bird, phoenix, or urban legend? The question of psychotherapy equivalence. *The Scientific Review of Mental Health Practice,* 1, 11–19.

Hróbjartsson, A. and Gøtzsche, P. (2001). Is the placebo powerless? An analysis of clinical trials comparing placebo with no-treatment. *New England Journal of Medicine,* 344, 1594–1602.

Ingelfinger, F.J. (1972). Informed (but uneducated) consent. *New England Journal of Medicine,* 287, 465–466.

Jablensky, A. (1987). Multicultural studies and the nature of schizophrenia: A review. *Journal of the Royal Society of Medicine,* 80, 162–167.

Jacob, J.S. (1996). *The behavior cycle as a framework for dynamic psychotherapy.* Gardner Press, Lake Worth.

Jacobs, M. (1999). *Psychodynamic counselling in action,* 2nd ed. Sage, London.

Janet, P. (1894). Histoire d'une idée fixe. *Revue Philosophique,* 37, 121–168.

Janet, P. (1889). *L'automatisme psychologique.* Alcan, Paris.

Janet, P. (1904). L'amnésie et la dissociation des souvenirs par l'émotion. *Journal Psychologique*, **4**, 417–453.

Janet, P. (1909). Problèmes psychologique de l'émotion. *Revue Neurologique*, **17**, 1551–1687.

Janet, P. (1925). *Psychological healing: A historical and clinical study*. E. Paul and C. Paul, trans. MacMillan, New York.

Jerome, J.K. (1889/1964). *Three men in a boat–to say nothing of the dog*. Time Incorporated, New York.

Jones, J.H. and Tusgekee Institute (1981). *Bad blood: The Tuskegee syphilis experiment*. Free Press, New York.

Jones, R.A. (1977). *Self-fulfilling prophecies: Social, psychological and physiological effects of expectations*. Erlbaum, New Jersey.

Jopling, D.A. (1996a). Sub-phenomenology. *Human Studies*, **19**, 153–173.

Jopling, D.A. (1996b). 'Take away the life-lie': Positive illusions and creative self-deception. *Philosophical Psychology*, **9**, 525–544.

Jopling, D.A. (1998). 'First do no harm': Over-philosophizing and pseudo-philosophizing in philosophical counselling. *Inquiry: Critical Thinking Across the Disciplines*, **17**, 100–112.

Jopling, D.A. (2000). *Self-knowledge and the self*. Routledge, New York.

Jopling, D.A. (2001). Placebo insight. *Journal of Clinical Psychology*, **57**, 19–36.

Kahneman, D., Slovic, P., and Tversky, A., eds. (1982). *Judgment under uncertainty: Heuristics and biases*. Cambridge University Press, New York.

Kaptchuk, T.J. (1998a). Powerful placebo: The dark side of the randomised controlled trial. *The Lancet*, **351**, 1722–1725.

Kaptchuk, T.J. (1998b). Intentional ignorance: A history of blind assessment and placebo controls in medicine. *Bulletin of the History of Medicine*, **72**, 389–433.

Kaptchuk, T.J. (2002). The placebo effect in alternative medicine: Can the performance of a healing ritual have clinical significance? *Annals of Internal Medicine*, **136**, 817–825.

Kazdin, A. (1981). Drawing valid inference from case studies. *Journal of Consulting and Clinical Psychology*, **49**, 183–192.

Keck, P.E. Jr., Welge, J.A., McElroy, S.L., *et al.* (2000). Placebo effect in randomized, controlled studies of acute bipolar mania and depression. *Biological Psychiatry*, **47**, 748–755.

Kendler, K.S., Walters, E.E. and Kessler, R.C. (1997). The prediction of length of major depressive episodes: Results from an epidemiological survey of female twins. *Psychological Medicine*, **27**, 107–117.

Khan, A., Warner, H.A., and Brown, W.A. (2000). Symptom reduction and suicide risk in patients treated with placebo in antidepressant clinical trials: An analysis of the Food and Drug Administration database. *Archives of General Psychiatry*, **57**, 311–317.

Kiene, H. (1993a). A critique of the double-blind clinical trial: Part 1. *Alternative Therapies*, **2(1)**, 74–80.

Kiene, H. (1993b). A critique of the double-blind clinical trial: Part 2. *Alternative Therapies*, **2(2)**, 59–64.

Kienle, G.S. and Kiene, H. (1997). The powerful placebo effect: Fact or fiction? *Journal of Clinical Epidemiology*, **50**, 1311–1318.

Kihlstrom, J.F. (2003). Expecting that a treatment will be given when it won't and knowing that a treatment is being given when it is. *Prevention and Treatment*, **6**(1), 4.

Kim, S. (2003). Benefits and burdens of placebos in psychiatric research. *Psychopharmacology*, **171**, 13–18.

Kirsch, I. (1985). Response expectancy as a determinant of experience and behavior. *American Psychologist*, **40**, 1189–1202.

Kirsch, I. (1997). Specifying nonspecifics: Psychological mechanisms of placebo effects. In A. Harrington, ed. *The placebo effect: An interdisciplinary exploration*, Harvard University Press, Cambridge, Mass. pp. 166–186.

Kirsch, I., ed. (1999). *How expectancies shape experience*. American Psychological Association, Washington, DC.

Kirsch, I. (2003). Hidden administration as ethical alternatives to balanced placebo design. *Prevention and Treatment*, **6**, Article 5. Available on the World Wide Web at: http://journals. apa.org/prevention/volume6

Kirsch, I. (2005). Placebo psychotherapy: Synonym or oxymoron? *Journal of Clinical Psychology*, **61**, 791–803.

Kirsch, I. and Baker, S.L. (1993). Clinical implications of expectancy research: Activating placebo effects without deception. *Contemporary Hypnosis*, **10**, 130–2.

Kirsch, I. and Sapirstein, G. (1998). Listening to Prozac but hearing placebo: A meta-analysis of antidepressant medication. *Prevention and Treatment*, **1**, Article 0002a. Available on the World Wide Web: http://www.journals.apa.org/prevention/volume1/pre0010002a.html#c22

Kirsch, I., Moore, T.J., Scoboria, A. and Nicholls, S.S. (2002). The emperor's new drugs: An analysis of antidepressant medication data submitted to the U.S. Food and Drug Administration. *Prevention and Treatment*, **5**, Article 23.

Kleinman, A., Guess, H.A. and Wilentz, J.S. (2002). An overview. In H.A. Guess, A. Kleinman, J.W. Kusek, and L. Engel, eds. *The science of the placebo: Towards an interdisciplinary research agenda*, BMJ, London. pp. 1–32.

Knight, R.P. (1952). An Evaluation of psychotherapeutic techniques. *Bulletin of the Menninger Clinic*, **16**, 113–124. Reprinted in R.P. Knight (1972). *Clinician and therapist: Selected papers of Robert P. Knight*. S.C. Miller, ed. Basic Books, New York.

Koehler, J.J. (1996). The base rate fallacy reconsidered: Descriptive, normative, and methodological challenges. *Behavioral and Brain Sciences*, **19**, 1–53.

Koocher, G.P. and Keith-Spiegel, P., eds. (1998). *Ethics in psychology: Professional standards and cases*, vol.3. Oxford University Press, New York.

Kotin, J. (1995). *Getting started: An introduction to dynamic psychotherapy*. Jason Aronson, Northvale.

Kottler, J.A. and Brown, R.W. (1999). *Introduction to therapeutic counseling: Voices from the field*, 4th ed. Brooks/Cole Thomson Learning, Belmont, CA.

Kramer, P. (1993). *Listening to Prozac*. Penguin, New York.

Kris, E. (1956). On some vicissitudes of insight in psycho-analysis. *International Journal of Psycho-Analysis*, **37**, 445–455.

Kubie, L.S. (1975). *Practical and theoretical aspects of psychoanalysis*. 2nd revised edition. International Universities Press, New York.

Lain Entralgo, P. (1970). *The therapy of the word in classical antiquity*. L.J. Rather and J.M. Sharp, trans. Yale University Press, New Haven.

Lambert. M.J. (2005). Early response in psychotherapy: Further evidence for the importance of common factors rather than placebo effects. *Journal of Clinical Psychology*,
61, 855–869.

Lambert, M.J. and Barley, D.E. (2001). Research summary on the therapeutic relationship
and psychotherapy outcome. *Psychotherapy*, **38**, 357–361.

Last, J.M., ed. (1988). *A dictionary of epidemiology*, 2nd ed. Oxford University Press, New York.

Leff, J. (1986). Epidemiology of mental illness across cultures. In J. Cox, ed., *Transcultural
psychiatry*, Croom Helm, London. pp. 23–36.

Lesse, S. (1980). Sources of individual and group decompensation in our future society:
a psychosocial projection. *American Journal of Psychotherapy*, **34**, 308–321.

Lévi-Strauss, C. (1963). *Structural anthropology*. Basic Books, New York.

Levine, J.D., Gordon, N.C. and Fields, H.L. (1978). The mechanism of placebo analgesia.
The Lancet, **2**, 654–657.

Lewis, J.A., Jonsson, B., Kreutz, G., Sampaio, C. and van Zwieten-Boot, B. (2002). Placebo-
controlled trials and the *Declaration of Helsinki. The Lancet*, **359**, 1337–1340.

Lewis, S. (1980). *Arrowsmith*. New American Library, Scarborough, ON.

Lieberman, L.R. and Dunlap, J.T. (1979). On O'Leary and Borkovec's conceptualization of
placebo: The placebo paradox. *American Psychologist*, **34**, 553–554.

Lilienfeld, S.O., Lynn, S.J. and Lohr, J.M., eds. (2003a). *Science and pseudo-science in clinical
psychology*. Guilford Press, New York.

Lilienfeld, S.O., Lynn, S.J. and Lohr, J.M. (2003b). Science and pseudoscience in clinical
psychology. In S.O. Lilienfeld, S.J. Lynn, and J.M. Lohr, eds. *Science and pseudo-science
in clinical psychology*, Guilford Press, New York. pp. 1–14.

Lin, K.-M. and Kleinman, A. (1988). Psychopathology and clinical course of schizophrenia:
A cross-cultural perspective. *Schizophrenia Bulletin*, **14**, 555–567.

Linde, C., Gadler, F., Kappenberger, L., and Ryden, L. (1999). Placebo effect of pacemaker
implantation in obstructive hypertrophic cardiomyopathy. PIC Study Group. Pacing in
cardiomyopathy. *American Journal of Cardiology*, **83**, 903–907.

Loftus, E. and Fries, J.F. (1979). Informed consent may be hazardous to health. *Science*, **204**, 11.

Loftus, E. (1993). The reality of repressed memories. *American Psychologist*, **48**, 518–537.

Loftus, E, Donders, K., Hoffman, H.G. and Schooler, J.W. (1989a). Creating new memories
that are quickly accessed and confidently held. *Memory and Cognition*, **17**, 607–616.

Loftus, E., Korf, N. and Schooler, J.W. (1989b). Misguided memories: Sincere distortions of
reality. In J. Yuille, ed. *Credibility assessment: A theoretical and research perspective*,
Kluwer, Boston. pp. 155–74.

Loftus, E. and Ketchum, K. (1994). *The myth of repressed memory: False memory and
allegations of sexual abuse*. St. Martin's Press, New York.

Luborsky, L., Singer, B. and Luborsky, L. (1975). Comparative studies of psychotherapies:
Is it true that 'Everyone has won and all must have prizes'? *Archives of General
Psychiatry*, **32**, 995–1008.

Luborsky, L., Crits-Christoph, P., Mclellan, A.T., *et al.* (1986). Do therapists vary much in
their success? Findings from four outcome studies. *American Journal of
Orthopsychiatry*, **56**, 501–511.

Ludwig, A.M. (1966). The formal characteristics of therapeutic insight. *American Journal
of Psychotherapy*, **20**, 305–318.

Mahrer, A. (1989). *The integration of psychotherapies*. New York, Human Sciences Press.

Malcolm, J. (1980). *Psychoanalysis: The impossible profession*. Picador, London.

Marlatt, G.A. and Rohsenow, D.J. (1980). Cognitive processes in alcohol use: Expectancy and the balanced placebo design. In N.K. Mello, ed. *Advances in substance abuse: Behavioral and biological research*, JAI Press, Greenwich, CT. pp. 159–199.

Marmor, J. (1962). Psychoanalytic therapy as an educational process. In J. Masserman, ed. *Psychoanalytic education*, Grune and Stratton, New York. pp. 286–289.

Marmor, J. (1970). Limitations of free association. *Archives of General Psychiatry,* **22**, 160–165.

Marmor, J. (1980). Recent trends in psychotherapy. *American Journal of Psychiatry*, **137**, 409–416.

Marshall, M.F. (2004). The placebo effect in popular culture. *Science and Engineering Ethics*, **10**, 37–42.

Martin, M., ed. (1985). *Self-deception and self-understanding: New essays in philosophy and psychology*. University of Kansas Press, Lawrence, KS.

Mays, D.T. and Franks, C.M. (1985). *Negative outcomes in psychotherapy*. Springer, New York.

McDonald, C.J., Mazzuca, S.A. and McCabe, G.P. (1983). How much of the placebo effect is really statistical regression? *Statistical Medicine*, **2**, 417–427.

McLaughlin, B.P. and Rorty, A.O., eds. (1988). *Perspectives on self-deception*. University of California Press, Berkeley, CA.

McLeod, J.D., Kessler, R.C. and Landis, K.R. (1992). Speed of recovery from major depressive episodes in a community sample of married men and women. *Journal of Abnormal Psychology*, **101**, 227–286.

Medawar, P. (1967). *The art of the soluble*. Methuen, London.

Meehl, P. (1953). *Clinical versus statistical prediction: A theoretical analysis and a review of the evidence*. University of Minnesota Press, Minneapolis, MN.

Meehl, P.E. (1955). Psychotherapy. *Annual Review of Psychology*, **6**, 357–78.

Meehl, P.E. (1978). Theoretical risks and tabular asterisks: Sir Karl, Sir Ronald, and the slow progress of soft psychology. *Journal of Consulting and Clinical Psychology*, **46**, 806–834.

Meehl, P.E. (1983). Subjectivity in psychoanalytic inference: The nagging persistence of Wilhelm Fliess's Achensee question. In J. Earman, ed. *Testing scientific theories: Minnesota studies in the philosophy of science*, **10**, University of Minnesota Press, Minneapolis, MN. pp. 349–411.

Meehl, P.E. (1990). Appraising and amending theories: The strategy of Lakatosian defense and two principles that warrant it. *Psychological Inquiry* **1**, 108–141.

Meehl, P.E. (1995). Commentary: Psychoanalysis as science. *Journal of the American Psychoanalytic Association*, **43**(4), 1015–1021.

Mele, A. (1997). Real self-deception. *Behavioral and Brain Sciences*, **20**, 91–136.

Melmed, R.N., Roth, D., Beer, G. and Edelstein, E.L. (1986). Montaigne's insight: Placebo effect and symptom anticipation are two sides of the same coin. *The Lancet*, **20/27**, 1448–1449.

Mendel, W. (1964). The phenomenon of interpretation. *American Journal of Psychiatry*, **24**, 184–189.

Messer, S.B. and Warren, C.S. (1995). *Models of brief psychodynamic therapy: A comparative approach*. Guilford Press, New York.

Messer, S.B. and McWilliams, N. (2007). Insight in psychodynamic therapy: Theory and assessment. In L.G. Castonguay and C. Hill, eds. *Insight in psychotherapy*, American Psychological Association, Washington, DC. pp.9–29.

Moerman, D.E. (1983). General medical effectiveness and human biology: Placebo effects in the treatment of ulcer disease. *Medical Anthropology Quarterly*, **14**, 13–16.

Moerman, D.E. (2002a). *Meaning, medicine and the 'placebo effect.'* Cambridge University Press, Cambridge.

Moerman, D.E. (2002b). The meaning response and the ethics of avoiding placebos. *Evaluation and the Health Professions*, **25**, 399–409.

Moerman, D.E. and Jonas, W.B. (2002c). Deconstructing the placebo effect and finding the meaning response. *Annals of Internal Medicine*, **136**, 471–476.

de Montaigne, M. (2003). *The complete essays*. M.A. Screech, trans. Penguin, London.

Montgomery, G. and Kirsch, I. (1996). Mechanisms of placebo pain reduction: An empirical investigation. *Psychological Science*, **7**, 174–176.

Moore, B.E. and Fine, B.D., eds. (1968). *A glossary of psychoanalytic terms and concepts*. American Psychoanalytic Association, New York.

Morgan, R.W., Luborsky, L., Crits-Christoph, P., *et al.* (1982). Predicting the outcomes of psychotherapy using the Penn Helping Alliance rating method. *Archives of General Psychiatry*, **39**, 397–402.

Moseley, J.B., O'Malley, K., Petersen, N.J., *et al.* (2002). A controlled trial of arthroscopic surgery for osteoarthritis of the knee. *New England Journal of Medicine*, **347**, 81–88.

Murray, C.J.L. and Lopez, A.D. (1996). *The global burden of disease: A comprehensive assessment of mortality and disability from diseases, injuries, and risk factors in 1990 and projected to 2020*. Harvard University Press, Cambridge, Mass.

Murray, C.J.L. (1996). Rethinking DALYs. In C.J.L. Murray and A.D. Lopez, *The global burden of disease: A comprehensive assessment of mortality and disability from diseases, injuries, and risk factors in 1990 and projected to 2020*. Harvard University Press, Cambridge, Mass.

Naftulin, D., Donnelly, F. and Wolkon, G. (1975). Four therapeutic approaches to the same patient. *American Journal of Psychotherapy*, **29**, 66–71.

Nau, S., Caputo, J. and Borkovec, T. (1974). The relationship between therapy credibility and simulated therapy response. *Journal of Behavioral Therapy and Experimental Psychiatry*, **5**, 129–133.

Neisser, U. ed. (1987). *Concepts and conceptual development: Ecological and intellectual factors in categorization*. Cambridge University Press, New York.

Neisser, U. (1988). Five kinds of self-knowledge. *Philosophical Psychology*, **1**, 35–59.

Neisser, U. ed. (1994a). *The perceived self*. Cambridge University Press, New York.

Neisser, U. (1994b). Self-narratives: True and false. In U. Neisser and R. Fivush, eds. *The remembering self: Construction and accuracy in the self-narrative*, Cambridge University Press, New York. pp. 1–18.

Neisser, U. and Fivush R., eds. (1994). *The remembering self: Construction and accuracy in the self-narrative*. Cambridge University Press, New York.

Neisser, U. and Jopling, D.A., eds. (1997). *The conceptual self in context: Culture, experience, self-understanding*. Cambridge University Press, New York.

Neu, J. (1977). *Emotion, thought, and therapy*. Routledge and Kegan Paul, London.

Neuberger, M. (1932). *The doctrine of the healing power of nature throughout the course of time*. L.J. Boyd, trans. *Journal of the American Institute of Homeopathy*, **25**.

Nichols, M. and Paolino, T. (1986). *Basic techniques of psychodynamic psychotherapy*. Jason Aronson, Northvale, NJ.

Nietzsche, F. (1886/1966). *Beyond good and evil*. W. Kaufmann, trans. Vintage Press, New York.

Nietzsche, F. (1968). *The will to power*. W. Kaufmann and R.J. Hollingdale, trans. Vintage Press, New York.

Nies, A. (1990). Principles of therapeutics. In A.G. Gilman, T.W. Rall, A.S. Nies and P. Taylor, eds. *Goodman and Gilman's The pharmacological basis of therapeutics*, 8th ed. Pergamon Press, New York.

Nisbett, R.E. and Wilson, T.D. (1977). Telling more than we can know: Verbal reports on mental processes. *Psychological Review*, **84**, 231–259.

Nisbett, R.E. and Ross, L. (1980). *Human inference: Strategies and shortcomings of social judgement*. Prentice Hall, Englewood Cliffs, NJ.

Nussbaum, M. (1994). *The therapy of desire: Theory and practice in Hellenistic ethics*. Princeton University Press, Princeton, NJ.

Ober, K.P. (2003). *Mark Twain and medicine: Any mummery will cure*. University of Missouri Press, MO.

O'Brian, P. (1998). *The Hundred Days*. W.W. Norton, New York.

O'Donohue, K. and Ferguson, K.E., eds. (2003). *Handbook of professional ethics for psychologists: Issues, questions, controversies*. Sage, Thousand Oaks, CA.

Oh, V.M.S. (2004). The placebo effect: Can we use it better? *British Medical Journal*, **309**, 69–70.

O'Leary, K.D. and Borkovec, T.D. (1978). Conceptual, methodological, and ethical problems of placebo groups in psychotherapy research. *American Psychologist*, **33**, 821–830.

O'Neill, E. (1946). *The iceman cometh*. Vintage Books, New York.

O'Neill, O. (1989). Paternalism and partial autonomy. In P.Y. Windt, P.C. Appleby, M.P. Battin *et al*., eds. *Ethical issues in the professions*. Prentice Hall, Englewood Cliffs, NJ.

Paris, J.A. (1843). *Pharmacologia: Being an extended inquiry into the operations of medicinal bodies, upon which are founded the theory and art of prescribing*. 9th ed. Samuel Highley, London.

Parloff, M.B. (1986a). Frank's 'common elements' in psychotherapy: Nonspecific factors and placebos. *American Journal of Orthopsychiatry*, **56**, 521–530.

Parloff, M.B. (1986b). Placebo controls in psychotherapy research: A sine qua non or a placebo for research problems? *Journal of Consulting and Clinical Psychology*, **54**, 79–87.

Park, L.C. and Covi, L. (1965). Nonblind placebo trial: An exploration of neurotic outpatients' response to placebo when its inert content is disclosed. *Archives of General Psychiatry*, **12**, 336–345.

Pascal, B. (1966). *Pensées*. A.J. Krailsheimer, trans. Penguin, Harmondsworth, U.K.

Paul, G.L. (1966). *Insight versus desensitization in psychotherapy*. Stanford University Press, Stanford.

Paul, I.M., Yoder, K.E., Crowell, K.R. *et al*. (2004). Effect of dextromethorphan, diphenhydramine, and placebo on nocturnal cough and sleep quality for coughing children and their parents. *Pediatrics*, **114**, 85–90.

Percival, T. (1803/1975). *Medical ethics*. Robert Krieger, New York.

Peters, D, ed. (2001). *Understanding the placebo effect in contemporary medicine*. Churchill Livingstone/Harcourt, London.

Pennebaker, J.W. (1997). *Opening up: The healing power of expressing emotions*. Revised edition. Guilford Press, New York.

Pfeffer, A.Z. (1959). A procedure for evaluating the results of psychoanalysis. *American Journal of Psychoanalysis*, 3, 418–458.

Phares, E.J. (1980). *Clinical psychology: Concepts, methods, and profession*. 3rd ed. Dorsey Press, Chicago.

Piatelli-Palmerini, M. (1994). *Inevitable illusions: How mistakes of reason rule our minds*. John Wiley, New York.

Piper, W.E., Joyce, A.S., McCallum, M. and Azim, H.F. (1998). Interpretive and supportive forms of psychotherapy and patient personality variables. *Journal of Consulting and Clinical Psychology*, 66, 558–567.

Plato (1961). *Charmides*. B. Jowett, trans. In E. Hamilton and H. Cairns, eds., *The complete dialogues of Plato*. Princeton University Press, Princeton.

Pocock, S. (2002). The pros and cons of non-inferiority (equivalence) trials. In H.A. Guess, A. Kleinman, J.W. Kusak, and L.W. Engel, eds. *The Science of the Placebo: Toward an interdisciplinary research agenda*, BMJ, London. pp. 236–248.

Pope, K.S., Melba, J. and Vasquez, T. (2001). *Ethics in psychotherapy and counselling: A practical guide*. Jossey Bass/John Wiley, San Fransisco.

Popper, K. (1963). *Conjectures and refutations*. Routledge and Kegan Paul, London.

Prentice, D.A., Gerrig, R.J., and D.S. Bailis (1997). What readers bring to the processing of fictional texts. *Psychonomic Bulletin and Review*, 4: 416–420.

Prentice, D.A. and Gerrig, R.J. (1999). Exploring the boundary between fiction and reality. In S. Chaiken and Y. Trope, eds. *Dual process theories in social psychology*. Guilford, New York.

Prioleau, L., Murdock, M. and Brody, N. (1983). An analysis of psychotherapy versus placebo studies. *Behavioral and Brain Sciences*, 6, 275–310.

Radden, J. (2000). From melancholic states to clinical depression. In J. Radden, ed. *The nature of melancholy*, Oxford University Press, Oxford. pp. 3–51.

Rangell, L. (1981). From insight to change. *Journal of the American Psychoanalytic Association*, 29, 119–141.

Rangell, L. (1992). The psychoanalytic theory of change. *International Journal of Psycho-Analysis*, 73, 415–428.

Rawlinson, M.C. (1985). Truth-telling and paternalism in the clinic: Philosophical reflections on the use of placebos in medical practice. In L. White, B. Tursky and G.E. Schwartz, eds. *Placebo: Theory, research, and mechanisms*, Guilford Press, New York. pp. 403–418.

Rich, B. (2003). A placebo for the pain: A medico–legal case analysis. *Pain Medicine*, 4, 366–372.

Richfield, J. (1954). An analysis of the concept of insight. *Psychoanalytic Quarterly*, 62, 553–571.

Ricoeur, P. (1970). *Freud and philosophy: An essay in interpretation*. D. Savage, trans. Yale University Press, New Haven, CT.

Roback, H. (1974). Insight: A bridging of the theoretical and research literatures. *Journal of the Canadian Psychologist*, 15, 61–89.

Roberts, L.W., Lauriello, J., Geppert, C. and Kieth, S.J. (2001). Placebos and paradoxes in psychiatric research: An ethics perspective. *Biological Psychiatry*, 49, 887–893.

Robinson, L.A., Berman, J.S. and Neimeyer, R.A. (1990). Psychotherapy for the treatment of depression. *Psychological Bulletin*, 108, 30–49.

Rorty, A.O. (1975). Adaptivity and self-knowledge. *Inquiry,* **18,** 1–22.

Rorty, A.O. (1988). The deceptive self: Liars, layers, and lairs. In B.P. McLaughlin and A.O. Rorty, eds. *Perspectives on self-deception,* University of California Press, Berkeley, CA. pp. 11–28.

Rorty, A.O. (1994). User-friendly self-deception. *Philosophy,* **69,** 211–228.

Rosen, R.D. (1977). *Psychobabble: Fast talk and quick cure in the era of feeling.* Atheneum, New York.

Rosenthal, D. and Frank, J.D. (1956). Psychotherapy and the placebo effect. *Psychological Bulletin,* **53,** 294–302.

Rosenthal, R. and Fode, K.L. (1963). The effect of experimenter bias on the performance of the albino rat. *Behavioral Science,* **8,** 183–189.

Rosenthal, R. (1976). *Experimenter effects in behavioral research.* Enlarged edition. Irvington, New York.

Rosenberg, N.K., Mellergard, M., Rosenberg, R., Beck, P. and Ottoson, J.O. (1991). Characteristics of panic disorder patients responding to placebo. *Acta Psychiatrica Scandinavia Supplement,* **365,** 33–38.

Ross, M. and Olson, J.M. (1981). An expectancy-attribution model of the effects of placebo. *Psychological Review,* **88,** 408–437.

Rothman, K.J. and Michels, K.B. (1994). The continuing unethical use of placebo controls. *New England Journal of Medicine,* **331,** 394–398.

Rothman, K.J. and Michels, K.B. (2002). When is it appropriate to use a placebo arm in a trial? In H.A. Guess, A. Kleinman, J.W. Kusak and L.W. Engel, eds. *The science of the placebo: Toward an interdisciplinary research agenda,* BMJ, London. pp. 227–235.

Rutan, J.S. and Stone, W.N. (1993). *Psychodynamic group psychotherapy.* 2nd ed. Guilford Press, New York.

Sartorious, N., Jablensky, A., Korten, A., *et al.* (1986). Early manifestations and first-contact incidence of schizophrenia in different cultures. *Psychological Medicine,* **16,** 909–928.

Sartre, J.P. (1943/1969). *Being and nothingness.* H. Barnes, trans. Methuen, London.

Schachter, S. and Singer, J.E. (1962). Cognitive, social, and physiological determinants of emotional state. *Psychological Review,* **69,** 379–399.

Schumaker, J.F., ed. (1991). *Human suggestibility: Advances in theory, research, and application.* Routledge, New York.

Schafer, R. (1981). *Narrative actions in psychoanalysis.* Clark University Press, Worcester, MA.

Schafer, R. (1992). *Retelling a life: Narration and dialogue in psychoanalysis.* Basic Books, New York.

Schwartz, N. (1999). Self-reports: How the questions shape the answers. *American Psychologist,* **54,** 93–105.

Schwartz, H. and Sudman, S., eds. (1992). *Context effects in social and psychological research.* Springer Verlag, New York.

Schwartz, H. and Sudman, S. (1994). *Autobiographical memory and the validity of retrospective reports.* Springer Verlag, New York.

Schwartz, H. and Sudman, S. (1996). *Answering questions: Methodology for determining cognitive and communicative processes in survey research.* Jossey Bass, San Francisco, CA.

Segal, H. (1962). The curative factors in psychoanalysis. *International Journal of Psychoanalysis,* **43,** 212–217.

Senn, S.J. (1988). How much of the placebo 'effect' is really statistical regression? *Statistics in Medicine*, **7(11)**, 1203.

Shapiro, A.K. (1964). Etiological factors in placebo effect. *Journal of the American Medical Association*, **187**, 712–715.

Shapiro, A.K. (1968). Semantics of the placebo. *Psychological Quarterly*, **42**, 653–695.

Shapiro, A.K. (1969). Iatroplacebogenics. *International Pharmacopsychiatry*, **2**, 215–248.

Shapiro, A.K. (1971). Placebo effects in medicine, psychotherapy, and psychoanalysis. In A.E. Bergin and S.L. Garfield, eds. *Handbook of psychotherapy and behavior change: An empirical analysis*, Wiley, New York. pp. 439–473.

Shapiro, A.K., Shapiro, E., Bruun, R., and Sweet, R. (1978). *Gilles de la Tourette syndrome*. Raven Press, New York.

Shapiro, A.K. and Morris, L. (1978). The placebo effect in medical and psychological therapies. In S. Garfield and A. Bergin, eds. *Handbook of psychotherapy and behavior change: An empirical analysis*. 2nd ed., John Wiley, New York. pp. 369–410.

Shapiro, A.K. and Shapiro, E. (1997a). The placebo: Is it much ado about nothing? In A. Harrington, ed. *The placebo effect: An interdisciplinary exploration*, Harvard University Press, Cambridge, Mass. pp. 12–36.

Shapiro, A.K. and Shapiro, E. (1997b). *The powerful placebo: From ancient priest to modern physician*. Johns Hopkins University Press, Baltimore and London.

Shaw, G.B. (1911/1941). *The Doctor's Dilemma*. Dodd, Meed, New York.

Simmons, B. (1978). Problems in deceptive medical procedures: An ethical and legal analysis of the administration of placebos. *Journal of Medical Ethics*, **4**, 172–181.

Singer, M.T. and Nievod, A. (2003). New age therapies. In S.O. Lilienfeld, S.J. Lynn and J.M. Lohr, eds. *Science and pseudoscience in clinical psychology*, Guilford Press, New York. pp. 176–204.

Skinner, B.F. (1971). *Beyond freedom and dignity*. Bantam Books, New York.

Smith, M.L., Glass, G.V. and Miller, T.I. (1980). *The benefits of psychotherapy*. Johns Hopkins University Press, Baltimore, MD.

Snyder, C., Shenkel, R. and Lowery, C. (1977). Acceptance of personality interpretations: The 'Barnum effect' and beyond. *Journal of Consulting and Clinical Psychology*, **45**, 104–114.

Sokal, A. (1996). Transgressing the boundaries: Towards a transformative hermeneutics of quantum gravity. *Social Text*, **46/47**, 217–252.

Sokal, A. and Bricmont, J. (1998). *Fashionable nonsense: Postmodern intellectuals' abuse of science*. Picador, New York.

Spence, D. (1982). *Narrative truth and historical truth: Meaning and interpretation in psychoanalysis*. W.W. Norton, New York.

Spinoza, B. (1677/1992). *The ethics; Treatise on the emendation of the intellect; and selected letters*. S. Shirley, trans. Hackett, Indianapolis, IN.

Strachey, J. (1934). The nature of the therapeutic action of psycho-analysis. *International Journal of Psychoanalysis*, **15**, 127–159.

Strawson, G. (2004). Against narrativity. *Ratio, XVII*, **4**, 428–452.

Strupp, H.H. (1972a). Needed: A reformulation of the psychotherapeutic influence. *International Journal of Psychiatry*, **10**, 114–120.

Strupp, H.H. (1972b). On the technology of psychotherapy. *Archives of General Psychiatry*, **26**, 270–278.

Strupp, H.H. (1973). 'Spontaneous' remission and the nature of the therapeutic influence. (*What is Psychotherapy? Proceedings of the 9th International Congress of Psychotherapy, Oslo*). *Psychotherapy Psychosomatics,* **24,** 389–393.

Strupp, H.H. (1979). Specific versus non-specific factors in psychotherapy. *Archives of General Psychiatry,* **36,** 1125–36.

Strupp, H.H. and Luborsky, L., eds. (1962). *Research in psychotherapy.* American Psychological Association, Washington, D.C.

Strupp, H.H., Hadley, H. and Gomes-Schwartz, B. (1977). *Psychotherapy for better or worse: The problem of negative effects.* Aronson, New York.

Strupp, H.H. and Binder, J.L. (1984). *Psychotherapy in a new key: A guide to time-limited dynamic psychotherapy.* Basic Books, New York.

Suh, C.S., O'Malley, S., Strupp, H.H., and Johnson, M.E. (1989). The Vanderbilt psychotherapy process scale (VPPS). *Journal of Cognitive Psychotherapy,* **3,** 123–53.

Sullivan, B.S. (2001). Christina. In D. Wedding and R.J. Corsini, eds. *Case studies in psychotherapy.* 3rd edition, F.E. Peacock, Itasca, IL. pp. 49–56.

Sundberg, N.D. (1966). The acceptability of 'fake' versus bona fide personality test interpretations. *Journal of Abnormal Social Psychology,* **50,** 145–147.

Sundland, D.M. (1977). Theoretical orientations of psychotherapies. In A.S. Gurman and A.M. Razin, eds. *Effective psychotherapy: A handbook of research,* Pergamon, New York. pp. 189–219.

Svartberg, M. and Stiles, T. (1991). Comparative effects of short-term psychodynamic psychotherapy: A meta-analysis. *Journal of Consulting and Clinical Psychology,* **59,** 704–714.

Talbot, M. (2000). The placebo prescription. *New York Times Magazine,* 1. September, 34–43.

Taylor, S. and Brown, J. (1988). Illusion and well-being: A social–psychological perspective on mental health. *Psychological Bulletin,* **103,** 193–210.

Taylor, S. (1989). *Positive illusions: Creative self-deception and the healthy mind.* Basic Books, New York.

Temple, R.J. (2002). Placebo controlled trials and active controlled trials. In H.A. Guess, A. Kleinman, J.W. Kusak, and L.W. Engel, eds. *The science of the placebo: Toward an interdisciplinary research agenda,* BMJ, London. pp. 209–226.

Thomä, H. (1977). 'Psychanalyse und Suggestion'. *Zeitschrift für psychosomatische medizin und psychoanalyse,* **23,** 35–56.

Tolor, A. and Reznikoff, M. (1960). A new approach to insight. *Journal of Nervous and Mental Disease,* **130,** 286–296.

Torrey, E.F. (1980). *Schizophrenia and civilization.* Aronson, New York.

Torrey, E.F. (1986). *Witch doctors and psychiatrists: The common roots of psychiatry and its future.* Harper and Row, New York.

Torrey, E.F. (1987). Prevalence studies in schizophrenia. *British Journal of Psychiatry,* **150,** 598–608.

Tversky, A. and Kahneman, D. (1974). Judgment under uncertainty: Heuristics and biases. *Science,* **184,** 1124–1131.

Tversky, A. and Kahneman, D. (1982). Judgments of and by representativeness. In D. Kahneman, P. Slovic and A. Tversky, eds. *Judgment under uncertainty: Heuristics and biases,* Cambridge University Press, New York. pp. 84–98.

Ulrich, R., Stachnik, T., and Stainton, R. (1963). Student acceptance of generalized personality interpretations. *Psychological Reports*, **13**, 831–834.

U.S. Food and Drug Administration (2002). *Guidance for industry: E10 choice of control group and related issues in clinical trials*. Available on the World Wide Web at: http://www.fda.gov/cder/guidance/4155fnl.htm#P498_68732

Valenstein, A.F. (1962). The psychoanalytical situation: Affects, emotional reliving, and insight in the psycho-analytic process. *International Journal of Psychoanalysis*, **43**, 315–24.

van der Kolk, B., Brown, P., and van der Hart, O. (1989a). Pierre Janet on post-traumatic stress. *Journal of Traumatic Stress*, **2**, 365–378.

van der Kolk, B., and van der Hart, O. (1989b). Pierre Janet and the breakdown of adaptation in psychological trauma. *American Journal of Psychiatry*, **146**, 1530–1540.

van der Hart, O., Brown, P., and van der Kolk, B. (1989c). Pierre Janet's treatment of post-traumatic stress. *Journal of Traumatic Stress*, **2**, 379–395.

van Rillaer, J. (1991). Strategies of dissimulation in the pseudosciences. *New Ideas in Psychology*, **9**, 235–244.

Vaughan, S.C. (1997). *The talking cure: The science behind psychotherapy*. G.P. Putnam's and Sons, New York.

Veatch, R.M. (1972). Models for medical ethics in a revolutionary age. *Hastings Center Reports*, **2**, 5–7.

Veatch, R.M. (1982). *A theory of medical ethics*. Basic Books, New York.

Vogel, A.V., Goodwin, J.S., and Goodwin, J.M. (1980). The therapeutics of placebo. *American Family Physician*, **22**, 105–109.

Wachtel, P. (1977). *Psychoanalysis and behavior therapy: Towards an integration*. Basic Books, New York.

Waelder, R.S. (1962). Review of *Psychoanalysis, scientific method and philosophy*, S. Hook, ed. *Journal of the American Psychoanalytic Association*, **10**, 617–637.

Wallerstein, R.S. and Robbins, L.L. (1956). Concepts: The psychotherapy research project of the Menninger foundation. *Bulletin of the Menninger Clinic*, **20**, 239–262.

Wallerstein, R.S. (1995). *The talking cures: The psychoanalyses and the psychotherapies*. Yale University Press, New Haven.

Walsh, B.T., Seidman, S., Sysko, R. and Gould, M. (2002). Placebo response in studies of major depression. *Journal of the American Medical Association*, **287**: 1844.

Waring, D. and Glass, K.C. (2006). Legal liability for harm to research participants: The case of placebo controlled trials. In T. Lemmins and D. Waring, eds. *Law and ethics in biomedical research: Regulation, conflict of interest, and liability*, University of Toronto Press, Toronto. pp.206–227.

Watters, E. and Ofshe, R. (1999). *Therapy's delusions: The myth of the unconscious and the exploitation of today's walking wounded*. Scribner, New York.

Waxler, N. (1977). Is mental illness cured in traditional societies? A theoretical analysis. *Culture, Medicine, and Psychiatry*, **1**, 233–253.

White L, Tursky, B. and Schwartz, G.E. (1985). *Placebo: Theory, research and mechanisms*. Guilford Press, New York.

Wilentz, J.S. and Engel, L. (2002). The research and ethical agenda. In H.A. Guess, A. Kleinman, J.W. Kusek, and L. Engel, eds. *The science of the placebo: Toward an interdisciplinary research agenda*, BMJ, London. pp. 283–5.

Wilkes, K.V. (1988). *Real people: Personal identity without thought experiments.* Oxford University Press, Oxford.

Wilkes, K.V. (1990). Analyzing Freud. *Philosophical Quarterly,* **40,** 241–254.

Wilson, T.D. (1985). Strangers to ourselves: The origins and accuracy of beliefs about one's own mental states. In J.H. Harvey and G. Weary, eds. *Attribution: Basic issues and applications,* Academic Press, Orlando, FL. pp. 9–36.

Wilson, T.D. (2004). *Strangers to ourselves.* Belknap Press, Cambridge, Mass.

Wisdom, J.O. (1967). Testing an interpretation within a session. *International Journal of Psychoanalysis,* **48,** 42–52.

Wittgenstein, L. (1982). Conversations on Freud: Excerpt from 1932–33 lectures. In R. Wollheim and J. Hopkins, eds. *Philosophical essays on Freud,* Cambridge University Press, Cambridge, U.K. pp.1–12.

Wollheim, R. (1993). *The mind and its depths.* Harvard University Press, Cambridge, Mass.

Woods, S.M., Natterson, J. and Silverman, J. (1966). Medical students' disease: Hypochondriasis in medical education. *Journal of Medical Education,* **41,** 785–790.

World Health Organization (1997). *The global burden of disease.* Harvard University Press, Cambridge, Mass.

World Medical Association (2000). *Declaration of Helsinki: Ethical principles for medical research involving human subjects. Journal of the American Medical Association,* **284,** 3043–3035. Available on the World Wide Web at: http://www.wma.net/e/policy/b3.htm

World Medical Association (2002). *Declaration of Helsinki: Ethical principles for medical research involving human subjects.* Available on the World Wide Web at: www.wma.net/e/policy/b3.htm#note1

Yalom, I. (1989). *Love's executioner and other essays.* Basic Books, New York.

Yapko, M. (1994). *Suggestions of abuse: True and false memories of childhood sexual trauma.* Simon and Schuster, New York.

Young, S.N. and Annable, L. (1996). The use of placebos in psychiatry: A response to the draft document prepared by the Tri-Council Working Group. *Journal of Psychiatry Neuroscience,* **21,** 235–238.

Young, S.N. and Annable, L. (2002). The ethics of placebo in clinical psychopharmacology: The urgent need for consistent regulation. *Journal of Psychiatry Neuroscience,* **27,** 319–321.

Name Index

Subject Index